SEXUALITY
AND OCCUPATIONAL THERAPY

Strategies for Persons With Disabilities

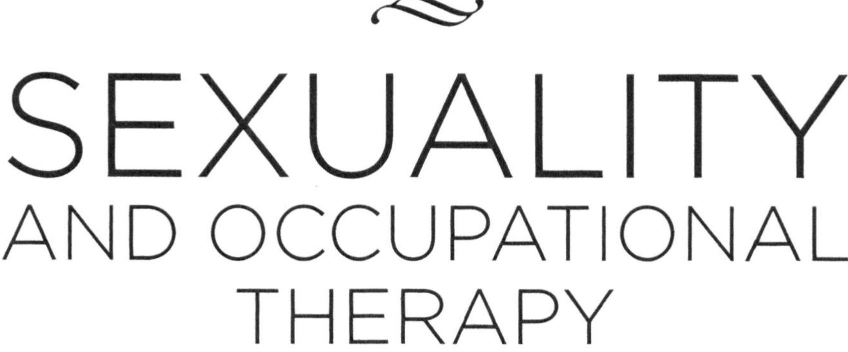

Edited by Bernadette Hattjar, DrOT, MEd, OTR/L, CWCE

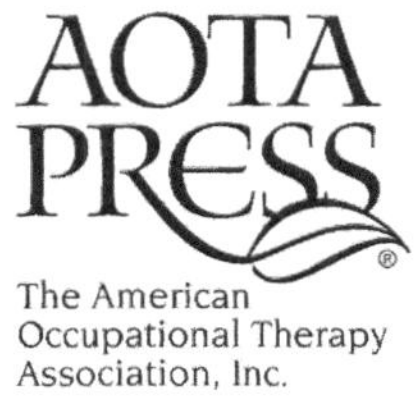

AOTA Centennial Vision
We envision that occupational therapy is a powerful, widely recognized, science-driven, and evidence-based profession with a globally connected and diverse workforce meeting society's occupational needs.

Mission Statement
The American Occupational Therapy Association advances the quality, availability, use, and support of occupational therapy through standard-setting, advocacy, education, and research on behalf of its members and the public.

AOTA Staff
Frederick P. Somers, *Executive Director*
Christopher M. Bluhm, *Chief Operating Officer*

Chris Davis, *Director, AOTA Press*
Ashley Hofmann, *Development/Production Editor*
Victoria Davis, *Production Editor/Editorial Assistant*

Beth Ledford, *Director, Marketing*
Amanda Fogle, *Marketing Specialist*
Emily Zhang, *Technology Marketing Specialist*
Jennifer Folden, *Marketing Specialist*

American Occupational Therapy Association, Inc.
4720 Montgomery Lane
Bethesda, MD 20814
Phone: 301-652-AOTA (2682)
TDD: 800-377-8555
Fax: 301-652-7711
www.aota.org
To order: 1-877-404-AOTA or store.aota.org

Disclaimers
This publication is designed to provided accurate and authoritative information in regard to the subject matter covered. It is sold or distributed with the understanding that the publisher is not engaged in rendering legal, accounting, or other professional service. If legal advice or other expert assistance is required, the services of a competent professional person should be sought.
—*From the Declaration of Principles jointly adopted by the American Bar Association and a Committee of Publishers and Associations*

It is the objective of the American Occupational Therapy Association/AOTA Press to be a forum for free expression and interchange of ideas. The opinions expressed by the contributors to this work are their own and not necessarily those of the American Occupational Therapy Association/AOTA Press.

ISBN: 978-1-56900-308-4

Library of Congress Control Number 2012935515

Cover Artwork "Passionate Kiss" by Rabi Khan. Used with permission.
Cover Design by Debra Naylor, Naylor Design, Inc., Washington, DC
Composition by Manila Typesetting Company, Manila, Philippines
Printed by Automated Graphic Systems, Inc., White Plains, MD

Contents

About the Editor

Bernadette Hattjar, DrOT, MEd, OTR/L, CWCE, is chairperson of the Occupational Therapy Program at Gannon University, Erie, PA, where she is also a tenured assistant professor. Dr. Hattjar has over 27 years of experience in academic and clinical arenas. Her areas of expertise and interest include pediatric psychiatry, job analysis and ergonomics, and the effect of chronic disease on occupational roles and occupational performance. Dr. Hattjar has headed several research projects and is a widely published author of journal articles, informational articles, and textbook chapters. Her interest in the topic of sexuality was spurred by her students' inquisitiveness about sexual activity and chronic disease and by clinical patients who did not know whom to talk to about this personal and intimate topic.

Contributors

Bernadette Hattjar, DrOT, MEd, OTR/L, CWCE
Chairperson and Assistant Professor
Gannon University
Erie, PA

Ashley Hofmann, MA
Development/Production Editor, AOTA Press
American Occupational Therapy Association
Bethesda, MD

Tammy L. Kordes, PhD
Neuropsychologist
Northshore Psychological Associates
Erie, PA

Constance Lappa, MSW, LCSW, Diplomate of Sex Therapy
Certified Sex Therapist and Licensed Social Worker
Private Practice
Pittsburgh
Professor
Robert Morris University
Moon Township, PA

Christine Linkie, MS, OTR/L
Occupational Therapist and Educational Consultant
Adjunct Instructor
Gannon University, Erie, PA
Doctoral Candidate
Texas Woman's University, Dallas

Michelle Mioduszewski, MS, OTR/L
Occupational Therapist and Owner
Niagara Therapy, LLC
Erie, PA

Vicki Pritchard, OTR/L
Senior Occupational Therapist
HealthSouth Rehab Hospital of Erie
Erie, PA

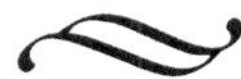

List of Case Examples, Exhibits, Figures, Tables, and Appendixes

Figures

Tables

Appendixes

Introduction

Bernadette Hattjar, DrOT, MEd, OTR/L, CWCE

When one considers the intrinsic elements of being human, such as the *physical* act of doing or engaging in something of a sexual nature, and the *psychological* component of how we feel and experience ourselves and others in relation to sexual activities, the topic of this textbook is far-reaching in relation to the profession of occupational therapy.

Sex is considered to an activity of daily living (ADL) by the American Occupational Therapy Association's (2008) *Occupational Therapy Framework: Domain and Process,* which defines *sexual activity* as "engaging in activities that result in sexual satisfaction" (p. 631). Occupational therapy practitioners must be prepared to address this important ADL with their clients.

Despite being an ADL, sexual activity is not typically or regularly addressed in the clinical or educational settings of occupational therapy, and as such, there is little research on this topic. This book is intended for occupational therapy clinicians, educators, and students who seek to acquire greater understanding of how to approach, assess, and address sexuality concerns in occupational therapy practice. Other health care professionals dealing with the populations included in this book will also find the information accessible, practical, and valuable.

This text is intended to provide a basic level of understanding about how to address, evaluate, and intervene with occupational therapy clients who experience difficulty with sexual activity.

It is an introductory conversation on a complex and often-overlooked topic. It is important to remember that occupational therapists are not sex therapists or physicians and must refer clients to the appropriate professionals as appropriate. Because occupational therapy practitioners deal with a wide variety of client populations and diagnoses, the specific diagnosis and age groups identified in text chapters are presented due to the frequency they are seen in clinical practice and focused on in therapist educational programs.

Occupational therapy endeavors to treat the "whole person," and this book reflects that holistic spirit of the profession. Sexual activity is a valued occupation among many people, and a client who experiences an injury or disease is still entitled to pursue such occupation. But how does an occupational therapy practitioner go about addressing sexuality? This text seeks to fill the void in clinical practical and occupational therapy education courses on the topic of sexuality, equipping the practitioner to effectively assess and intervene with various populations facing challenges in sexual activity.

Although much of the information presented in this publication can be equally applied to heterosexual or same-sex relationships, information is limited to a general framework of heterosexual relationships. Additionally, topics such as contraception or reproduction after illness or injury is discussed as appropriate.

It is hoped that this book will foster greater discussion and inclusion of topics related to sexuality in clinical and educational settings and encourage others to research and publish on this topic.

How This Book Is Organized

This book is structured and organized to be consistent and user-friendly from chapter to chapter. The first chapter provides a clear and concise history and review of what has been researched in the past half-century. Although much recent discussion has transpired in relation to sexual activity and spinal cord injury, much of it deals with technological developments, social changes, and improvements in medical interventions. In the past 20 years, a closer tie-in with emotional issues and sexual activity has been researched, and this has resulted in, perhaps, a clearer understanding and ability to critically think about how a disability affects sexuality (Verschuren, Enzlin, Dijkstra, Geertzen, & Dekker, 2010). However, occupational therapy still does not address this ADL with consistency or with the spirit or comfort in which we address other ADLs.

Following the literature review, the chapters are diagnosis-specific and cover the following conditions and areas:

- Arthritis
- Cancer
- Diabetes
- Spinal cord injury

- Cardiovascular disease
- Traumatic brain injury
- Stroke
- Mental disorders
- Adolescents with disabilities.

As previously mentioned, diagnoses selected for inclusion in this book were determined by the editor and chapter contributors to be diagnosis groups frequently seen in the clinical practice of occupational therapy. Significant focus is placed on diagnoses that are more common in the adult population, such as arthritis, cardiovascular disease, diabetes, and stroke. This was determined to be appropriate because the population in the United States is aging. The Baby Boomer generation is entering its sixth decade of life, and this generation is 80 million strong (Lyons, 2010). By 2030, over 20% of the total population in America will be 65 years of age or older, and 30% will be 50 years of age or older (Centers for Disease Control and Prevention & Merck Company Foundation, 2007). However, persons of any age can acquire many of the conditions discussed in this text.

Each diagnosis-specific chapter includes demographics; typical signs and symptoms of the disease, disability, or illness; sexual activity issues related to the specific diagnosis; the focus of occupational therapy, including evaluation; intervention suggestions; a case study with questions to consider; and in some cases, a handout for the clinician to use as appropriate.

Finally, two appendixes provide additional, valuable information. Appendix A offers illustrations of the various sexual positions mentioned throughout text. Appendix B presents a sample of a practical questionnaire that practitioners can use to realistically determine a client's comfort with sexuality and to facilitate more open communication between the client and practitioner.

Sexuality is something that is necessary to address in occupational therapy professional practice, in our educational institutions, and among ourselves as health care providers and human beings. By addressing this part of human life in the clients we serve and students we educate, occupational therapy practitioners can better and more effectively assist people in living full, meaningful lives.

References

American Occupational Therapy Association. (2008). Occupational therapy framework: Domain and process (2nd ed.). *American Journal of Occupational Therapy, 62,* 625–683. doi: 10.5014/ajot.62.6.625

Centers for Disease Control and Prevention, & Merck Company Foundation. (2007). *The state of aging and health in America, 2007*. Whitehouse Station, NJ: Merck Company Foundation.

Lyons, E. (2010). *Examining baby boomers: Statistics, demographics, segments, and predictions*. Retrieved October 20, 2010, from http://www.sparxoo.com

Verschuren, J., Enzlin, P., Dijkstra, P., Geertzen, J., & Dekker, R. (2010). Chronic disease and sexuality: A generic conceptual framework. *Journal of Sex Research, 47*, 153–170.

Disclaimer

Participation by the authors in this publication does not imply endorsement by Gannon University.

1

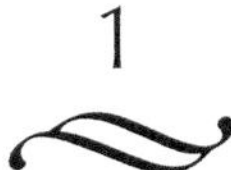

Overview of Occupational Therapy and Sexuality

Bernadette Hattjar, DrOT, MEd, OTR/L, CWCE

Key Terms and Concepts

- Assertive communication
- Caregiver role
- Intimacy
- PLISSIT Model
- Sexual activity
- Sick role.

"Sex is an emotion in motion."

—Mae West (as cited in Fitzhenry, 1993, p. 412)

"While a person does not give up on sex, sex does not give up on the person."

—Gabriel Garcia Marques (as cited in Fitzhenry, 1993, p. 414).

These two very different quotes represent the continuum of sex and sexual activity. On the one hand, sex and sexual activity is probably one of the most powerful expressions of emotions and feelings that humans possess. To those in love, sex can represent the culmination of a relationship and a way to demonstrate strong feelings in a physical and intimate manner. On the other hand, to those with different emotions as desires, sex can be a way simply to be with another person and to attain another "notch" on their headboard of conquests. To people in troubled relationships or in the cases of nonconsensual sex, sex can take on a negative, angry, and fear-producing connotation and provide great distress. To those who have experienced disappointment or loss, sex might be a memory—a memory that might be too painful or upsetting to delve into. Regardless of how and what sex and sexual activity mean to an individual, emotions and physicality figure prominently in the act of sex.

Occupational therapists take into account the physical and psychological arenas; development areas; daily, common, or usual activities; cognition; the power of activity and engagement; and the motor components that comprise activity "doing." Occupational therapists also consider the emotional and feelings aspect of engagement in activities, which are important in the realm of sexual activity and sexuality.

When a chronic disability or illness is superimposed upon sexuality or sexual activity, the entire picture changes for an individual. Any chronic condition has unique and individual physical and psychological issues attached to its presence. On an individual level, the client might feel that he or she is no longer physically desirable or physically capable of enduring sex or assuming positions for intercourse. Some individuals fear involvement in sexual activity because they think that they might die while engaging in the activity itself. An individual might feel that he or she cannot "flirt" or be seductive with another person because of his or her chronic condition. Because of this, the individual might become depressed, angry, or anxious at the thought of having—or not having—a significant other in his or her life or of not having any opportunity for sexual release or satisfaction.

These issues can make any assessment or intervention related to sexual activity a difficult task for a health care professional. The client might not want to address his or her concerns regarding sexuality and sexual activity and, conversely, the therapist might never broach this topic with a client. If a therapist comprehends the magnitude and the impact of sexual activity and sexuality for individuals' quality of life, the reasons the subject is not addressed on a regular basis are confounding.

Chronic Disability

For individuals with a chronic disability, the mind might be willing, but the body might struggle with becoming involved in sexual activity. With chronic disabilities, the body and mind might be in two very different places and domains when sexual activity is desired or considered. If a disability is newly diagnosed, an individual might be experiencing an upheaval of emotions and a restriction in his or her daily routines. The person might wonder whether his or her life will ever be the same and if he or she will ever be the same. He or she might be unsure of how this diagnosis will affect his or her life, relationships, and life roles. If a disability is ongoing, the individual might sublimate desires into another area, give up on having sex, or feel as though he or she is responding in a perverted manner to his or her innate desire if he or she wants to become intimate with another person.

However, with chronic disability, sexual activity can be one consistent activity that provides comfort and solace. In fact, sex is one of the most normal and typical activities of daily living (ADLs). Relationship and sexual satisfaction are important boosters of quality of life (QoL) in chronically ill, adult populations. Sex and sexual activity can become a primary source of "comfort, pleasure and intimacy, and an affirmation of gender when other gender roles have been stripped away" (McInnes, 2003, p. 264). When many common occupations are taken away by a chronic illness, injury, or disability, sex and sexual activity might provide one way of feeling "normal" or connected with another person.

Where Is Occupational Therapy?

Although the *Occupational Therapy Practice Framework: Domain and Process* (*Framework*; American Occupational Therapy Association [AOTA], 2008) identified *sexual activity* as an ADL, along with dressing, grooming, bathing, hygiene, household management, it is not routinely addressed by occupational therapists and other health care professionals.

For many reasons, sexual activity is not consistently addressed in occupational therapy. The prominent reasons across the illness continuum include

- Therapist discomfort with the subject;
- Therapist lack of educational preparedness for addressing sexual activity and sexuality;
- The assumption that another health care discipline is addressing the subject; and,
- Today, when productivity in health care is crucial, not having enough time to address sexual activity (Hattjar, 2007).

These shortcomings reduce sexual activity to another ADL and eliminates the special and unique qualities that comprise sexual activity and intimacy. The divergence between more common and, perhaps "safe and not uncomfortable to address" ADLs like dressing or grooming are assessed on a very consistent basis. However, the ADL of sexual activity is not addressed with any regularity by the profession of occupational therapy, and it is not given the attention that it deserves.

Chronic illness tends to progress slowly, and the progression of the illness, disability, or injury might equate to increasing limitations, including the ability to become engaged in sexual activity (Kazan, 1990; Pitzele, 1995). It always amazes me when a chronically ill client's understanding of his or her medication schedule, restrictions in mobility, safety precautions and techniques, dietary requirements or restrictions, home exercise programs, and pain reduction techniques—all of which are specific to his or her diagnosis—is thorough, yet his or her understanding of the impact of his or her chronic condition on sexuality and sexual activity is inaccurate, incorrect, or totally absent. In other words, the individual does not secure information from the therapist on one crucial ADL but is well versed (or at least much better versed) in other ADL areas. Why are occupational therapy practitioners not addressing this aspect of "human-ness"?

Another confounding issue is the way that occupational therapists and health care providers have a tendency to place clients in a "sick role," as opposed to an active, engaged role in relation to rehabilitation areas like sexual activity, even though occupational therapists identify with being a "client-centered" profession. Sociologist Talcott Parsons (1975) proposed the "sick role," suggesting that illness was a dysfunctional deviance comprised of four specific norms:

- The individual is not responsible for his or her illness.
- The individual's normal obligations become excusable.
- Illness is undesirable.
- The ill should seek professional help (Hughes, 1994).

The client is placed into or assumes the sick role until social reintegration (comprised of rehabilitation, the absence of disease, or wellness) is attained. The sick role might be a passive role in which the health care provider takes control of the situation, or it might be a shared decision-making process (Stiggelbout & Kiebert, 1997) where the health care provider and the client work cooperatively, thereby promoting client empowerment within the specific situation. The *sick role* is defined as a client role that is aligned with the traditional medical model of care in which the amelioration of the disease or illness is the primary focus of care. However, LaRue and Huebner (2001) expanded on the total definition of the sick role, saying that it is comprised of the physical, psychological, and sexual self for all clients who receive occupational therapy services. By aligning ourselves with this broader concept, we address the whole person, not merely components of the whole.

Occupational therapy purports to be a holistic and client-centered discipline. If we consider the idea that the client is the only true expert on his or her personal situation and if we adopt a client-centered approach to evaluation and intervention without addressing this subject, we miss two intrinsic components of being human: sexuality and sexual activity. Sexuality and sexual activity also consist of intimacy, closeness with another individual, and sensuality.

Understanding Terminology

To understand the concepts included in this textbook, you must understand the terminology that surrounds the topic. The *Framework* (AOTA, 2008) defined *sexual activity* as "engaging in activities that result in sexual satisfaction" (p. 631). *Taber's Cyclopedic Medical Dictionary* (2005) defined *sexuality* as "the constitution and life of an individual as related to sex; all the dispositions related to intimacy, whether associated with the sex organs or not" (p. 1982).

In this text, *intimacy* is closeness with another individual. *Closeness* might relate to proximity, tenderness, familiarity, and a sense of another person being special and unique and someone to be cherished. Pope John Paul II defined *sensuality* as simply "tenderness" (Sri, 2007). Along with tenderness, sensuality is comprised of the information we interpret and process through all of our senses (*Taber's Cyclopedic Medical Dictionary*, 2005). Our interpretation of incoming sensory information can provide pleasure and excitement when we are with the "right" person, in the "right mood," or in the "right" situation.

Important Concepts in Sexuality and Occupational Therapy

The Annon Model for Permission, Limited Information, Specific Suggestions, and Intensive Therapy (PLISSIT)

To broach the subject of sexual activity or sexuality with any client appropriately, professionally, and maturely, the use of a structure or set of guidelines can substantiate addressing this personal topic and can provide an objective method or format for addressing this topic. The PLISSIT Model (Annon, 1976) will be mentioned throughout this text because of its thoroughness and structure. The PLISSIT Model provides occupational therapists with an organizing context by which they can address sexual activity with their clients.

Psychologist Jack Annon (1976) developed the PLISSIT Model to facilitate health care providers' ability and likelihood to address sexuality and sexual activity with clients on a regular basis. PLISSIT is an acronym for *permission, limited information, specific suggestions,* and *intensive therapy,* as detailed below:

- *P: Permission.* Permission relates to the client opening the lines of communication about the topic of sexual activity or sexuality. The therapist might accomplish such communication by asking the client about the topic, by providing a questionnaire that addresses sexual activity or relationships in general (see Appendix B), or by including sexual activity in the occupational therapy evaluation process. The client must grant permission before any further discourse on sexual activity can occur. It is a very personal and private topic, so no coercion may occur. Additionally, and perhaps especially with this topic, confidentiality is of paramount importance.

- *LI: Limited information.* Once the client permits discussion of sexual activity, the therapist should provide general information, which is usually considered limited in scope. The therapist might provide this through a one-to-one discussion with the client or through a review of handouts or articles. The overall scope of the discussion should be comfortable and not stressful for both the therapist and client.

- *SS: Specific suggestions.* This relates to suggestions concerning sexual activity components like positioning for comfortable sex, the use of alternative positions for sexual activity, alternative methods of gratification in lieu of sexual intercourse related to the clients' limitations or fears, and the addition of the partner in this process. The therapist might want to include the client's partner to help him or her gain a greater understanding of the clients' physical and psychological situation as it is affected by the illness, injury, or disability. Including the partner at this point might also help with discussion and communication about sexual activity between the two individuals and help to determine whether difficulties are anticipated or present. If relationship and sexual problems are of an ongoing nature, a referral to more intensive therapy might be warranted. This PLISSIT component is generally thought not to be under the domain of the profession of occupational therapy.

- *IT: Intensive therapy.* In the case of ongoing sexual or relationship issues, a referral, made by the occupational therapist, should occur. It is prudent to refer these types of cases to a psychologist or a licensed and certified sex therapist. *It is important to remember that occupational therapists are not sex therapists.*

Communication

Open communication is essential for any constructive and positive interpersonal relationship. In the case of intimate relationships, honest, positive, constructive, and assertive communication skills are crucial components in relationship building. Introducing the concept of assertive communication can provide, perhaps, a new and constructive way for the client and partner to interact.

Assertive communication is the best and most effective, whereas non-assertive and aggressive communication is less effective.

Assertive communication

Assertive communication involves being honest with feelings and wishes, making "I feel" statements, being verbally open, actively listening and hearing what is being said, responding instead of reacting, maintaining good eye contact, assuming a comfortable body language stance, and talking at a normal tone of voice. Being assertive means that the individual respects the rights of the other person.

Nonassertive communication

Nonassertive communication involves passivity, information withholding, being indirect, talking softly, internalizing feelings and wishes for fear of retribution or confrontation, not hearing what is being said because of listening to internal messages or recording in the mind, maintaining little if any eye contact, maintaining a closed-off body language, or being fidgety when talking (e.g., being distracted).

Aggressive communication

Aggressive communication is displayed when a person responds in an angry or spiteful or hurtful manner, talks loudly or yells, shows physicality in response to the other individuals' verbal productions, is easy to anger, acts in a hostile manner, is rude or flippant, does not listen or tries to "talk over" the other person, stares or glares at the other individual, assumes an aggressive body language stance (e.g., stands if the other person is sitting), does not let the other individual maintain his or her own safe "body space" (usually considered to be a distance of about 2–3 feet around the body), "gets in the other person's face," storms out of the room, or throws objects.

Mental Health

When dealing with a chronic illness, disability, or injury, learning to live with the limitation can promote unrelenting stress and concern. The client might not understand the ramifications of the situation and might question how his or her future will unfold. Of concern to many clients is how their family, friends, and close relationship will be sustained. These feelings are normal but usually resolve with time and, possibly, counseling.

Included in this book are questionnaires or scales to assist therapists in addressing some of the mental health issues that chronic populations confront. The Beck Depression Inventory (2nd ed.; Beck, Steer, & Brown, 1996) is referenced frequently throughout the chapters of this book. This particular scale is well known to those who work with mental health problems. It has sustained the test of time and has good application to a variety of clients at various ages and stages in adulthood. The assessment provides a well-rounded review of a variety of problem-causing concepts and sets the stage for further intervention and counseling needs. It has been used for over 30 years to assess and identify depressive symptoms in adults.

Also mentioned in this book is the Hospital Anxiety and Depression Scale (HADS; Zigmond & Snaith, 1983). This scale was designed to measure the level and causes of anxiety in hospitalized individuals. When an individual with a chronic disability is hospitalized, feelings and issues surface that are distress producing. This scale can highlight suspect areas and provide a venue for the health care professional to intervene.

Although neither of these items specifically addresses the area of sexual activity or sexuality, this important occupational role and its components are alluded to by many of the questions included in these, and other, questionnaires, screens, or scales in this book.

Manner in Which Care Is Provided

One aspect of the occupational therapy constellation of service provision that is limitedly addressed is that of the role of the caregiver. Within the context of this book, the *caregiver role* is defined as the primary care provider, the partner, the spouse, or the significant other. Although these words might conjure up very different ideas of the level and type of involvement in relation to the client, the common thread associated with all of these roles is the connection or relatedness to the client. Caregiving can be provided in a variety of ways, and the manner of caregiving directly relates to the functional level (both real and supposed or imagined) of the client. Superimposing the concepts of sexual activity and sexuality on the caregiver–client relationship provides an additional layer of intimacy to the caregiving scenario. The levels of care giving include

- *Active engagement:* Includes constructive problem solving between the caregiver and the client.

- *Protective buffering:* Consists of both parties hiding concerns and denying worries from the other.

- *Overprotection:* Refers to an underestimation of the client's capabilities by the caregiver or to the client's underestimation of their own abilities (Vilchinsky et al., 2010).

When one considers how the type of caregiving that the client receives plays into an intimate relationship that includes sexual activity, one understands how other problems in the relationship are quite likely to surface—except in the case of active and engaging caregiving. *Active caregiving* represents an open, honest, and assertive style of giving care and personal interaction. Active caregiving also reflects a mature and respectful way of the caregiver relating with the client and the client relating with the caregiver.

Physical Symptoms and Prognosis Status

Disease chronicity means that, whatever the problem is, it is of a long-standing duration and has most likely developed over time (with the exception of spinal cord or traumatic brain injuries). Whatever the problems are, they will not magically disappear; they will be with the client for the duration of his or her life and might cause or contribute to his or her death. This situation can be best described by a past client, who said, regarding her arthritis, "It's like a little black cloud that will not go away. It's always with me. Sometimes it affects me more, sometimes it doesn't seem to affect me at all, but it's always there in the back of my mind."

The magnitude of symptoms and the extent of disability contribute to the client's health QoL—not only how satisfied the client is overall with all the facets of his or her life but also how satisfied he or she is regarding his or her health, wellness, and health care. Some diagnoses presented in this book offer myriad symptoms and the need to adopt a different type of day-to-day living experience. Other diagnoses in this book might present with internal and psychological manifestations and few (if any) physical symptoms. Some diagnoses mandate self-monitoring, an ongoing need to evaluate energy and food intake, and physical activity to maintain mobility or, at least, to improve joint integrity. Regardless of the impact of the chronic disease, illness, or injury, coping with it becomes an integral part of the client. The client as a sexual being can be affected in a multitude of ways—as many ways as there are clients. Therefore, addressing sexual activity and sexuality becomes a very personal experience for each client.

References

American Occupational Therapy Association. (2008). Occupational therapy practice framework: Domain and process (2nd ed.). *American Journal of Occupational Therapy, 62,* 625–683. doi: 10.5014/ajot.62.6.625

Annon, J. S. (1976). The PLISSIT model: A proposed conceptual scheme for the behavioral treatment of sexual problems. *Journal of Sex Education and Therapy, 2,* 1–15.

Beck, A., Steer, R., & Brown, G. K. (1996). *Beck Depression Inventory* (2nd ed.). San Antonio, TX: Psychological Corporation.

Fitzhenry, R. I. (Ed.). (1993). *The Harper book of quotations* (3rd ed.). New York: HarperCollins.

Hattjar, B. (2007). *Occupational therapy practitioners' perspectives related to addressing sexual activity with chronic, physically disabled clients.* Unpublished Capstone Project, Fort Lauderdale–Davie, FL: Nova Southeastern University.

Hughes, J. (1994). *Approaches to the doctor–patient relationship.* Retrieved August 3, 2007, from http://www.changesurfer.com/Hlth/DPReview.html

Kazan, L. (1990). Chronic illness and sexuality. *American Journal of Nursing, 90*(1), 54–59.

LaRue, A., & Huebner, R. (2001). The influence of the sick role on health in rehabilitation. *Physical Disabilities Special Interest Section Quarterly, 24*(2), 1–4.

McInnes, R. A. (2003). Chronic illness and sexuality. *Medical Journal of Australia, 179*(5), 263–266.

Parsons, T. (1975). The sick role and the role of the physician reconsidered. *Milbank Memorial Fund Quarterly Health and Society, 53*(3), 257–278.

Pitzele, S. (1995). Chronic illness, disability, and sexuality in people older than fifty. *Sexuality and Disability, 13*(4), 309–325.

Sri, E. (2007). Men, women, and tenderness. *Lay Witness, 24–25,* 43. Retrieved September 4, 2007, from http://catholiceducation.org/articles/sexuality/se0134.htm

Stiggelbout, A. M., & Kiebert, G. M. (1997). A role for the sick role: Patient preferences regarding information and participation in clinical decision-making. *Canadian Medical Association Journal, 157*(4), 383–389.

Taber's cyclopedic medical dictionary (20th ed.). (2005). Philadelphia: F. A. Davis.

Vilchinsky, N., Haze-Filderman, L., Leibowitz, M., Reges, O., Khaskis, A., & Mosseri, M. (2010). Spousal support and cardiac patients' distress: The moderating role of attachment orientation. *Journal of Family Psychology, 24*(4), 508–512.

Zigmond, A. S., & Snaith, R. P. (1983). The Hospital Anxiety and Depression Scale. *Acta Psychiatrica Scandinavica, 67*(6), 361–370.

2

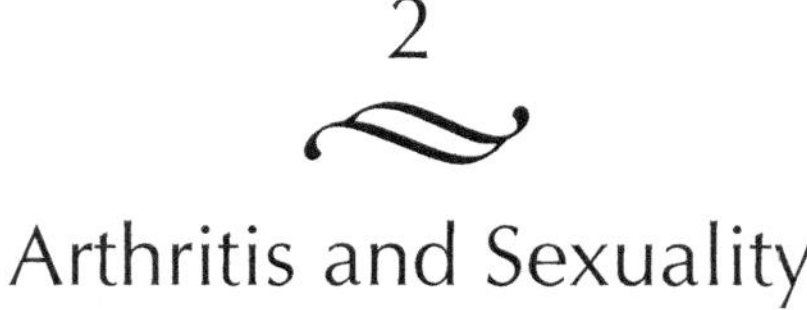

Arthritis and Sexuality

Bernadette Hattjar, DrOT, MEd, OTR/L, CWCE

Key Terms and Concepts

- Autoimmunity
- Energy conservation
- Fibromyalgia
- Gout
- Joint protection
- Mind–body connection
- Modalities
- Osteoarthritis
- Quality of life
- Rheumatoid arthritis.

Upon completion of this chapter, readers will be able to

- Recognize common symptoms associated with arthritis;
- Identify modalities that decrease arthritis symptoms;
- Understand the importance of energy conservation and joint protection in regard to sexual activity and the client with arthritis;
- Select appropriate screen or assessment tools to enhance client assessment, client needs, and occupational therapy goal development;

- Synthesize screen or evaluation results into meaningful and appropriate client interventions; and

- Incorporate the PLISSIT Model into evaluation and interventions with arthritic clients.

Introduction

Arthritis means inflammation (*-itis*) of a joint (*arthro-*; Willis, 2008). Arthritis has and continues to be a chronic disease factor. Arthritis was found in the skeleton of "The Ice Man" Otzi, a mummified male body dating from approximately 3,000 B.C. that was found frozen in ice near the border of Italy and Austria (Arthritis Basics, 2009). Egyptian mummies also show evidence of arthritic joint changes.

Although many forms of arthritis exist, the common thread in all forms of arthritis is that joint or tissue destruction or deformity is present. Arthritis is not a selective disease, for it can affect people from birth to death.

Demographics

An estimated 46 million adults in the United States reported being told by a physician that they had some form of arthritis ("arthritis" here refers to osteoarthritis), rheumatoid arthritis (RA), gout, lupus, or fibromyalgia, and 1 in 5 adults in the United States report having physician-diagnosed arthritis (Centers for Disease Control and Prevention [CDC], 2008). Although arthritis can affect individuals of any age, the incidents of diagnosed arthritis increase proportionately with age. In 2004–2005, half of all adults ages 65 years or older reported an arthritis diagnosis.

The CDC (2008) reported that that the most common form of arthritis, osteoarthritis, is followed in order of occurrence by other rheumatic conditions including RA, gout syndrome, and fibromyalgia. The incidents of arthritis in adults reported include the following numbers:

- *Osteoarthritis:* 27 million

- *RA:* 1.3 million

- *Gout:* 3 million

- *Fibromyalgia:* 5 million (CDC, 2008).

Arthritis in all of its forms tends to be more prevalent in women, obese individuals, and individuals who do not regularly participate in physical activities or exercise (CDC, 2008). Women are more prone to certain types of arthritis, especially systemic forms like RA, and are affected 2.5 times more frequently than men, especially women between 40–50 years of age (Yasuda, 2008). This might be because of genetic predisposition, hormonal fluctuations, child bearing, or dietary issues.

Obesity is often cited as being a contributing factor to the development of arthritis, especially arthritis that affects the weight-bearing joints, which occurs in osteoarthritis (CDC, 2011). An obese individual experiences greater joint stress and wear and tear that can compromise joint integrity. An obese person might also have difficulty with gross-motor activities and exercise, which can lead to a sedentary lifestyle. Lack of physical exercise can contribute to the development of arthritis because joints function better and function longer when regularly challenged with weight-bearing exercise and range of motion (ROM).

The most frequently identified daily living limitations caused by arthritis are

- Physical limitations
- Financial difficulties
- Decreased satisfaction with current life situation
- Less optimism about the future (National Academy on an Aging Society, 2000).

Arthritis symptoms impede the ability to fulfill personal life roles and cause a decrease in the client's perceived overall quality of life (QoL). Therefore, one area that arthritis affects is the ability to pursue and fulfill intimate relationships.

Arthritis Signs and Symptoms

Osteoarthritis

Osteoarthritis is the most common form of arthritis and is sometimes referred to as a *degenerative joint disease*. In osteoarthritis, joint changes are directly related to the progressive loss of the articular cartilage and synovium that results from inflammation. As the bones attempt to mend or remold, bone spurs *(osteophytes)* are formed. This stage is followed by joint pain, stiffness, ROM limitations, and joint deformity (Porth, 2004).

Arthritis is usually thought to be a disease of old age because of the joint wear-and-tear associated with daily living. When people are adolescents or young adults (ages 30 years or younger), a joint is sustained by adequate synovial fluid, ROM, and appropriate joint articulation. As an individual ages, the synovium provides less of a cushioning effect because of the typical daily joint wear-and-tear, a lifetime of potential mechanical problems, or injury. Osteoarthritis is commonly associated with the aging process, and the majority of individuals ages 40 years or older have some type of osteoarthritis.

Pain is commonly identified in the weight-bearing joints, including the hips, knees, ankles or feet, and spine. Pain or joint pain is usually related to a body position (e.g., flexion at the waist) or specific activity. Pain decreases or diminishes participation in activities that the client deems to be meaningful. Pain increases and is usually noted after activity or at the end of the day. Pain often decreases with rest. However, as osteoarthritis progresses, pain is present most of the time, even during periods of rest. Pain is persistent; therefore, sleep patterns and periods of truly restful and replenishing sleep become less frequent, and this disrupts daily engagement in meaningful occupations. Stiffness after periods of rest is very common, although stiffness usually dissipates after gentle movement and light activity or gentle ROM.

Osteoarthritis includes the following common symptoms:

- Joint stiffness after rest
- Joint crepitus (usually described by clients as "creaking," "crunching," or "snapping")
- Joint deformity (usually in the later stages of osteoarthritis)
- Limited active range—and sometimes passive range—of motion because of joint pain limitations
- Joint tenderness, occasional swelling, and joint pain (Porth, 2004).

Rheumatoid Arthritis

RA, a systemic and virulent form of arthritis, is more likely to affect women between the ages of 40–60 years. RA is the result of *autoimmunity*, in which the individual's own body creates antibodies that destroy or damage synovial joint linings. The affected joint linings become thick and craggy, and this thickness impedes tendon and ligament gliding. As tendons and ligaments stretch to accommodate motion, they become weakened and compromised. Joint destruction, boney deformities, and bone destruction might result as the disease progresses.

RA tends to affect smaller joints (e.g., joints in the hands, wrists, elbows, jaw); however, as the disease progresses, other joints can be involved (Yasuda, 2008).

RA includes the following common symptoms:

- Joint pain
- Joint swelling
- Joints that are tender to the touch
- Puffy, red hands
- Firm bumps (rheumatic nodules) located under the skin.
- Fatigue
- Morning stiffness that lasts for longer than 1 hour
- Weight loss
- Feeling of malaise (Mayo Clinic, 2011).

RA clients have not only to deal with the physical, autoimmune disease process, but they also are more likely to experience psychological problems such as depression, anxiety, and a diminished QoL (Doeglas et al., 2004). In fact, people with RA are twice as likely to experience depression compared to the general population (Dickens & Creed, 2001). It is difficult to determine whether depression highlights pain symptoms, or whether having pain and functional limitations contributes to feelings of depression (Ryan, 2009).

Gout

Gout is characterized by sudden, abrupt, severe, and acute attacks of pain, redness, and joint tenderness, which usually begin at night after excessive exercise; certain medications, food, or alcohol intake; or dieting. It is reported that the pain associated with the gout syndrome is so excessive that even the negligible weight of a bed sheet touching the great toe can cause unbearable pain. The gout syndrome manifests as a *monoarticular* (one-joint) event and usually affects the *metatarsaophalangeal joint* (the base of the great toe; Porth, 2004). Gout can also attack the tarsal joints, instep of the foot, ankles, heels, knees, wrists, fingers, and elbows.

Residual effects of a gout attack include joint tenderness, development of *gouty tophi* (round or curved bubble-like projections that develop at the site of the gout attack), and redness that lasts from a few days to a few weeks. An attack will occur and then subside for months or even years in the early stages of this disease. As the disease progresses, joint changes occur and become permanent. Men are affected by gout earlier (around ages 40–50 years), but after women reach menopause, incidents of gout are essentially equal between the sexes.

Gout is frequently attributed to a rich, fatty diet, along with underlying medical conditions such as untreated high blood pressure, high cholesterol, diabetes, and atherosclerosis (Primatesta, Plana, & Rothenbacher, 2011). Gout usually occurs concurrently with other diagnoses; therefore, occupational roles and responsibilities might be dually affected because of the gout symptoms and the other issues that the client might experience.

During a *gouty exacerbation,* a period in which gout symptoms (extreme pain and sensitivity to even the lightest of touch, redness, and swelling) abruptly increase, and function and daily performance of activities is curtailed or decreased because of pain and discomfort, occupational role limitations and work limitations are common because of the acute and incredibly painful nature of the incident. Once the episode diminishes, the ability to reengage in life roles and responsibilities resumes in most cases.

Fibromyalgia

Fibromyalgia is a chronic condition characterized by widespread pain in muscles, tendons, and ligaments, as well as unrelenting fatigue and diffuse tender points throughout the body, usually occurring in a symmetrical dispersion pattern. The pain associated with fibromyalgia is often described as a continual dull ache, arising from muscles (Mayo Clinic, 2011). The common pain dispersion is located at the back of the head, on the sides of the neck, between the scapulae or dispersed over the trapezius muscles, over the top of the shoulders, at the upper chest, at the lateral elbows, at the upper hip below the waist, at the outer hip (usually close to the widest part of the hip), on the side of the legs, and at the inner knees. Fatigue after hours of rest or sleep is common because fibromyalgia is sometimes associated with restless leg syndrome or sleep apnea (Hallberg & Bergman, 2011; Mayo Clinic, 2011).

Conditions that frequently coexist with fibromyalgia include depression, chronic fatigue syndrome, sleep disorders, restless leg syndrome, headaches, irritable bowel syndrome, and endometriosis (Mayo Clinic, 2011).

Once a client receives the diagnosis of fibromyalgia, he or she might be emotionally relieved because of the diffuse and varied symptom presentation of this disease. Medical tests do not always confirm an illness or disease; therefore, many times, these clients have been told that nothing is wrong with them. The occupational role and responsibility devastation that fibromyalgia inflicts can be extremely detrimental to clients' self-esteem, family and intimate relationships, compensated employment and work roles, and work relationships.

Sexual Activity Issues Related to Arthritis

Arthritis reduces an individual's overall QoL and inflicts physical and psychological problems concerning sexual activity, sexuality, and sensuality. The physical problems presented by arthritis concerning intimacy and sexual activity include general pain or discomfort, specific joint pain, joint swelling, or stiffness (Newman, 2007).

Psychological components associated with arthritis include depression, anxiety, lowered self-esteem (Eustice & Eustice, 2009), and a potential for body image distortion because of physical changes. Consideration of these overriding problems highlights the issues that arthritis can cause. The specific issues that a client has will directly relate to his or her prediagnosis personality. In this case, arthritis usually magnifies problems, quirks, and issues, and this magnification can provide disruption in overall QoL, engagement, and fulfillment.

Quality of Life

A client's overall QoL might be challenged by any chronic disease, including arthritis. *QoL* is a broad term that includes life satisfaction, self-esteem, well-being, happiness, health, the value and meaning of life, functional status, and adjustment (Carr, Thompson, & Kirwan, 1996). A client's occupational performance, physical abilities and limitations, psychosocial health, and occupational engagement—all of which apply to QoL—can be assessed and addressed within the occupational therapy domain of practice. Because sexual activity is an activity of daily living (ADL; American Occupational Therapy Association [AOTA], 2008), addressing it as part of QoL is appropriate.

Social Support

Clients with arthritis might experience a disruption or change in social support systems because of their symptoms (e.g., pain, stiffness, fatigue, depression), which are the result of the disease process. For example, clients might not feel like attending a social or family event because they do not feel well or energetic. They might curtail their social interactions because they feel they are burdening others by their limitations. They might be embarrassed by their appearance or because of difficulty moving freely and independently in their environment and not want to ask for assistance.

Social support systems buffer stress for any individual, and this is magnified in the cases of individuals with chronic illnesses, including arthritis (Doeglas et al., 2004). The proponents of the stress-buffering hypothesis held that the impact of stress on mental health is stronger under conditions of low stress. Although indirect, this effect means that a person who has or receives social support during low or no stress periods will be better prepared to deal with higher stress incidents because he or she will have a firmer self-esteem level and the presence of a support system. Social support availability will result in a lower vulnerability or susceptibility to high-stress situations, like chronic diseases such as arthritis, because of a stronger level of self-esteem and self-worth.

Sense of Self-Esteem

An individual's sense of self, as measured by esteem and worth, is also a prominent component of close and intimate relationships. Humans connect at many levels with other individuals, but those who are closest to each other are, for the most part, valued, cherished, and loved the most. Chronic illness or disease can compromise this situation. Arthritis, in any of its forms, can be unpredictable and ambiguous (Doeglas et al., 2004). The uncertainty of what the future holds is a potent defeater and deflator of self-esteem and self-worth. Lower self-esteem and self-worth provide the stage for a variety of psychosocial problems, including a decreased sex drive or libido and a diminished sense of attractiveness and desirability.

Mind–Body Connection

The *mind–body connection* refers to a holistic connection between one's mind (how one feels emotionally) and body (how one feels physically). Arthritis is a disease that reflects a strong mind–body connection, as physical and psychological limitations or problems affect social and personal interactions and affect the ability to engage in personally meaningful occupations. Social worker Max Schwartz (2010) stated, "The mental, physical, and spiritual planes all penetrate and overlap one another. An impact on one plane has immeasurable effect on the others." In relation to arthritis, decreased physical ability, emotional distress, or social limitations should be considered major evaluation and intervention areas in health care, including occupational therapy.

Occupational Therapy Assessment

A paucity of current literature exists concerning how occupational therapists and other health care professionals intervene with sexual activity issues with arthritic clients. Although arthritis affects the sexual lives of a substantial number of patients, sexuality is a subject that is difficult for many professionals to present or discuss with clients (Abdel Nasser & Ali, 2006; Law, 2001). McAlonan (1996) reported that occupational therapists felt that sexual rehabilitation was an important component in a rehabilitation environment, but few therapists actually addressed this topic with patients.

The transformation of *meaning perspectives,* such as personal values, beliefs, feelings, and knowledge, is identified as being a proactive method to redefine occupational involvement for clients with RA (Dubouloz, Laporte, Hall, Ashe, & Smith, 2004). If consideration is given to sexual activity's inclusion as an ADL, it is identified in *Occupational Therapy Practice Framework: Domain and Process* (AOTA, 2008), which stated that addressing sexual activity as a part of a client's treatment plan is logical. Although sexual activity is a typical ADL, this topic is a "missing ADL" (Linder, 2007, p. 47) because it is not usually addressed.

Canadian Occupational Performance Measure

Occupational therapy is a client-centered profession. In being truly client centered, a therapist should seek information about the client, including the client's sexual activity issues. According to psychologist Carl Rogers (1980), if a therapist adopts a client-centered approach, the therapist must realize that the client is the only real expert on his or her situation. Rogers's person- (or client-) centered approach to psychotherapy relates to both *interaction* (with another person) and *introspection* (what are my needs or feelings?). These client-centered concepts and constructs form the basis for humanistic and client-centered interaction with a client.

In keeping with the spirit of this approach, the use of the Canadian Occupational Performance Measure (COPM; Canadian Association of Occupational Therapy [CAOT], 1996) is an appropriate tool for client-centered and occupationally based assessment or reassessment. This assessment enables the client to identify questions and concerns relating to his or her status, ability or disability, fears, needs, issues concerning any areas of concern or interest, and sexual activity and sexuality. This option is exercised at the discretion of the interviewee (client), not the interviewer (therapist). When addressing a subject like sexuality or sexual activity, the COPM provides a viable and usable method for permission, by the client, to discuss this personal and intimate subject.

The COPM is an individualized, client-centered measure designed to detect change in a client's self-perception of occupational performance over time. It is designed to use as an outcome measure for clients with a variety of disabilities and across all developmental stages (CAOT, 1996). The measure, designed as a semi-structured interview, can be completed in about 20–30 minutes. This client-driven measure uses open-ended inquiry (questions) concerning client performance, satisfaction, and importance of ADLs and occupational performance areas. The COPM provides a venue for addressing sexual activity components, as it can seek "permission" to talk about sexual activity issues based on open-ended inquiry. If the client does not state the topic of sexual activity, the therapist can ask in general, "Are there any other areas or activities that you would like occupational therapy to address?" or more specifically, "Are there any personal areas or activities that you would like to work on or discuss in therapy?" or very targeted, "Have you thought about more personal areas you believe are important to address? Consider things like your personal, sexual, or family relationships" (Hattjar, Parker, & Lappa, 2008). By asking questions in this manner, the therapist permits the client to broach sexual activity without questioning the client in a prying or intrusive manner.

Beck Depression Inventory

Psychosocial issues figure prominently when dealing with arthritis and occur as a means of dealing with the disease and the diagnosis (Rogers, Liang, & Partridge, 1982). In turn, these issues can negatively affect sexuality, contributing to decreased libido and sexual dysfuntion (Shabsigh, Zakaria, Anastasiadis, & Seidman, 2001). Psychological issues are influenced by the client's premorbid personality, but the most common psychological issues identified with arthritis as it progresses or exacerbates include anger, sadness, anxiety, frustration, and depression (Rogers et al., 1982). To address those symptoms that are related to loss of function and the chronic disease process, therapists can use the Beck Depression Inventory, 2nd Edition (BDI–II; Beck, Steer, & Brown, 1996).

The BDI–II consists of 21 questions. The questionnaire is composed of items that relate to depressive symptoms such as hopelessness; irritability; feelings of being punished; and physical symptoms including fatigue, weight loss, and a lack of interest in sex. Participants who use the BDI–II are asked to rate how they have been feeling over the past 2 weeks. The client rates the 21 questions on a 0–3 scale. The lower a client's overall score, the less likely that depression is a major illness component.

Center for Epidemiological Studies–Depression Scale and Hospital Anxiety Depression Scale

Limitations of the BDI–II relate to the presence of physical illness. It is determined that, in the presence of a physical illness, BDI–II scores might be inflated because of the physical illness symptoms rather than depression. In this case, it is suggested that additional and alternative measures be used, including the Center for Epidemiological Studies–Depression Scale (CES–D; Radloff, 1977) or the Hospital Anxiety and Depression Scale (HADS; Zigmond & Snaith, 1983). These questionnaires provide additional layers of information concerning daily living tasks, including sexual activity.

The CES–D (Radloff, 1977) was created in conjunction with the National Institute of Mental Health. This scale is composed of a questionnaire and a 4-point scale ranging from how a client has felt in the last 0–3 weeks to how a client has felt during the past week. The items include common depressive symptoms like loss of appetite, feeling "blue," concentrating on problems, having sleep problems, and having a general sense of not feeling well. Sexual activity is not directly referred to, but inclusion components in the CES–D are representational of things that comprise a healthy sexual persona: feeling confident or good about the self, feeling healthy, having motivation, being focused, attending to tasks, and achieving satisfaction from one's occupational performance in daily activities.

The HADS (Zigmond & Snaith, 1983) measures the severity of anxiety and depression separately. It can be used with clients from adolescence throughout the adult lifespan who are service recipients in any type of health care setting. This assessment provides separate scores for depression and anxiety and additionally provides an indication of the severity of anxiety and depression. This scale measures the effect of more or less negative or detrimental feelings on an individual's perceived QoL and his or her ability to benefit or be comfortable with health care services.

Using the COPM (CAOT, 1996), BDI–II (Beck et al., 1996), CES–D (Radloff, 1977), and HADS (Zigmond & Snaith, 1983), or other screens should not be considered the sole occupational therapy evaluation. These measures can be used to augment a traditional occupational therapy evaluation that focuses on occupational performance and performance components and contexts. However, the COPM, BDI–II, or other assessments can provide useful information for intervention planning purposes for clients with arthritis.

The use of a questionnaire related to sexual activity (see Appendix B) can be used alone, or it can be added to augment information as appropriate.

Physical Measures

Sexual activity has strong physical components concerning initiation, execution, and completion of the act of intercourse or any sexual activity, including masturbation and oral sex. Within the physical realm of occupational therapy, measurements of ROM, grip and prehension strength, balance and mobility, and the presence of pain should be assessed to clearly understand physical abilities and limitations, including those that figure prominently in sexual activity and including whole body and extremity strength, balance, endurance, and the experience of pain.

A visual assessment of joint deformity should occur as a means of documenting the disease effects. This will vary from client to client because the course of arthritis is individual. Additionally, an assessment of client independence in the usual ADLs (e.g., dressing, bathing, grooming, ambulation and mobility, homemaking tasks) and a review of compensated or volunteer work should occur because arthritis can disrupt occupational roles. The client's perception of pain or discomfort should also be evaluated. The manner in which a client approaches activities and the energy that he or she expends when performing an activity can provide evidence of his or her ability to use *joint protection* (i.e., using joints in a way that avoids excessive stress) and work or *energy conservation* techniques (i.e., planning and doing activities so less effort is necessary and fatigue is reduced) that occupational therapists frequently recommend for intervention purposes. All of these items figure prominently in the execution of a sexual act.

Occupational Therapy Interventions

Addressing sexual activity with clients with arthritis has both physical and psychological components. Physical symptoms can influence the psychological well-being of a client, and the psychological issues can influence how the client feels physically, illustrating the mind–body connection. The arthritis symptoms might increase and decrease as the disease progresses, and this tends to provide a level of concern for these clients in their day-to-day lives, as they might not be able to predict how they will feel from day to day or hour to hour. In short, clients with arthritis cannot assume they will feel well enough in the immediate future to engage in sexual activity, or any other activity.

Components of activity pacing (Murphy, Smith, & Alexander, 2008), joint protection, and task or work simplification are identified as areas in which occupational therapists provide intervention for clients with arthritis (Palmer & Simons, 1991). However, no literature exists to clearly identify how and what occupational therapists can do to intervene with sexual activity deficits or perceived deficits for clients with arthritis.

Occupational therapy interventions that might be used to address sexual activity will most likely be a secondary result of primary or typical interventions. Occupational therapists would typically address issues pertaining to energy conservation, joint protection techniques, ROM, mobility and functional ambulation, focus and attention, and pain management. This chapter discusses energy conservation, joint protection techniques, and use of thermal agents, as these interventions have great application to sexual activity and consideration of any of them as a primary intervention method would have secondary effects of improving the comfort and motion necessary for sexual activity (as shown in Case Example 2.1). Occupational therapy interventions directly related to sexuality, including positioning, devices, and communication, will also be discussed.

Energy Conservation

Energy conservation techniques ensure that a client will have enough energy to engage in any task and involves the client simplifying, planning, and organizing his or her daily activities. In essence, it is important for the client to have enough energy to do the activities that need to be done and to have enough energy to do the activities that the client wants to do. Energy conservation might be indirectly related to a consistent medication schedule. For example, if medication is taken and safe participation in tasks occurs, pain and discomfort could be less likely, and the energy level and energy reserve would permit engagement of the tasks of daily living.

Case Example 2.1. Margie: RA

Margie, age 58 years, was diagnosed with RA almost 8 years ago. Since the time of her diagnosis, she has gone through menopause and has experienced an increase of RA symptoms, including fatigue and joint pain, resulting joint deformity, and a significant decrease in her overall activity tolerance level and libido. Margie used to work 40–50 hours each week as a cake and cookie decorator at a local bakery but has had to reduce her work hours to less than 20 hours per week. She also reports "feeling wiped out" on the days that she does work. This fatigue results in her not being able to interact and socialize with her husband, family, and friends. Margie and her husband have two grown children and one grandchild. Her children and grandchild used to visit her and her husband almost daily. However, Margie has fatigue and discomfort; therefore, family visits occur infrequently. Margie also reports that she is usually too tired to "even think about having sex." She reports "feeling depressed" over the status of her marital relationship.

Margie was referred to occupational therapy to help her improve her involvement in and tolerance for work-related, leisure, social, and family activities. After completing a comprehensive evaluation, the occupational therapist developed a daily, customized schedule for Margie. The major focus of the schedule is to maximize daily work and leisure or social involvement during Margie's "best time of day," which is usually the late morning to early afternoon. To help Margie work and maintain her pre-diagnosis QoL, the energy conservation schedule includes

---

(*Continued*)

Case Example 2.1. Margie: RA (*cont.*)

1. Taking medication after breakfast (rather than "whenever," as Margie used to do)
2. Performing gentle stretching exercises after the morning warm shower or bath (as opposed to stretching after activity when she was already fatigued)
3. Taking short breaks as necessary to assist with task completion (whereas Margie would not take breaks and force herself to keep working)
4. Using a tall kitchen stool to decorate cookies and cakes while in a sitting position (rather than standing) during work and personal kitchen activities
5. Using a rolling kitchen cart to move items from one side of the kitchen to another (as opposed to Margie's previous method of walking back and forth) at work and at home
6. Scheduling work and personal activities during times when energy is highest and disease symptoms are lowest
7. Developing a schedule of daily work and leisure or social activities
8. Use of padded or ergonomically correct tools for work-related tasks
9. Use of pillows or bolsters to increase comfort at home and in bed
10. Consistently using energy conservation principles both at work and at home.

Using general principles of energy conservation will help Margie resume her pre-diagnosis life roles and assume the responsibility for engagement in those roles. By her development of and adherence to a daily schedule, she will attain a reserve of energy that will enable her to become reengaged in work and personal roles at a level that is more acceptable to her standards. Frequently, joint protection techniques are linked to energy conservation principles because an individual uses less energy when joints are used and positioned in a less physically stressful manner.

Joint Protection

Joint protection principles include the following:

1. Respect pain as a signal to stop the activity.
2. Maintain muscle strength and joint ROM.
3. Use each joint in its most functional anatomical and functional plane of motion.

4. Avoid positions of deformity and forces in their direction.
5. Use the largest and strongest joints available for the job.
6. Ensure correct patterns of movement.
7. Avoid staying in one position for long periods.
8. Avoid starting an activity that cannot be stopped immediately if it proves to be beyond capability.
9. Balance rest and activity.
10. Reduce the force exerted on joints using ergonomics, body mechanics, and work simplification strategies (Yasuda, 2008).

Using the example of Margie in Case Example 2.1, Margie can use joint protection principles in a variety of settings. For example, if Margie uses appropriate joint positioning in bed using pillows or bolsters, her sleep will become more rejuvenating, and pain or discomfort will be decreased. In work or kitchen activities, if she uses ergonomically appropriate tools or modified tools, the stress on her hands and elbows will be lessened, and she will use less joint force, decreasing pain and minimizing position of deformity (e.g., ulnar deviation when cutting, static positioning during activity, sustained and forceful grip or pinch). If Margie follows her daily schedule, she will have the opportunity to take breaks or stop an activity if pain occurs because of time allotments for work and rest.

Thermal Agents

To ensure that motion is comfortable, especially in the upper extremities, hips, knees, and low back, the use of thermal agents (in this situation the use of heat or cold) can be presented to the client. Thermal agents can increase overall comfort and improve tolerance for any activity if used safely and correctly. Taking a warm shower or bath prior to engaging in sex might increase the client's level of comfort and improve ROM in joints. The use of *modalities* like moist heat or something cold might also be a good inclusion before engaging in sex. Note that some clients with arthritis get greatest relief from symptoms with heat, whereas some individuals prefer cold.

Therapists frequently discover that clients are already incorporating the use of thermal agents in their daily routines. However, it is a good idea to stress the safe use of any thermal agent with a client. Thermal agents should be thought of as a precursor to any activity, including sexual activity. Safety rules for thermal agents include

1. Use safe and recommended devices like gel packs or heating pads with Underwriters Laboratories approval.

2. Provide layers of skin protections via the use of a terrycloth towel. There should be at least 2–3 layers of "insulation" between the thermal device and the client's skin.

3. Use a timer to ensure that the thermal device is not left on the skin area for too long. Generally, it is prudent to leave hot or cold devices on for no longer than 15 minutes.

4. Instruct the client to immediately remove the device if it is uncomfortable or a burning or stinging sensation occurs.

5. Follow the use of thermal modalities with gentle ROM to the affected joint or joints.

6. Make certain the skin area returns to its normal color within 5–10 minutes after removing the thermal agent. If skin blanching (whiteness) or redness does not go away within this time, discontinue use of the thermal agent, and consult with the therapist or physician (Cameron, 2008).

Positioning Suggestions for Sexual Activity

It is important to stress to a client that there is no right or wrong way to engage in sexual intercourse. There really are no rules as to what sex is, looks like, sounds like, or smells like (Silverberg, 2006), so long as it involves only consenting adults.

The client with arthritis might find that the common position for sexual activity, with one partner on his or her back and the other partner on the top, might be uncomfortable, especially if one partner has arthritis that affects the hips, knees, or spine. In this case, the therapist can suggest alternative positions for sex (see suggested positions for more comfortable sexual activity Appendix A). Having sexual intercourse in a side-lying position (Figures A.1 and A.2) is generally considered a safe and more comfortable position, as joint stress is minimized in this position. Additionally, the use of any position that decreases joint stress to affected joints is suggested while stronger or unaffected joints assist with body stability.

The use of positioning aids like pillows or bolsters can also make positioning for sex more comfortable. For example, a "J" pillow, which looks like an upside down "J" and the head and neck are supported by the hook and the back is supported by the stem of the "J," are available in various sizes and shapes and can be used to support the head and neck and arms or legs. Bolster pillows can be used to promote side laying or hip and knee flexion.

Some clients also prefer the use of a mattress warmer (covered by a fitted or top sheet) if they are lying on their backs. A bed or mattress warmer provides a gentle heat source from the bottom, as opposed to warmth provided by an electric blanket, where warmth is on top of the individual. Bed or mattress warmers can be purchased through a variety of discount stores and marts and are generally available for less than \$50. They come in mattress sizes from twin-sized through king-sized. Because a mattress warmer provides a neutral heat source, covering or partially covering the body with a blanket during cool or cold weather might not be necessary. Additionally, not using a blanket to cover oneself increases unrestricted motion and mobility (University of Washington, 2009).

Devices

If pain or discomfort precludes involvement in sexual intercourse, alternate ways to gain sexual or sensual pleasure can be employed. The client's partner can provide gentle massage and sensual touch. Cuddling, hugging, or laying close to each other can provide a sense of security and closeness. The use of devices is also an appropriate option. Note that some clients might accept the use of devices, and others might not. Again, the use of the PLISSIT Model (Annon, 1976; see also Chapter 1) provides the therapist with structure and guidelines to broach this subject with a client. Additionally, it is important to stress that the use of devices or alternate positions for sex is quite normal and is a natural expression of human sexuality and intimacy. If oral stimulation is preferred in lieu of sexual intercourse, the positioning of the partners' bodies should be comfortable and supportive of weight and painful joints. If the temporal mandible joint (TMJ) is affected by arthritis, providing oral stimulation might be difficult because the TMJ might become fatigued and uncomfortable during the stimulation.

There are a variety of vibrators and dildos available if the client is unable to become involved in sexual intercourse. Vibrators or dildos can be held in the client's hand or in the partner's hand. Vibrators can also be used for self-stimulation, as this decreases forces on the fingers and hands.

If arthritis affects the clients' hands, a Velcro® hand strap can be used to facilitate placement in the hand and the use of the device. Vaginal lubrication might be insufficient for comfortable intercourse, especially if the client is taking higher doses of medication or is diagnosed with a systemic form of arthritis. In this case, vaginal, gel-based lubricants (e.g., K–Y™ jelly) are available to increase lubrication and comfort during sexual activity.

Communication

Good communication skills are crucial to any relationship. When sexual activity is problematic or difficult, good communication between partners is essential (see Case Example 2.2). The client should be encouraged to be clear and direct when speaking about sexual difficulties with his or her partner (see Exhibit 2.1). Presenting issues in an assertive manner is the most honest and direct method of communication. If the client is hesitant to speak to his or her partner because he or she is embarrassed or shy, assertive behavioral role-play can be conducted with general topics. Many individuals do not assert themselves outside of the bedroom, let alone in the bedroom. The occupational therapist can intervene by providing suggestions and role-play for assertive communication.

Once the client practices and integrates assertive skills, with the permission of the client, the therapist can broach issues related to sexual activity. For example, if a client is too tired or fatigued to engage in sexual activity and his or her partner is interested in having sex, the client can say,

> I understand that you want to have sex now, and I'm glad you want to and that you find me desirable. My day has been stressful, and I'm having a lot of pain in my hips and low back now. Can we cuddle or maybe wait until tomorrow?

By phrasing needs in this manner, the client shares honest information without acquiescing to having sex or responding in an aggressive manner. Please note that assertive role-playing might not be within the comfort zone of the therapist and, if this is so, a referral to another health care professional is appropriate.

Case Example 2.2. Carol: Fibromyalgia

Carol is a 53-year-old client diagnosed with fibromyalgia. She is married and has one college-aged child living at home. She resides with her husband and daughter in a two-story home in the suburbs. Carol has been teaching elementary school for the past 25 years. She currently is assigned to teach sixth grade at a school located about 3 miles from her home. Carol's husband works as a high school teacher. Her daughter is a college junior at a local university.

Carol was diagnosed with fibromyalgia 3 years ago. Carol states, "I thought I was just getting old—going through menopause—with a lot of aches and pains." Carol also reports that she and her husband have had marital difficulties for the last 10 years because, "Things aren't like they were when I felt better."

Concerning daily living activities, Carol is independent in dressing, bathing, and grooming. She cooks and "tidies up" daily after working from 8:00–3:30 as a teacher. She was active in local church and community organizations but has had to curtail involvement because of fibromyalgia symptoms of fatigue, diffuse pain and discomfort, and, from her report, "just feeling like I can't do much more than I am doing. I'm tired all the time."

(Continued)

Case Example 2.2. Carol: Fibromyalgia (*cont.*)

Carol reports that her husband "is usually off doing something during the evenings, so I'm at home by myself or with my daughter—if she is free." Carol indicates that she and her husband used to have "a regular sex life" but indicates that they no longer have sex because of her symptoms, her fatigue, and "my husband's indifference to me. He just doesn't think I'm attractive, or like my daughter would say, I'm not 'a hottie.'"

Carol has gained approximately 30 pounds over the past 2 years, and this is a source of concern for her. Carol states that her husband does not want to talk about their marital problems and thinks "that all of this is in my head."

Questions to Consider

1. What are common symptoms associated with fibromyalgia?
2. What problems does this client experience overall?
3. What issues regarding sexual activity does this client report?
4. What interventions can occupational therapy provide?

Exhibit 2.1. Assertive Communication Suggestions

Communication is a key element in personal interaction. Communication channels with a significant other must be open, honest, and clear. The following represent a few helpful hints designed to maintain good communication:

1. Maintain eye contact.
2. Use statements beginning with words like "*I feel (state feelings) when you (state behavior or action)*."
3. Do not be accusatory.
4. Maintain a calm voice tone.
5. If you find yourself becoming angry, state this. If you need to stop the communication, you can return to it when you are calmer. Let the other person know your intent.
6. Treat the other person with respect and speak with him or her in a respectful manner.
7. Speak or talk *with* the other person. Don't talk or speak *to* or *at* the other person.

Summary

Arthritis affects millions of adults and can profoundly affect sexuality, especially as clients battle pain and fatigue. Occupational therapy interventions that acknowledge sexual activity as an ADL and the unique challenges that clients with arthritis face can allow clients to participate in sexuality activity and experience greater well-being.

References

Abdel-Nasser, A., & Ali, E. (2006). Determinants of sexual disability and dissatisfaction in female patients with rheumatoid arthritis. *Clinical Rheumatology, 25*(6), 822–830.

American Occupational Therapy Association. (2008). Occupational therapy practice framework: Domain and process (2nd ed.). *American Journal of Occupational Therapy, 62,* 625–683. doi: 10.5014/ajot.62.6.625

Annon, J. S. (1976). The PLISSIT model: A proposed conceptual scheme for the behavioral treatment of sexual problems. *Journal of Sex Education and Therapy, 2,* 1–15.

Arthritis Basics. (2009). *History of arthritis.* Retrieved December 13, 2009, from http://arthritis.ygoy.com/history-of-arthritis/

Beck, A., Steer, R., & Brown, G. K. (1996). *Beck Depression Inventory* (2nd ed.). San Antonio, TX: Psychological Corporation.

Cameron, M. M. (2008). *Physical agents in rehabilitation* (3rd ed.). Philadelphia: Saunders Press.

Canadian Association of Occupational Therapy. (1996). *Canadian Occupational Performance Measure.* Ottawa, ON: Author.

Carr, A., Thompson, P., & Kirwan, J. (1996). Quality of life measures. *British Journal of Rheumatology, 35,* 275–281.

Centers for Disease Control and Prevention. (2008). *Data and statistics: Arthritis related statistics.* Retrieved November 26, 2008, from http://www.cdc.gov/arthritis/data_statistics_related_stats.htm

Centers for Disease Control and Prevention. (2011). Arthritis as a potential barrier to physical activity among adults with obesity: United States, 2007 and 2009. *Morbidity and Mortality Weekly Report, 60,* 614–618.

Dickens, C. M., & Creed, F. (2001). The burden of depression in patients with rheumatoid arthritis. *Rheumatology, 40,* 1327–1330.

Doeglas, D. M., Suurmeijer, T., van den Heuvel, W. J. A., Krol, B., van Rijswick, M. H., van Leeuwen, M. A., et al. (2004). Functional ability, social support, and depression in rheumatoid arthritis. *Quality of Life Research, 13*(6), 1053–1065.

Dubouloz, C., Laporte, D., Hall, M., Ashe, B., & Smith, C. D. (2004). Transformation of meaning perspectives in clients with rheumatoid arthritis. *American Journal of Occupational Therapy, 58,* 398–407. doi: 10.5014/ajot.58.4.398

Eustice, C., & Eustice, R. (2009). *Signs and symptoms of osteoarthritis.* Retrieved January 17, 2009, from http://osteoarthritis.about.com/od/osteoarthritissymptoms/a/signs_symptoms.htm

Hallberg, L. R., & Bergman, S. (2011). Minimizing the dysfunctional interplay between activity and recovery: A grounded theory on living with fibromyalgia. *International Journal of Qualitative Studies on Health and Well-Being, 6*(2). doi:10.3402/qhw.v6i2.7057

Hattjar, B., Parker, J., & Lappa, C. (2008). Addressing sexuality with adult clients with chronic disabilities: Occupational therapy's role. *OT Practice, 13*(1), CE1–CE8.

Law, C. (2001). Sexual health and the respiratory patient. *Nursing Times, 97*(12), 11.

Linder, S. (2007). The missing activity of daily living. *Advance for Occupational Therapy Practitioners, 22*(17), 47.

Mayo Clinic. (2011). *Rheumatoid arthritis symptoms*. Retrieved June 3, 2011, http://www.mayoclinic.com/health/rheumatoid-arthritis/DS00020/DSECTION=symptoms

McAlonan, S. (1996). Improving sexual rehabilitation services: The patient's perspective. *American Journal of Occupational Therapy, 50,* 826–834. doi: 10.5014/ajot.50.10.826

Murphy, S. L., Smith, D. M., & Alexander, N. B. (2008). Measuring activity pacing in women with lower-extremity osteoarthritis: A pilot study. *American Journal of Occupational Therapy, 62,* 329–334. doi:10.5014/ajot.62.3.329

National Academy on an Aging Society. (2000). *Arthritis: A leading cause of disability in the United States*. Retrieved January 25, 2012, from http://www.agingsociety.org/agingsociety/pdf/arthritis.pdf

Newman, A. M. (2007). Arthritis and sexuality. *Nursing Clinics of North America, 42*(4), 621–630.

Palmer, P., & Simons, J. (1991). Joint protection: A critical review. *British Journal of Occupational Therapy, 54,* 453–458.

Porth, C. M. (2004). *Essentials of pathophysiology: Concepts of altered health states*. Philadelphia: Lippincott Williams & Wilkins.

Primatesta, P., Plana, E., & Rothenbacher, D. (2011). Gout treatment and comorbidities: A retrospective cohort study in a large U.S. managed-care population. *BMC Musculoskeletal Disorders, 12*(1), 103.

Radloff, L. S. (1977). The CES–D Scale: A self-report depression scale for research in the general population. *Applied Psychological Measurement, 1*(3), 385–401.

Rogers, C. R. (1980). *A way of being*. New York: Houghton Mifflin.

Rogers, M., Liang, M., & Partridge, J. (1982). Psychological care of adults with rheumatoid arthritis. *Annals of Internal Medicine, 96*(3), 344–348.

Ryan, S. (2009). *The psychological and social implications of rheumatoid arthritis*. Retrieved December 18, 2009, from http://www.library.nbs.uk/musculoskeletal/ViewResource.aspx?resID=5218

Schwartz, M. (2010, January 23). A shift of mind: Rethinking the way we live: Beyond the mind–body connection. *Psychology Today.* Retrieved December 2, 2011, from http://www.psychologytoday.com/blog/shift-mind/201001/beyond-the-mind-body-connection

Shabsigh, R., Zakaria, L., Anastasiadis, A. G., & Seidman, S. N. (2001). Sexual dysfunction and depression: Etiology, prevalence, and treatment. *Current Urology Reports, 2*(6), 463–467.

Silverberg, C. (2006). *Sexuality and disability.* Retrieved January 10, 2012, from http://sexuality.about.com/od/disability/p/disability_sex1.htm?p=1

University of Washington. (2009). *Sex and arthritis: Body positions and techniques.* Retrieved December 19, 2009, from http://www.orthop.washington.edu/uw/livingwith/tabID_3376?ItemD_99/PageID_15_

Willis, M. C. (2008). *Medical terminology: The language of healthcare* (2nd ed.). Philadelphia: Lippincott Williams & Wilkins.

Yasuda, Y. (2008). Rheumatoid arthritis, osteoarthritis, and fibromyalgia. In M. Radomski & C. Latham (Eds.), *Occupational therapy for physical dysfunction* (6th ed., pp. 1214–1243). Philadelphia: Lippincott Williams & Wilkins.

Zigmond, A. S., & Snaith, R. P. (1983). The Hospital Anxiety and Depression Scale. *Acta Psychiatrica Scandinavica, 67*(6), 361–370.

3

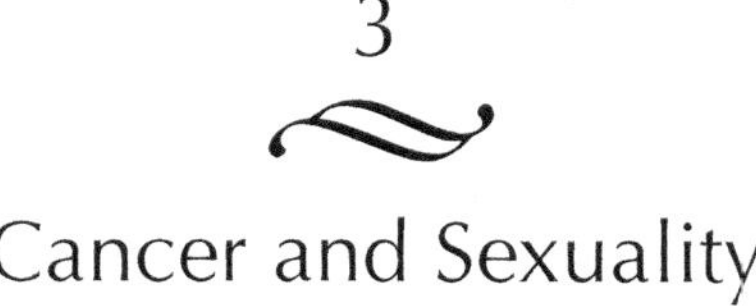

Cancer and Sexuality

Constance Lappa, MSW, LCSW, Diplomate of Sex Therapy

Key Terms and Concepts

- BETTER Model
- Body image
- Cancer
- PLISSIT Model
- Quality of life
- Sexual health.

Upon completion of this chapter, readers will be able to

- Recognize common symptoms associated with the major forms of cancer that affect quality of life,
- Understand how to assess the physical and psychological effects of cancer on a particular individual,
- Identify specific sexual side effects of cancer and the treatment of cancer,
- Identify strategies to manage the sexual side effects of cancer and its treatment,
- Use either the PLISSIT Model or the BETTER Model to assess and intervene to improve sexual functioning in clients with cancer.

Cancer and Sexual Health

Cancer occurs when "abnormal cells divide without control and can invade nearby tissues" (National Cancer Institute [NCI], 2011). Cancer cells may also travel and invade other areas of the body, including the reproductive, digestive, and urinary systems. Both males and females of all ages may experience the impact of cancer. Like many illnesses, cancer is diagnosed in various stages, from early to late, and it may or may not progress or reoccur. Each form of cancer, stage, and treatment has different physical and psychological effects. In addition, factors unique to each individual such as their prior state of health, availability of social supports, and emotional resilience can lessen or intensify the physical and psychological consequences of the diagnosis of cancer.

As the population of older adults increases and cancer treatments improve, residual effects and disabilities in clients with cancer are increasing the need for occupational therapy (Cooper, 2006). People coping with cancer and its aftermath often must deal with physical and emotional changes. These changes, which have the potential to significantly affect the body and self-image, can also negatively affect the person's sexual health. *Body image,* or "a person's perceptions, thoughts, and feelings about his or her body" (Grogan, 2008, p. 3), might be affected by the changes brought about by cancer and its treatment.

Cancer affects both physiological and psychological health; therefore, it affects sexual health. According to the World Health Organization (WHO; 2002), *sexual health* is

> the experience of the ongoing process of physical, psychological, and socio-cultural well-being related to sexuality. Sexual health is evidenced by the free and responsible expressions of sexual capabilities that foster harmonious personal and social wellness, enriching individual and social life. It is not merely the absence of dysfunction, disease, or infirmity. For sexual health to be attained and maintained, it is necessary that the sexual rights of all people be recognized and upheld. (p. 1)

WHO includes sexual health as part of a person's overall health; therefore, anything that affects an individual's physical or psychological health could affect sexuality. Because cancer affects both the physical and psychological realms, it can affect sexual health. Persons with cancer might have changes in their physical functioning (e.g., difficulty with the bowels or bladder, fatigue, vaginal atrophy or narrowing) that create barriers to sexual functioning. Such persons might also experience the loss of body parts (e.g., breasts, ovaries, testicles, prostate) that can affect patterns of sexual arousal. Clients might feel that their bodies have failed them or that they are no longer attractive;

although these feelings are not uncommon, they can affect psychological functioning and cause the person to withdraw from sexual contact.

Oncologists do not always know exactly which cancerous cells will become deadly (e.g., some cancer cells die off or stay local without causing major trouble or death), but for some cancers, survival rates are increasing as more cancers are found that would never have gone on to cause death (Esserman, Shieh, & Thompson, 2009). More cancers are being found; therefore, more are being treated (American Cancer Society [ACS], 2010). Although precise causes for decreased mortality are widely debated (Paneth, Vande Woude, & Kort, 2010), aggressive intervention for early-stage breast or prostate cancer (e.g., mastectomy, prostatectomy) might dramatically affect a client's sexuality, when less aggressive intervention (e.g., watchful waiting, active surveillance) might offer the same mortality rate (Esserman et al., 2009).

At initial diagnosis, survival issues naturally take precedence over sexual concerns, but as the shock lessens, quality of life (QoL), including sexuality, becomes a part of recovery. *Quality of life* "measures the difference, at a particular moment in time, between the hopes and expectations of the individual and that individual's present experiences" (Calman, 1984, p.125). Although research on the sexual effects of cancer is still lacking in many areas, enough has been done to demonstrate that cancer affects the quality of sexuality for most clients (Rustoen & Begnum, 2000) and that clients want more information to restore function in this area (Feldman-Stewart et al., 2000).

Demographics

Over a million Americans are diagnosed with cancer each year (ACS, 2010). With improvements in diagnosis and treatment, more people are surviving cancer and hoping to return to their daily activities, including sexual functioning. The incidence of cancer increases with age, and sexuality issues are certainly paramount to younger clients (along with fertility issues), but an occupational therapy practitioner cannot assume that women who have already passed through menopause do not have sexual challenges from cancer or treatment. Likewise, practitioners cannot assume that older men with prostate cancer are not as worried about impotence as younger men are.

The three most common cancers diagnosed in women are (1) breast, (2) lung, and (3) colorectal. The most common types of cancers diagnosed in men are (1) lung, (2) prostate, and (2) colorectal. In addition, incidence of colorectal cancers in both men and women ages 50 years or younger is increasing (Edwards et al., 2009; Siegel, Jemal, & Ward, 2009). Certain cancers, for example, those in the breast, prostate, testes, penis, gynecological areas (e.g., cervix, uterus, vagina, vulvae), bladder, and colon–rectum, have a more profound effect on sexuality. Recent statistics for the numbers of cancer survivors include the following statistics: There were over 11 million Americans living with a history of cancer in at least one site as of 2008 (Surveillance, Epidemiology, and End Results Program [SEER], 2011).

- The median age at diagnosis was 66 years of age, according to SEER[1] incidence data from 2004 to 2008.

- It was estimated that over 207,000 women would be diagnosed with breast cancer in 2010 (NCI, 2010).

- It was estimated that over 217,000 men would be diagnosed with prostate cancer in 2010 (NCI, 2010).

Cancer Signs and Symptoms

The signs and symptoms of cancer vary widely, depending on its type, location, and stage. Most cancers do not cause pain in the earlier stages; however, in later stages, pain is often a symptom. Table 3.1 describes types of cancer-related pain. Symptoms may include

- A thickening or lump in the breast or any other part of the body

- A new mole or a change in the appearance of an existing mole

- A sore that does not heal

- Hoarseness or a cough that does not go away

- Changes in bowel or bladder habits

- Discomfort after eating

- Difficulty with swallowing

- Weight gain or loss with no attempt to lose or gain weight

- Unusual bleeding or discharge from a body orifice

- Feeling very weak or very tired.

The most common forms of cancer—of the breast, prostate, colon-rectum, and lung—present with a variety of symptoms. Exhibit 3.1 lists specific types of cancer and the common symptoms associated with them.

---

1. *Note.* SEER is a report of the most recent cancer statistics for incidence, prevalence, survival, lifetime risk, and mortality. It is published by the National Cancer Institute, a branch of the U.S. National Institutes of Health. The most recent year report available at the time this book was published was used by the author.

Table 3.1. Cancer-Related Pain

Type of Pain	Descriptors	Possible Etiology	Exam
Neuropathic pain	• Tingling • Burning • Numbness • Shock-like • Intermittent • Constant	• Tumor adjacent to or adhered to peripheral nerves • Vertebral collapse causing nerve compression • Radiation fibrosis causing tissue adherence to nerve	• Motor weakness • Altered sensation • (+) neural tension tests • Pain along a myotome or dermatome • Numbness/tingling in distal fingertips and toes
Skeletal pain	• Sharp • Intermittent or constant • Escalating back pain • Pain in supine • Pain with ambulation • Pain in groin with standing	• Altered bone stability • Cord compression • Avascular necrosis	• Pain with weight-bearing • Pain with joint compression • Pain that radiates to groin or anterior thigh with weight-bearing • Pain in a band across chest • Pain with coughing
Joint pain	• Pain with functional activity • Ache	• Tumor encroaching joint space • Neupogen pain • Arthralgia syndrome associated with Taxanes	• Possible palpation of tumor • Pain with passive and active ROM
Postsurgical pain	• Pain with coughing • Pain with mobility • Sharp • Constant ache • Intermittent or chronic	• Positioning during surgery • Manipulation of nerves during surgery • Altered biomechanics from nerve palsy • Muscle spasm from positioning	• Pain along surgical site • Tingling along nerve distribution • Pain with deep inspiration
Soft tissue pain	• Ache • Stiffness with movement	• Radiation fibrosis • Soft tissue changes from graft-versus-host disease • Contracture from immobility • Protective muscle spasm	• Reproduction of symptoms with passive stretching • Decreased skin elasticity • (+) trigger points • Decreased passive or active ROM

Note. From "Oncological Diseases and Disorders," by L. Packel. In D. L. Malone and K. L. B. Lindsay (Eds.), *Physical Therapy in Acute Care: A Clinician's Guide*, Thorofare, NJ: Slack. Copyright © 2006, by SLACK, Inc. Used with permission.
ROM = range of motion.

Exhibit 3.1. Selected Cancers and Symptoms

Lung Cancer

- A cough that doesn't go away and gets worse over time
- Consistent chest pain
- Coughing up blood
- Shortness of breath, wheezing, or hoarseness
- Repeated problems with pneumonia or bronchitis
- Swelling of the neck or face
- Fatigue
- Loss of appetite or weight loss.

Colorectal Cancer

- A change in bowel habits such as diarrhea, constipation, or narrowing of the stool that lasts for more than a few days
- A feeling of urgency to have a bowel movement that is not relieved by doing so
- Rectal bleeding, dark stools, or blood in the stools
- Cramping or abdominal pain
- Weakness and fatigue.

Breast Cancer

- A lump or thickening in or near the breast or in the underarm area
- A change in the size or shape of the breast
- Dimpling or puckering in the skin of the breast
- A nipple turned inward into the breast
- Discharge (fluid) from the breast, especially if it is a bloody discharge
- Scaly, red, or swollen skin on the breast, nipple, or *areola* (the dark area of skin at the center of the breast surrounding the nipple). The skin may have ridges or pitting so that it looks like the skin of an orange.

(Continued)

Exhibit 3.1. Selected Cancers and Symptoms (*cont.*)

Prostate Cancer

- Urinary problems, including (1) not being able to pass urine; (2) having a hard time starting or stopping urine flow; (3) needing to urinate often, especially at night; (4) weak flow of urine; (5) urine flow that starts and stops; or (6) pain or burning during urination
- Difficulty having an erection
- Blood in the urine or semen
- Frequent pain in the lower back, hips, or upper thighs.

Note. From National Cancer Institute (2011).

In addition to the physical symptoms of cancer, the client must cope with the psychological issues that come with a diagnosis of cancer. The psychological factors include (1) facing mortality, (2) changing self-esteem, (3) changing or losing occupational roles, (4) addressing effects on relationships, (5) addressing financial pressures, and (6) addressing altered body image. These psychological effects can lead to depression, anxiety, grief, and anger. All of these issues can have a negative impact on sexuality and sexual activity.

Treatment for cancer varies, depending on the type, location, and stage of the detected cancer. Treatments might include removal of a body part, surgical alternation of the usual appearance or functioing of the body (e.g., shortening the vagina), chemotherapy, hormonal therapy, and radiation therapies. Treatment for cancer might cause difficulties, including

- Postoperative pain
- Joint pain
- Loss of or change in appearance of body parts (e.g., breast, prostate)
- Loss of fertility
- Changes in bodily function (e.g., colostomy, vaginal atrophy, erectile dysfunction)
- Nausea and vomiting
- Hair loss or baldness

- Hormonal changes (e.g., decreased estrogen or testosterone)
- Fatigue
- Numbness (because of surgery, radiation, or chemotherapy).

Physical Changes

Physical changes that often occur with cancer can negatively affect sexuality for both males and females. These changes might be attributed to the cancer itself and to the treatment of the cancer, and they affect sexuality in multiple ways. The hormonal treatments for prostate cancer cause a decrease in testosterone, which lowers a man's libido and compromises his ability to become aroused. Women who have had radical hysterectomies for cervical cancer often have shortened vaginas, and follow-up radiation treatments can lead to vaginal scarring. Both treatments can make vaginal intercourse painful. People with lung cancer are often short of breath and might want to avoid sexual exertion. Prostate surgery, even if nerve sparing, can lead to nerve damage that affects the ability to have an erection. Women who lose a breast or clitoris to cancer might feel they have lost a critical part of their sexual arousal pattern (Katz, 2007).

Sometimes physical changes are temporary, but some changes are permanent and require exploring new patterns of arousal. For example, a woman may be able to find alternative ways to become aroused through the stroking of other body parts such as the inside of the thighs; kissing the neck; or stimulation of the tissue of the *legs of the clitoris,* which are areas of erectile tissue that descend from the clitoral bulb under the labia (O'Connell, Sanjeevan, & Hutson, 2005). For most men, the ability to have an erection is not immediately possible post-surgery for prostate cancer, but after 18 months to 2 years, erectile ability often returns (Wittman, Montie, Hamstra, Sandler, & Wood, 2009). Radiation therapy gradually causes a loss of erectile functioning as the treatment proceeds over time.

Hormonal Challenges

The loss or suppression of a key male or female hormone because of treatments such as radiation, hormonal agents, or chemotherapy compromises hormonal function, creating significant changes in sexuality. In women, the ovaries produce *estrogen,* which is responsible for the ability of the vagina to stretch and to lubricate, making vaginal intercourse comfortable. The ovaries also produce testosterone in women, which plays an important role in their sexual desire and ability to become aroused (Mayo Clinic, 2009). *Testosterone* is produced in the testicles in men and is responsible for both sexual desire and arousal, such as the ability to have an erection. Chemotherapy and radiation may damage the ovaries or testicles, causing them to lower or cease the production of estrogen and testosterone (Katz, 2007). Hormonal treatments for cancer lower the production of testosterone in men and estrogen in women for those people who have cancers that are dependent on those hormones, such as prostate or breast cancers.

Hormonal decline might lead to a decrease or loss in desire for sexual activity, difficulty in getting aroused, problems attaining orgasm, and impaired fertility in men and women. Hormonal changes or fluctuations in women can also lead to hot flashes, vaginal atrophy, and vaginal pain and dryness in women (symptoms are similar to those of menopause). Men may experience difficulty in getting or maintaining an erection.

Neurological Challenges

Nerve damage from surgery, chemotherapy, or radiation may cause a decrease or loss in arousal and orgasm. During surgery, even when performed by a skilled physician, nerves are often cut or traumatized, leading to an interruption in the signals sent between the genitals or breasts and the brain that tell the body to become aroused (NCI, 2010). Chemotherapy and radiation also have the potential to damage nerves with the same results. Therefore, clients might have decreased sensation, which makes it more difficult to become aroused. These losses often lead to frustration and decreased satisfaction with sexual activity; in turn, they can lead to a decrease in desire.

Circulatory Challenges

Damage to the genital area in men and women during surgery or because of radiation therapy can cause the arteries, which carry blood to the genital area, to become less flexible and to slow the blood flow. Impairment in blood flow impairs *vasocongestion,* the swelling of the tissue in the genital areas, which allows the areas to feel pleasurable by causing the spongy tissues in the penis and clitoris to become erect. The reduction in vasocongestion leads to a decrease or loss of arousal and orgasm, difficulty with erections for men, and decreased lubrication in women. Again, this can lead to decreased desire for sexual intimacy.

Structural Challenges

Loss or alteration of body parts (e.g., breast, uterus, ovaries, testicles, penis, prostate, vagina, clitoris) can lead to losses in desire, arousal, and orgasm. Breasts, for example, might be an important source of arousal for women, and the loss of or change in their breasts can create difficulty in arousal. Changes in functioning because of bowel or bladder removal can make spontaneous sexual encounters difficult. Similarly, a man who loses his penis loses a primary source of sexual arousal. The ovaries and testicles produce sex hormones, and once removed, the effect of that loss on sexual functioning as described above is immediate.

Other Physical Changes

Nausea, fatigue, pain, incontinence, and hair loss all play a part in creating obstacles to returning to former levels of sexual functioning. It is difficult to have interest in sexual activity when you are so fatigued, nauseated, or in such pain that it is difficult to move. Often, clients must decide what activities they can tolerate at a given time, for basic needs such as walking to the bathroom or attending a doctor's appointment take priority over sexual activity. Incontinence can occur during sexual activity, especially for men recovering from prostate surgery, which might lead to embarrassment and avoidance of sexual activity (Wittmann, Foley, & Balon, 2011). Similarly, changes (e.g., loss of hair) can cause a decrease in body image and the fear of being seen without hair during sexual activity may lead to avoidance.

Psychological Changes

Psychological changes have a less tangible but no less real effect on sexual activity for people with cancer. When someone is diagnosed with cancer, he or she is forced to face his or her own mortality. Uncertainty about the future, loss of control, and the loss the ability to participate in meaningful occupations can cause great emotional distress (Smith-Gabai, 2011).

Clients with cancer often experience a sense of vulnerability, even after the initial shock begins to fade. Being sexual also involves a certain amount of vulnerability and openness. In a situation where vulnerability is present (e.g., being sexual), the additional feeling of vulnerability stemming from the diagnosis of cancer might prove to be "too much." The client might be afraid to return to sexual activity until he or she can regain more confidence. In this situation, clients often lack information about what sexual changes to expect and do not know how to cope with these changes. They do not feel prepared to address their own or their partner's reactions to the changes. Anxiety about treatment or the prognosis might also weigh heavily on them. These feelings can tremendously dampen sexual desire and energy.

Treatment may also challenge a client's view of his or her masculinity or femininity, which is often tied to his or her sexual self-image. For a woman, the loss of her uterus, breasts, or part of her vulva to cancer may make her feel like less of a woman, as these body parts are associated with femininity

(Katz, 2007). Such loss can negatively affect her self-image and sexuality, leading to feelings of shame and avoidance of sexual contact. For a man, the loss of his testicles, the lack of ejaculate (caused by removal of the prostate gland), and problems with erection can symbolize a loss of masculinity, which might also lead to a poor self-image and negatively affect sexuality. Men and women who become infertile (i.e., unable to reproduce) as a result of treatment may experience damage to their masculine or feminine identities, in addition to grief over the loss of the ability to reproduce.

Often, treatment and recovery from cancer involves (1) taking time from work or family responsibilities and activities, (2) physical limitations, and (3) concern about a compromised immune system. These issues can affect a client's ability to perform in his or her previous roles at work, within his or her family, and with friends. The loss or change in roles can diminish self-esteem or self-image. This is often exacerbated by feelings of guilt ("This must be punishment for something I did in the past") or anger ("I always tried to keep myself healthy").

Sadness, anxiety, and frustration are common reactions to the diagnosis of cancer (NCI, 2009). These emotions can cause people to lose interest in sexual activity. Anger about their diagnosis might cause clients to push others away, including intimate partners. The client's intimate partner also goes through a range of emotions and often feels helpless to assist his or her partner through this crisis. Perhaps neither person knows what to say. He or she might fear upsetting the other person; thus, nothing is stated, and the feelings go unheard. Under these circumstances, it is common for communication problems to develop from misunderstandings or avoidance. If communication difficulties existed prior to diagnosis, the situation will frequently worsen without professional intervention. Because sexuality is an area many people are uncomfortable discussing, general communication difficulties compound the problem and make a bad situation worse.

Intimacy Assessment for Clients With Cancer

As identified by the *Occupational Therapy Practice Framework: Domain and Process* (American Occupational Therapy Association, 2008), sexual activity is an activity of daily living (ADL) and should be considered as such for the purpose of a thorough and comprehensive occupational therapy assessment. This can be accomplished by including an intimacy history (Hattjar, Parker, & Lappa, 2008) as a component of the initial evaluation or by using a questionnaire (see Appendix B) as an adjunct to the initial evaluation.

An *intimacy assessment* consists of questions about sexual concerns initiated by the client or occupational therapist within the framework of inquiring about other ADLs. The questions should be added to the customary evaluation and "align[ed] with physical, psychosocial and sensory issues that fall within the domain of occupational therapy practice" (Hattjar et al., 2008, p. CE5). Including questions about sexuality as well as questions about ADLs sends the message that sexuality is considered to be a normal part of life and is acceptable to discuss. Once sexuality concerns are brought out and clarified, they can be addressed as part of the overall care of the client. Although some clients may bring up sexual concerns themselves in the course of the occupational therapy evaluation, if they do not, the therapist should introduce the topic and then respect the client's level of interest in pursuing it.

The following guidelines help to establish the appropriate atmosphere in which to ask questions about intimacy.

- *The therapist must be comfortable initiating a discussion about sexuality.* This includes comfort with sexual terminology, a variety of sexual practices, and sexual orientation. It is not necessary to have complete comfort as long as the therapist is sincere in his or her desire to assist the client in this area and is respectful of any differences in values.

- *The therapist must understand the importance of sexuality in daily life and be comfortable with the variety of ways sexuality can be expressed.* The ways sexuality might manifest in daily life would include flirtatious touching, kissing, oral sex, or intercourse.

- *A behavioral rehearsal for the therapist with coworkers or friends can increase comfort in discussing sexual concerns.* Practicing the part of the assessment that addresses asking questions about sexual concerns with coworkers or friends can help the therapist become more comfortable using sexual terminology and addressing concerns in a calm, respectful manner that will increase the client's comfort level.

- *The therapist must have adequate knowledge of the illness.* Know the typical effects of cancer treatments, and know strategies commonly used to address sexual concerns resulting from these treatments.

- *The therapist must ensure confidentiality and privacy when intervening with concerns of a sexual nature.* Assuring the client that discussion of his or her sexual concerns will remain strictly confidential can increase the client's trust and openness.

- *The therapist must be aware of his or her body language and eye contact with the client.* A consistent stare may intimidate the client, while no eye contact may lead the client to believe that something negative or suspicious is occurring. Crossed arms can indicate that the therapist is not open to discussing the topic, while sitting too closely while discussing intimacy may make the client uncomfortable.

- *The therapist must project a nonjudgmental attitude.* Individuals express their sexuality in various ways, and people might hesitate to bring up their concerns if they feel that they will be judged, criticized, or ridiculed. It is important to convey that any question the client has is important. The goal is to give him or her information. Facial expressions should be kept neutral, and there should be no comments on the activity itself that could be interpreted by the client as judgmental.

- *The therapist should use language that is commonly understood.* Eliminate medical jargon that the client might not understand and be embarrassed to ask about. For example, instead of saying radiation can lead to "vaginal atrophy," the client could be told that the effects of radiation can lead to "vaginal dryness and a loss of stretchiness."

- *The therapist must be aware that not all clients are heterosexual.* Sensitivity must be expressed to homosexual or transgendered clients.

Sexual Assessment and Intervention Methods

Two models of intervention for sexual concerns might be used with clients who have cancer: the PLISSIT (Annon, 1976) or the BETTER Model (Mick, Hughes, & Cohen, 2003). Either model may be used after the therapist introduces the topic of sexuality as a part of life normalcy and QoL. This gives the client "permission" to speak about sexuality and sexual activity.

PLISSIT Model

PLISSIT (Annon, 1976) is an acronym for obtaining *P*ermission for the client to discuss sexual concerns, providing *L*imited *I*nformation needed by the client to function sexually, giving *S*pecific *S*uggestions for the individual to enable him or her to proceed with sexual relations, and providing referrals for *I*ntensive *T*herapy surrounding the issues of sexuality as they relate to the client.

Giving permission

Clients are often unsure when and if it is acceptable to discuss sexual concerns. Bringing up the topic of sexual activity along with other ADLs in a nonjudgmental way helps the client know that it is acceptable. In the process, making global statements such as "many people with cancer have concerns about their sexual functioning" normalizes the client's concerns about sexual issues and opens the door to future inquires.

Providing limited information

Clients might have questions about the changes they are experiencing in sexual functioning and might be anxious that nothing can be done to improve it. They might have been focused on survival and now believe that the sexual changes are something they just must accept as a tradeoff for survival. Providing information can help them understand the changes, which ones might be improved, and provide realistic hope for an improved QoL.

Giving specific suggestions

Clients might be at a loss about how to improve their sexual functioning; thus, specific suggestions tailored to their concerns are usually quite welcome. Perhaps they never used lubricants before their cancer diagnosis but now have significant vaginal dryness and could benefit from the suggestion of using them. The suggestions might also encourage the client to ask for further information related to their sexual functioning.

Providing intensive therapy

At times, specific suggestions are not sufficient, so the client needs to be referred to his or her physician for an examination or prescription or to a sex therapist for more intensive therapy. The diagnosis of cancer, combined with other stressful events (e.g., recent divorce), might cause the client to become quite depressed and anxious about future romantic and sexual relationships. It could be beneficial to refer him or her to a mental health–sex therapist who can address these concerns in psychotherapy. A man who has tried pills for erectile dysfunction to no avail might need an exam by a urologist and a prescription for another option such as a vacuum pump.

BETTER Model

The *BETTER* Model (Mick et al., 2003) is an acronym that encourages health care professionals to *B*ring up sexual issues with the client, *E*xplain the fact that sexual functioning is a QoL issue, *T*ell the client that resources are available, be aware of the importance of *T*iming in addressing sexual issues, *E*ducate clients about how the treatment they have received might affect their sexual functioning, and *R*ecord the intervention.

Bring up intimacy issues

Bringing up the topic of sexuality along with other issues of ADL gives the client assurance that sexual concerns are acceptable to discuss.

Explain

Verbally stating that sexuality is a part of normal, daily living normalizes it for the client and helps to make them more comfortable.

Tell

Telling clients that you are prepared to offer information and resources to address their concerns about sexual functioning will often encourage them to accept the information and ask further questions that could aid in improving their situation.

Timing

It is important to bring up the discussion along with other issues of functioning in a private area and give the client time to respond.

Educating

Clients may not be aware of all the sexual side effects of cancer treatment. For example, they may attribute their loss of desire to other reasons. It is helpful for them to recognize when the changes they are experiencing in their sexual functioning may be a result of their treatment.

Recording

It may be helpful to record some notes to assist the therapist in remembering to check back in with the client about the progress in restoring their sexual functioning while being careful to maintain as much privacy as possible. Extensive notes are not necessary in this situation.

There is some overlap in the two methods, as both address the issues of (1) normalizing the topic of sexuality as an appropriate concern to bring up, (2) providing education, and (3) offering suggestions for improving sexual functioning. The BETTER Model notes the importance of timing and specifically identifies sexual functioning as a QoL issue. Both models recognize the importance of other resources being available, although the BETTER Model places more focus on this area. The BETTER Model is more specific about some of the statements to use, such as telling the patient about resources that are available, while the PLISSIT Model is more open-ended. The differences between the models are not marked enough to recommend one over the other; therefore, therapists should use the method with which they feel most comfortable.

Further Assessment

If the client indicates an interest in discussing sexual issues further, the occupational therapist may choose to use one of several approaches to obtain a more detailed assessment of the sexual concerns. Information that is more specific can be gleaned through a conversational approach, starting with questions such as those suggested in "Addressing Sexuality With Adult Clients with Chronic Disabilities: Occupational Therapy's Role" (Hattjar et al., 2008) or the Kingsberg Brief Assessment (Kingsberg, 2006), to assess client concerns about sexuality.

The questions listed in Hattjar et al.'s (2008) article begin with a general inquiry about the client's physical status as related to his or her feelings of desirability and gradually to move into areas that are more sensitive. The questions are more detailed, although open ended, allowing the client to elaborate his or her answer.

The Kingsberg (2006) questions are very brief and open-ended, enabling the client to give additional information rather than simply a "yes" or "no" answer. Using the Kingsberg assessment, the therapist would start by asking whether the client was sexually active with anyone at the present time, which gender their partner(s) are, and inquiring in more detail about sexual problems if the client expresses concerns. The Kingsberg assessment is more specific and may be more or less comfortable for a particular therapist.

Either assessment can be used as part of a general occupational therapy assessment, or the therapist can add or subtract questions, depending on the client's level of interest and responses. As part of the psychosocial assessment, it is important to assess whether clients have concerns about depression or anxiety that could affect their overall functioning, including sexual functioning.

- If symptoms of depression are evident, administer the Beck Depression Inventory, 2nd Edition (BDI–II; Beck, Steer, & Brown, 1996), which has been validated in cancer populations (Vodermaier, Linden, & Siu, 2009).
- If symptoms of anxiety are evident, administer the Burns Anxiety Checklist (Burns, 1999).

Note. The BDI–II and the Burns Anxiety Checklist are administered to determine the degree that these psychological issues are affecting the individual and, conversely, the client's involvement in sexual activity and his or her personal sense of sexuality and gender.

Intervention

This section discusses how to intervene with a client who is experiencing any type of sexual dysfunction or sexual issue related to cancer. First, address depression, anxiety, relationship concerns, and other psychological issues through referrals to a counselor or physician. Using the LI (Limited Information) and the SS (Specific Suggestions) components of the PLISSIT Model (Annon, 1976), intervene with information and suggestions addressing the clients' concerns. Many of these interventions require a referral to a physician.

Education

Begin with education about the sexual effects of cancer and treatment. Review the common sexual side effects of the type of treatment the client has received or the location of the cancer, and address his or her questions.

- *Assess physical side effects.* Assess physical side effects of the cancer and its treatment and manage these side effects, including fatigue, pain, and loss of function or body part. How do the physical side effects interfere with functioning, and to what degree? Are there situations when things are better or worse? What has the client tried so far to manage the side effects?

- *Assess psychological effects.* Assess psychological effects and the management of cancer and treatment side effects, including depression, anxiety, and grief. Normalize the feelings that commonly arise when someone is diagnosed with cancer, and use questions and psychological inventories to determine if a referral is needed.

- *Encourage creativity and flexibility.* Encourage creativity and flexibility in thinking patterns to accommodate the client's status. Inform the client that he or she might need to look for ways to improve his or her sexual functioning beyond his or her usual routines.

- *Improve communication.* Provide and support involvement in communication skill training as a means of enhancing verbalization and expression of needs. It can be difficult to communicate needs, especially sexual needs; thus, clients and their partners can benefit from some guidance in voicing their needs. First, clients should choose a time to talk when both people are relaxed and not rushed. Before stating a concern, advise clients to start the conversation with a positive statement, such as "I enjoy the closeness we have when we have sex." Then have clients bring up a concern in a constructive way that is not critical, such as "I think I would get more into sex if [fill in the blank]." Making specific suggestions, using the first person "I" instead of "you," and inviting feedback can lead to a more productive discussion.

Inhibited or Loss of Desire, Arousal, and Orgasm

Many options exist to address inhibited desire or loss of desire or arousal and orgasm in men and women alike.

- *Engage in fantasy or erotica.* Recalling past positive sexual experiences, engaging in fantasies either mentally or through role-play with a partner, and using written or visual erotica can stimulate desire and arousal.

- *Use of sex toys or vibrators.* Vibrators can be used by both men and women externally or internally (e.g., on the clitoris, vaginally, anally, on the penis or testicles) to increase arousal and orgasm. Penis rings can help maintain an erection, and those with small vibrators attached can arouse both partners. They come in all sizes, some with a variety of speeds or sensations, and are available via the Internet, at local shops, and even at drugstores. Other sex toys, such as restraints and blindfolds, are also available to add novelty, which can enhance arousal.

- *Use of teasing touch to increase arousal.* Taking time to slowly build arousal by starting sexual touching away from the genital or breast area and gradually working toward those areas; touching them and moving elsewhere before returning; and touching lightly at first, followed by more pressure as arousal increases, can intensify arousal.

- *Use of sensual arousal (e.g., sensate focus or massage, affection exercises, tantric methods).* Starting with nongenital touching that is relaxing and sensual can lead to increased comfort by giving more time for the client to relax, turn off his or her worries, and focus on pleasurable body sensations. Exercises using nonsexual types of affection (e.g., increasing kissing and handholding) can also provide a transition time that takes pressure off the sexual experience. Tantric methods of massage that involve slowly moving the hands over the partner's body also offer similar benefits.

- *Hormonal interventions* (Seek a physician's advice in this area). Some female clients may benefit from the addition of estrogen or testosterone applied locally to the genital areas, but this may be contraindicated in some cancers, so the client should consult a physician.

- *Medication changes and additions* (Discuss with physician). Certain antidepressant and hypertensive medications, as well as other medications, can have a more damaging effect on sexual functioning than others can. There are times when the client's physician may be able to offer an alternative medication that has fewer sexual side effects.

- *Creative scheduling for intimate moments.* Try scheduling intimacy for times when energy is greater and fatigue is low, or try taking a nap prior to intimacy. Have clients review the times of day, days of the week, or times between treatments that they have the most energy and the least physical discomfort to determine when would be a better time to have intimacy.

- *Trying new things.* Increasing a novelty element of intimacy can elevate excitement, and partners trying something new or playful together increases arousal. Such new things could include sex at a different location, use of sex toys, a different activity or position, or a game.

- *Self-exploration.* Clients can take part in self-exploration to learn how things have physically changed and to determine what feels good now. If the body doesn't feel or respond as it did in the past, exploring by touching the body without one's partner can help the client to learn about the changes without feeling any pressure or worrying about a partner getting bored. Clients can then share what they learned with their partner.

Decreasing Vaginal Pain for Women

To decrease vaginal pain in women, suggest

- *Lubricants.* Water- or silicone-based lubricants for sexual intimacy and the use of moisturizing formula lubricants several times a week help to maintain tissue moisture. This increases comfort, which can facilitate arousal.

- *Vaginal Renewal Program.* Suggest use of the Vaginal Renewal Program, which is a process of gently massaging the external vulvar and internal vaginal tissues with a lubricant to moisturize the tissues and stimulate circulation to improve blood flow to the genital area (A Woman's Touch, 2007). Consult a physician, especially for cervical cancer.

- *Dilators.* Dilators are plastic or silicone penis-shaped forms in graduated sizes. Working from small to larger sizes, clients can gently stretch tissue and decrease muscle spasms (Lancaster, 2004). With permission from their physician, clients can begin a dilation program. Using the smallest dilator first, after coating it with lubricant, the client should relax and slowly insert the dilator into her vagina. She should allow it to remain inside for about 10 minutes. Once it is painless to insert the dilator, she can move to the next size up and follow the same process with each dilator until she can comfortably insert the largest one. She should practice with the dilators 3 times a week in order to make progress, but she can take whatever time she needs to become comfortable before moving up to the next size.

- *Physical therapy and biofeedback.* Physical therapy can reduce muscle spasms that may be causing pain (Rosenbaum & Owens, 2008). With permission of a physician, clients can learn to relax their pelvic muscles and perform Kegel exercises, which can improve blood flow, through pelvic floor biofeedback. This form of biofeedback consists of inserting a tampon-like sensor into the vagina. The sensor is connected to a computer that measures how much a client tightens and relaxes her pelvic muscles when she performs Kegel exercises. This feedback assists clients in learning to relax her pelvic muscles (Rosenbaum & Owens, 2008).

- *Muscle massage.* Receiving whole-body massages can help the client to relax and feel more positive about his or her body.

- *Kegel exercises.* Both men and women can learn to do Kegel exercises by stopping the flow of urine briefly—the muscle used to stop is the muscle on which to focus. The client should contract the muscle for a few seconds, then relax it. This can be repeated as several sets of 10 a day. Clients can learn to do Kegel exercises at home, which can help with muscle relaxation and improve circulation to the genital area.

- *Relaxation training.* Use of relaxation training, guided imagery, and deep breathing prior to sexual activity can increase the likelihood of relaxation and calmness and decrease anxiety that can interfere with arousal. Relaxation techniques often improve QoL for clients with cancer (Hidderley & Holt, 2004; Wright, Courtney, & Crowther, 2002).

- *Positional variations.* Use positional variations to increase overall comfort or to control the extent of penetration. For example, the woman-on-top position allows her to better control the depth of penetration, which is helpful if she has a shortened vagina (see Figure A.3 in Appendix A). It can also be beneficial for the client who is fatigued to be the one on the bottom to expend less energy.

- *Pillows, bolsters, wedges.* Use pillows, bolsters, or wedges for sexual positioning and to increase comfort. Lying flat on the back may cause breathing difficulties for some clients with lung cancer, so the use of a wedge pillow under the back so he or she is sitting up more can be helpful. Leaning over a pillow can also give support in a rear-entry sexual position for those with less arm or leg strength.

- *Localized hormonal treatments* (seek a physician's advice in this area). Use of localized hormonal treatments, such as Vagifem, Esring, or estrogen cream, can improve the elasticity of the vaginal tissue and the ability to lubricate (A-Baqhdai & Ewies, 2009).

Erectile Difficulty

- *Oral medications.* Use of oral medications (e.g., Viagra, Cialis, Levitra) can improve blood flow to the penis, improving the quality of erections. They can be used just before sexual activity with an effective time that varies from 6 to 36 hours. Stimulation is still important to achieve an erection, and these medications do not directly affect desire. Recently, a lower daily dose of Cialis has become available to assist clients in being able to be more spontaneous and not have to wait for the pill to take effect. (Consult a physician for these prescription medicines.)

- *Hormones.* For some men with below-normal testosterone levels, testosterone gel, patches, pills, or injections can restore the ability to become aroused and to achieve an erection. However, use of hormones may be contraindicated in men with certain cancers, such as prostate cancer, so the client should consult a physician to discuss this option.

- *Penile injections.* Injections into the penis of a prescription drug that improves blood flow (i.e., a vasodilator) with an ultrafine needle can produce an erection in about 20 minutes. Consult a physician.

- *Pellets.* Pellets called *Muse* also contain a vasodilator and are available by prescription. The pellet is inserted into the end of the penis where it dissolves and improves blood flow to help the man achieve an erection. Consult a physician.

- *Vacuum devices.* Vacuum devices can be used to increase firmness of erection or to attain erection. Only available by prescription, these devices create an erection by using gentle vacuum suction to draw blood into the penis. A stretchy ring is then placed on the base of the penis to help the blood stay in the penis. Consult a physician.

- *Penile implants.* If other less invasive methods have not been successful in producing an adequate erection, a surgeon can place implants in the penis that can be filled with fluid through squeezing a pump, or be permanently inflated and just bent down when not needed.

- *Vibrators.* Vibrators can be used on the penis or testicles for external stimulation or anally for stimulation of the prostate gland or tissue in that area. The vibration can offer more intense stimulation that can improve arousal.

- *Experiment with outercourse.* Place the penis between the lubricated breasts or thighs, or use oral or manual stimulation. This does not require an erection and can still lead to orgasm.

- *Try different position for sexual activity.* Some men find it is easier to maintain an erection in certain positions, such as being on top, than in others (see Figure A.4 in Appendix A).

Premature Ejaculation

Use of Kegel exercises, as previously described, can be used to control ejaculation through muscular control (tense–relax techniques).

- *Stop–start techniques.* Using stop–start techniques during sexual activity can help with improving erectile problems because of performance anxiety after a period of not being sexual because of treatments. The client can ask his partner to stimulate him to achieve an erection, then to slow down or stop the stimulation and allow the erection to wane, and then to restart stimulation. This can be done several times. This technique can help the client to not panic when he begins to lose his erection and instead to be more comfortable with his level of erection.

- *Antidepressants.* In some cases, the use of antidepressants slows ejaculation time (consult a physician). Some men may experience premature ejaculation after a period of sexual inactivity or may have had lifelong difficulties with controlling ejaculation, and certain antidepressants can slow down ejaculation.

Painful Ejaculation

For painful ejaculation, encourage the client to seek a physician's advice. Ensure that he secures an examination, as pain may signal a postoperative complication from surgery, an infection, or an obstruction in the ejaculatory duct (Ilie, Mischianu, & Pemberton, 2007).

General Pain

For clients, male or female, who experience general pain because of cancer or treatment, the following interventions could alleviate some discomfort:

- Use of thermal agents (e.g., heat, ice)
- Stretching and tension–release exercises as tolerated
- Use of guided imagery and other relaxation techniques
- Use of a warm shower or bath as tolerated
- Use of positional changes to increase comfort.

For persistent sexual problems that do not respond to LI and SS, consider a referral to a physician, therapist, or sex therapist.

Summary

Sexual activity is a part of life and should be included in the assessment of occupational therapists along with other areas of functioning. By using appropriate questions, maintenance of privacy and a nonjudgmental attitude, a therapist can determine a client's needs for assistance with sexual concerns. The diagnosis and treatment of cancer can cause significant changes to a client's sexual functioning in both the physical and psychological realms. Being able to assist the client in regaining functionality in the sexual area of their lives by acknowledging sexuality as an issue, providing information, and offering suggestions and resources is an important role for the occupational therapist (see Case Example 3.1).

Case Example 3.1. Kim: Breast Cancer

Kim is a 34-year-old woman who has been diagnosed with Stage II breast cancer. She was diagnosed approximately 20 months ago and has subsequently undergone a bilateral mastectomy, reconstructive surgery, and chemotherapy. She recovered from her treatments and was attempting to return to her normal ADLs, including involvement in sexual activity. Six months ago, she was diagnosed with a lesion in her spinal cord after experiencing numbness and weakness in her right leg. Kim underwent surgery, which left her unable to walk without assistance from a walker. She also experienced left-side numbness, including numbness in her genital area. At this time, she is continuing with chemotherapy and rehabilitation.

Kim is married and has a 5-year-old son and a 2.5 year-old daughter. Prior to her most recent diagnosis, Kim worked as a school librarian. She is

(Continued)

Case Example 3.1. Kim: Breast Cancer (*cont.*)

now unable to work and is receiving disability payments. Kim's husband, Michael, is a local sales representative for a large company. Michael must occasionally travel for his work. Kim and Michael's families are supportive and provide child care and transportation when needed.

When Kim was first diagnosed after the birth of her daughter, she and her husband were devastated. Kim prided herself in leading an active and healthy lifestyle. She felt that her body betrayed her. Her husband was supportive and loving in relation to Kim's situation. Together, they made the difficult decision for Kim to have bilateral mastectomies to decrease the chances of the cancer's reoccurrence. After the surgery, Kim underwent 6 months of aggressive chemotherapy as further insurance against reoccurrence. Although the extensive chemotherapy was physically difficult, she felt that the experience was worth it. She was exhausted and nauseated, lost her hair, and had low ovary function during treatment, which caused her hormone levels to be lowered. This contributed to lower sexual desire, vaginal dryness, and inability to achieve orgasm. Kim stated, "I just didn't feel like a woman at that time. I had no hair, no breasts, and no hormones. It was hard on Michael, too. He is supportive and loving. We cuddled a lot, and I felt very close to him, even though we weren't having sex."

After the chemotherapy was completed, Kim underwent breast reconstruction, regrew her hair, and her menses returned. She began to feel more like a woman again, but she was self-conscious about the changes in her body. Gradually, her energy and interest in sex started to return, and she and her husband began to enjoy being sexual again. She took more time to become aroused and had to learn to adjust to the numbness in her breasts.

Then Kim noticed numbness and weakness in her right leg. After many evaluations, she was diagnosed with a lesion in her spine. Following surgery, she was unable to walk or control her bowels and bladder. She also had to undergo more chemotherapy. This situation placed stress on the marital relationship. Michael had to curtail travelling for his work, as the bulk of family responsibilities now rested on his shoulders. This change in work and home responsibilities added additional stress on the marital relationship. Michael and Kim became more distant. They not only stopped having sex but also stopped cuddling and kissing. Neither one felt they could talk to the other for fear of hurting the other person's feelings.

Gradually, Kim began to respond to the treatment and regained use of her bowels and bladder. She also began to ambulate with a walker. She regained energy and began to believe in her doctor's positive prognosis. How-

(Continued)

Case Example 3.1. Kim: Breast Cancer (*cont.*)

ever, because of the chemotherapy, she still experiences hormonal changes, and the emotional distance between her and her husband seems to have increased. Even when she had some sexual desire, she kept it to herself, thinking that, with the hormonal changes, intercourse would probably be painful, as her gynecological exam had been. She wondered about exploring for herself but was embarrassed to do this. Kim felt that Michael would not be attracted to her any longer, even though he was supportive of her situation.

Questions to Consider

1. What are some of the common symptoms Kim experienced with her first diagnosis?
2. How did initial treatment affect Kim's sexuality?
3. How is the second diagnosis and treatment affecting her? What are the differences?
4. What are some suggestions to make to Kim to help her restore her sexual functioning?

References

A-Baqhdai, O., & Ewies, A. A. (2009). Topical estrogen therapy in the management of postmenopausal vaginal atrophy: An up-to-date review. *Climacteric, 12*(2), 91–105.

American Cancer Society. (2010). *Cancer facts and figures.* Retrieved May 20, 2010, from http://www.cancer.org/Research/CancerFactsFigures/index

American Occupational Therapy Association. (2008). Occupational therapy practice framework: Domain and process (2nd ed.). *American Journal of Occupational Therapy, 62,* 625–683. doi:10.5014/ajot.62.6.625

Annon, J. S. (1976). The PLISSIT model: A proposed conceptual scheme for the behavioral treatment of sexual problems. *Journal of Sex Education and Therapy, 2,* 1–15.

Beck, A., Steer, R., & Brown, G. K. (1996). *Beck Depression Inventory–II.* San Antonio, TX: Psychological Corporation.

Burns, D. D. (1999). *The feeling good handbook.* New York: Plume.

Calman, K. C. (1984). Quality of life in cancer patients: An hypothesis. *Journal of Medical Ethics, 10,* 124–127.

Cooper, J. (2006). What is cancer? In J. Cooper (Ed.), *Occupational therapy in oncology and palliative care* (2nd ed., pp. 1–10). West Sussex, UK: Whurr.

Edwards, B. K., Ward, E., Kohler, B. A., Eheman, C., Zauber, A. G., Anderson, R. N., et al. (2009). Annual report to the nation on the status of cancer, 1975–2006, featuring colorectal cancer trends and impact of interventions to reduce future rates. *Cancer, 116*(3), 544–573. doi:10.10002/cncr.24760.

Esserman, L., Shieh, Y., & Thompson, I. (2009). Rethinking screening for breast cancer and prostate cancer. *JAMA, 302*(15), 1685–1692.

Feldman-Stewart, D., Brundage, M., Hayter, C., Groome, P., Nickel Curtis, J., Downes, H., et al. (2000). What questions do patients with curable prostate cancer want answered? *Medical Decision Making, 20*, 7–19.

Grogan, S. (2008). *Body image: Understanding body dissatisfaction in men, women, and children.* East Sussex, UK: Routledge.

Hattjar, B., Parker, J., & Lappa, C. (2008). Addressing sexuality with adult clients with chronic disabilities: Occupational therapy's role. *OT Practice, 13*(11), CE1–CE8.

Hidderley, M., & Holt, M. (2004). A pilot randomized trial assessing the effects of autogenic training in early-stage cancer patients in relation to psychological status and immune system responses. *European Journal of Oncology Nursing, 8*(1), 61–65.

Ilie, C. P., Mischianu, D. L., & Pemberton, R. J. (2007). Painful ejaculation. *British Journal of Urology International, 99*(6), 1335–1339.

Katz, A. (2007). *Breaking the silence on cancer and sexuality.* Philadelphia: Oncology Nursing Society.

Kingsberg, S. (2006). Taking a sexual history. *Obstetrics and Gynecology Clinics of North America, 33*(4), 535–547.

Lancaster, L. (2004). Preventing vaginal stenosis after brachytherapy for gynecological cancer: An overview of Australian practices. *European Journal of Oncology Nursing, 8*(1), 30–39.

Mayo Clinic. (2009). *Cancer treatment for women: Possible sexual side effects.* Retrieved January 14, 2011, from http://www.mayoclinic.com/health/cancer-treatment/SA00071

Mick, J., Hughes, M., & Cohen, M. (2003). Sexuality and cancer: How oncology nurses can address it BETTER. *Oncology Nursing Forum, 30*(Suppl. 2), 152–153.

National Cancer Institute. (2009). *Cancer topics: Depression.* Retrieved January 14, 2011, from http://www.cancer.gov/cancertopics/pdq/supportivecare/depression/Patient/

National Cancer Institute. (2010). *Sexuality and reproductive issues.* Retrieved May 18, 2010, from http://www.cancer.gov/cancertopics/pdg/supportivecare/sexuality/HealthProfessional

National Cancer Institute. (2011). *Dictionary of cancer.* Retrieved September 14, 2011, from http://www.cancer.gov/dictionary?expand=C

O'Connell, H. E., Sanjeevan, K. V., & Hutson, J. M. (2005). Anatomy of the clitoris. *Journal of Urology, 174*, 1189–1195.

Packel, L. (2006). Oncological diseases and disorders. In D. J. Malone & K. L. B. Lindsay (Eds.), *Physical therapy in acute care: A clinician's guide* (pp. 503–544). Thorofare, NJ: Slack.

Paneth, N., Vande Woude, G., & Kort, E. (2010). Screening and detection of breast cancer and prostate cancer [Letter]. *JAMA, 303*(11), 1032–1033.

Rosenbaum, T., & Owens, A. (2008). The role of pelvic floor physical therapy in the treatment of pelvic and genital pain–related sexual dysfunction. *Journal of Sexual Medicine, 5,* 513–523.

Rustoen, T., & Begnum, S. (2000). Quality of life in women with breast cancer: A review of the literature and implications for nursing practice. *Cancer Nursing, 23*(6), 416–421.

Surveillance, Epidemiology, and End Results Program. (2011). *Surveillance epidemiology and end results report, 2002–2006.* Retrieved May 18, 2010, from http://seer.cancer.gov/statistics

Siegel, R., Jemal, A., & Ward, E. (2009). Increase in incidence of colorectal cancer among young men and women in the United States. *Cancer Epidemiology, Biomarkers, and Prevention, 18,* 1695.

Smith-Gabai, H. (2011). Oncology. In H. Smith-Gabai (Ed.), *Occupational therapy in acute care* (pp. 407–442). Bethesda, MD: AOTA Press.

Vodermaier, A., Linden, W., & Siu, C. (2009). Screening for emotional distress in cancer patients: A systematic review of assessment instruments. *Journal of the National Cancer Institute, 101*(21), 1464–1488.

Wittmann, D., Foley, S., & Balon, R. (2011). A biopsychosocial approach to sexual recovery after prostate cancer surgery: The role of grief and mourning. *Journal of Sex and Marital Therapy, 37*(2), 130–144.

Wittmann, D., Montie, J. E., Hamstra, D. A., Sandler, H. , & Wood, D. P. (2009). Counseling patients about sexual health when considering post-prostatectomy radiation treatment. *International Journal of Impotence Research, 21*(5), 275–284.

A Woman's Touch. (2007). *Vaginal renewal.* Retrieved May 22, 2010, from http://www.awomanstouchonline.com/sex_counselor.php?articleID=3069

World Health Organization. (2002). *Working definition of sexual health.* Retrieved January 12, 2010, from http://www.cdc.gov/sexualhealth/

Wright, S., Courtney, U., & Crowther, D. (2002). A quantitative and qualitative pilot study of the perceived benefits of autogenic training for a group of people with cancer. *European Journal of Cancer Care, 11*(2), 122–130.

4

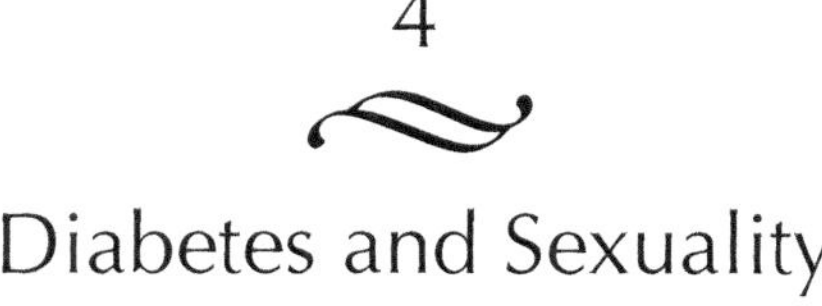

Diabetes and Sexuality

Bernadette Hattjar, DrOT, MEd, OTR/L, CWCE

Key Terms and Concepts

- Erectile dysfunction
- Gestational diabetes
- Health-related quality of life
- Neuropathy
- Obesity
- Retrograde ejaculation
- Type 1 diabetes
- Type 2 diabetes
- Yeast infection.

Upon completion of this chapter, readers will be able to

- Identify the signs and symptoms of diabetes,
- Understand the complications commonly associated with diabetes,
- Understand the differences between Type 1 and Type 2 diabetes,
- Know disease management and possible prevention strategies, and
- Know how diabetes affect sexual activity for males and females.

History

Diabetes is a chronic condition that can cause serious health complications, including unstable blood sugar levels termed *hypoglycemia* (low blood sugar levels) and *hyperglycemia* (high blood sugar levels). High blood sugar levels can lead to microvascular complications (damage to small blood vessels especially noted in the eyes, kidneys, and nerves) and damage to the large blood vessels (heart and brain; Leontis & Walker, 2011).

Diabetes and the health problems associated with diabetic conditions diminish quality of life (QoL) and increase the level of disability among those diagnosed with this disease. Diabetes has become a huge burden on the health care system because of the chronic nature of the disease and the multiple physical and psychological problems that are associated with it. It is expected that the health care burden associated with diabetes will increase as younger individuals are being diagnosed with Type 2 diabetes because of a lifestyle of poor nutrition, obesity, and little physical exercise and activity.

A Greek physician, Aretaeus of Cappadocia, called diabetes *diabanien,* which means *to siphon.* This terminology was related to the diabetic individual's condition of passing excessive amounts of urine (*polyuria*). The American Indians called diabetes "sweet urine disease" because they tested for diabetes by observing whether ants were attracted to the person's urine (positive for diabetes) or not. In 1750, William Cullen, a scientist added the word *mellitus,* a Latin word that means "honey sweet." Hence, we have the diagnosis name, *diabetes mellitus* (Sattley, 2008).

A better understanding of diabetes occurred with scientific discoveries. Paul Langerhans, in 1869, described the islet cells of the pancreas (now called the *islets of Langerhans*) and attempted to make a connection between pancreatic function or dysfunction and the presence of diabetes. In 1900, Dr. Josef von Mering and Dr. Oskar Minkowski verified that the pancreas plays an important role in the disease. In 1901, Eugene Opie substantiated that the function of islet cells in the pancreas—the cells responsible for making insulin—are directly correlated with the presence or absence of diabetes. In 1921, Frederick Banting and Charles Best discovered that the insulin hormone could be used to manage diabetic symptoms (Sattley, 2008).

Medications to help control and manage diabetes gained acceptance and effectiveness beginning in the 1940s. In 1942, the first class of antidiabetic drugs to help Type 2 diabetes was developed (sulfonylurea). In 1952, Lente Insulin was created using zinc. Oral medications of sulfonylurea were developed for persons with Type 2 diabetes in 1956. The first single-syringe insulin treatments were developed and marketed in the early 1960s, and the first portable glucose meter was marketed and used in the late 1960s. From the 1970s to the present, increasing research and better pharmacological management strategies have been supplemented by better testing procedures; improved monitoring procedures; and a stronger focus on prevention, diet, and exercise for those diagnosed with diabetes (Sattley, 2008).

Demographics

Approximately 800,000 new cases of diabetes are diagnosed each year. The occurrence of Type 2 diabetes, especially, is increasing in the United States. Some 18.8 million people have been diagnosed with diabetes, while 7 million people are estimated to have diabetes but are undiagnosed (Centers for Disease Control and Prevention [CDC], 2011b). Diabetes was listed as the underlying cause on over 71,000 death certificates and was listed as a contributing factor on an additional 160,022 death certificates in 2011 (American Diabetes Association, 2011a). As a disease entity, diabetes has remained the 7th-leading cause of death in the United States, primarily from underlying diabetes-related cardiovascular disease (CDC, 2011b). The presence of diabetes in premenopausal women is associated with an increase of cardiovascular disease that is 3–4 times greater than in women without diabetes. In the United States, diabetes is the leading cause of nontraumatic amputations (approximately 57,000 per year), blindness among working-age adults (approximately 20,000 per year), and end-stage renal disease (approximately 28,000 per year; U.S. Department of Health and Human Services [DHHS], 2010).

High-risk and vulnerable populations in the United States include African Americans, Hispanics, American Indians, Alaska Natives, Asians or Pacific Islanders, elderly persons, and economically disadvantaged persons. Several factors account for this chronic disease epidemic, including poor nutrition, decreased physical activity, obesity, the aging process, and the increased growth of the at-risk populations overall (DHHS, 2010).

Types of Diabetes

Type 1 Diabetes

Type 1 diabetes is an autoimmune disease of the insulin-producing beta cells in the pancreas. The pancreas cannot make the insulin necessary to transport sugar from the blood into other cells of the body for energy. Sugar, or glucose, builds up in the blood and, over time, can damage internal organs and blood vessels. Type 1 diabetes was previously referred to as *Type I diabetes, juvenile diabetes,* or *insulin-dependent diabetes mellitus.* Type 1 diabetes accounts for 5%–10% of all diagnosed cases of diabetes (CDC, 2011b).

Type 1 diabetes typically strikes children and young adults, although adults of any age can be diagnosed with Type 1 diabetes. The onset of this disease is rather quick. As insulin stops being produced, the blood sugar rises, causing hyperglycemia. Someone diagnosed with Type 1 diabetes must take insulin every day to survive. The individual must check his or her blood sugar level frequently throughout the day to inject himself or herself with the correct amount of insulin (or he or she must use a subcutaneous infusion insulin pump). The correct amount of insulin mimics the action of the pancreas in someone without diabetes. Individuals with Type 1 diabetes are encouraged to follow a healthy diet and exercise program in order to stabilize glucose levels and to remain in good health.

Type 2 Diabetes

Type 2 diabetes is often not diagnosed until serious health complications have occurred. This type of diabetes develops gradually, and about one-third of people who have this type of diabetes do not know they have it (National Diabetes Education Program, n.d.). Type 2 diabetes affects adults and adolescents, and Type 2 diabetes in adolescents is a growing phenomenon (CDC, n.d.). Individuals with this type of diabetes might take oral medications to stabilize blood sugar levels. As occurs with Type 1 diabetes, Type 2 diabetes blood sugar levels must be checked, and diet and exercise programs are usually recommended. Blood sugar–level checking is usually done once or twice each day, although this might be done more frequently when the client is newly diagnosed or when medication is being changed or stabilized.

Gestational Diabetes

Gestational diabetes is identified in pregnant women who have not been diagnosed with diabetes prior to their pregnancy. With gestational diabetes, the pancreas cannot make and use all the insulin needed for pregnancy, preventing glucose from leaving the blood (American Diabetes Association [ADA], 2012). A woman might not realize that she has gestational diabetes until she receives a glucose tolerance test between weeks 24–28 of pregnancy. The ADA (2011b) recommends that a full, 3-hour oral glucose tolerance test be given at 24–28 weeks of pregnancy to all pregnant women, while the American Congress of Obstetricians and Gynecologists (ACOG; 2011) continues to recommend a two-step approach, beginning with the 1-hour challenge test, followed by the 3-hour test if the first test results or other risk factors call for further testing.

A 3-hour glucose tolerance test includes a fasting blood draw to determine the baseline glucose level, followed by drinking a concentrated glucose solution. Blood draws are completed every hour for a total of 3 hours. The current ADA (2011b) standard of care is to make a diagnosis of gestational diabetes with only one abnormal blood draw.

Gestational diabetes can often be treated with diet, exercise, and close monitoring by a physician. In more serious cases, insulin injections might be required (ADA, 2012). This type of diabetes places both the mother and the baby at risk for complications; therefore, it cannot be ignored.

Diabetes Signs and Symptoms

Although categorized under the "diabetes" group of diagnoses, presenting symptoms for Type I, Type 2, and gestational diabetes are different. The onset of Type 1 diabetes is rapid. Diabetic ketoacidosis is often the first sign of Type 1 diabetes in people who do not yet have other symptoms. This occurs when the body cannot use glucose as a fuel source because there is no insulin or not enough insulin. Fat is used for fuel instead. As fats are broken down, acids (called *ketones*) build up in the blood and urine. At high levels, ketones are poisonous (MedlinePlus, 2011).

The symptoms associated with Type 1 diabetes and ketoacidosis include deep, rapid breathing; dry skin and mouth; flushed face; fruity smelling breath; nausea and vomiting; and stomach pain. Other symptoms that can occur are abdominal pain, breathing difficulty when lying down, decreased appetite, decreased consciousness, dulled senses that might worsen to a coma, fatigue, frequent urination or thirst that lasts for a day for longer, headache, muscle stiffness or aches, and shortness of breath (MedlinePlus, 2011).

In Type 2 diabetes, common symptoms include frequent thirst (*polydipsia*); frequent urination (*polyuria*) and hunger (*polyphagia*); weight loss; fatigue; blurred vision; slow healing sores or frequent infections; and areas of darkened skin, especially in skin fold and under arms (Mayo Clinic, 2011b). Other symptoms that are more frequently associated with Type 2 diabetes include

- Slow-healing cuts or sores
- Itching of the skin (around the groin or vagina)
- Frequent yeast infections in females
- Recent weight gains (not necessarily associated with over eating)

- Velvety, dark skin changes of the neck, armpits, groin
- Numbness or tingling of the hands or feet
- Decrease in vision
- Impotency in males (ADA, 2011a).

Psychological Considerations

Psychological problems are also associated with diabetes because it is a chronic metabolic disorder that requires constant monitoring, and it can affect numerous systems throughout the body, including sexual response. The psychological problems associated with diabetes are those that are frequently experienced by individuals with chronic diseases: increased frequency of somatic complaints (Nauert, 2010); depression (ADA, 2011c); and disengagement from life activities, roles, and responsibilities (Chapman, Perry, & Strine, 2005).

With diabetes, there is no "break" from its management—glucose testing, diet and exercise, and skin inspection are daily responsibilities with no respite. All of the daily and unrelenting effort that is required of a person diagnosed with diabetes can lead to a phenomenon called *diabetic burnout,* in which individuals grow tired of the effort required to safely manage their disease and stop their daily management activities. This might occur for a period of time or be ongoing, which will result in compromised health. Diabetic burnout can occur in isolation or be accompanied by psychological issues. The ebb and flow of glucose levels can affect one's mood, energy, and interest levels, resulting in depression (feeling overwhelmed), anxiety (fear of blood sugar peaks and valleys), and frustration (because of the unrelenting need to monitor the disease; ADA, 2011c).

Nerve Damage

Nerve damage, or *neuropathy,* is a common complication of diabetes. Nerve damage is caused by nerve fibers that are injured by high blood sugar levels. Neuropathy can occur throughout the body, but in the case of sexual activity, diabetic autonomic neuropathy (DAN) figures most prominently. The autonomic nervous system (ANS) governs the heart, bladder, lungs, stomach, intestines, sex organs, and eyes. When the ANS is involved, these can be symptoms of DAN can be present:

- Lack of awareness of low blood sugar level
- Bladder problems, including urgency or incontinence
- Constipation or diarrhea

- Nausea, vomiting, or loss of appetite

- Erectile dysfunction (ED) or retrograde ejaculation in men

- Vaginal dryness in women

- An increase or decrease in sweating (Mayo Clinic, 2011b; Vinik, Maser, Mitchell, & Freeman, 2003).

DAN affects the genitourinary tracts, including bladder dysfunction and sexual dysfunction (Vinik et al., 2003). For the client with diabetes, these symptoms might make engagement in sexual intercourse difficult (because of vaginal dryness in women and ED in men) or embarrassing (because of incontinence or voiding urgency). If symptoms of DAN are present, the client should speak with his or her health care professional for advice and medical interventions.

Diabetes Prevention

Taking a proactive stance might help to prevent the onset of diabetes. Strategies that can help to prevent the disease include living a well-balanced and healthy life.

- *Get physical activity.* Physical activity should include both aerobic exercise and strength or resistance training for maximal effectiveness and patient benefit.

- *Eat plenty of fiber.* The typical American diet is fiber-poor. Eating foods that are high in fiber helps to regulate and stabilize blood sugar levels, whereas highly processed and sugar-rich food cause blood sugar increases and decreases (commonly referred to as "sugar highs" and "sugar lows"). Eating whole grains and legumes not only decreases your risk of diabetes, but it also lowers the risk of heart disease. Fiber-rich foods tend to fill you up more quickly; thus, they promote weight loss and weight regulation. Foods that are high in fiber include whole grains, fruits, vegetables, beans, nuts, and seeds.

- *Eat plenty of whole grains.* As stated above, a diet rich in whole-grain foods tends to promote a stabilization of blood sugar levels. Breads, cereals, and pastas are all available in whole-grain varieties (Mayo Clinic, 2011b).

Obesity

Maintaining a normal weight level is important for individuals across the lifespan. *Obesity* is an excess of body fat. To determine whether an individual

---

Exhibit 4.1. Calculating BMI

Calculations are based on a 150-pound individual who is 5′5″ tall. To calculate BMI,

1. Divide the weight (pounds) by the height (inches).
2. Divide the result of Step 1 by the height (inches).
3. Multiply the result of Step 2 by 703.
4. Round the result of Step 3 to the second decimal place.

The entire calculation looks like this:

$$[150 : (65)2] \times 703 = 24.96$$

What does this mean? Compare your results to the BMI weight status chart:

BMI	WEIGHT STATUS
Below 18.5	Underweight
18.5–24.9	Normal or average weight
25.0– 29.9	Overweight
30.0 and above	Obese

Note. CDC (2011a).

---

is obese, health care professionals use a body mass index (BMI) test (Exhibit 4.1). A BMI assessment will identify whether and to what extent a client is obese. The BMI can provide the therapist with objective findings and can assist with a diet and exercise plan.

Obesity is present in 33.8% of adults in the United States (Flegal, Carroll, Ogden, & Curtin, 2010). Along with diabetes, obesity inflicts other health risks including, but not limited to, reproductive health consequences and additional chronic disease prevalence (including cardiovascular risks and arthritis–osteoarthritis risk among many other factors; Polotsky, 2011).

Occupational therapy practitioners can evaluate BMI, physical status, and the psychological and environmental issues and consider what the client deems to be important in order to decrease a weight problem. Occupational therapy practitioners' perspective on performance, as well as their knowledge of psychosocial, physical, environmental, and spiritual factors, help clients take on a structured approach for lifestyle change (American Occupational Therapy Association [AOTA], 2007).

Obesity creates additional positional problems for sexual activities. For both men and women, obesity promotes joint pain, especially in the hips, knees, and ankles, and 11% of obese women reported positional difficulties (Polotsky, 2011). Decreased mobility and body movement in obese individuals affect sexual positioning, and general physical problems are identified as a major problem when considering sexual activity in this group of clients. Because Type 2 diabetes is associated with the adult and older adult population, decreased muscle mass and strength are likely present.

The occupational therapist could assess physical range of motion, overall mobility and transfer skills, and endurance, as these factors contribute to the mechanical act of having sex. However, obese and overweight women do not report decreased frequency of sexual encounters when compared to their lean counterparts, and obese men report the ability to engage in sexual activity but cannot always achieve orgasm (Polotsky, 2011). Obese men might have up to a 30% higher risk of ED and impotency than nonobese men (Polotsky, 2011). The therapist can address sexual activity issues related to diabetes by using the PLISSIT Model (Annon, 1976) described in detail in Chapter 1.

Referral to Occupational Therapy

The client with diabetes would be referred to occupational therapy for education and treatment to "modify current habits and routines and develop new ones to promote a healthier lifestyle and minimize disease progression" (AOTA, 2011). The American Association of Diabetes Educators (AADE) views occupational therapists as part of the diabetes self-care team (AOTA, 2011). In this context, the occupational therapist would address activities within the professional domain, including sexual activity.

Diabetes affects all components of life and affects the individual's *QoL* and *health-related quality of life (HRQoL)*. Diabetes can provide both physical and psychological problems for a client of either sex with diabetes; therefore, the occupational therapist should consider the HRQoL of the patient important. HRQoL is concerned with physical and psychological health, social relationships, and the environmental domain and the overall satisfaction with treatment and intervention designed to improve client status and function (Odili, Ugboka, & Oparah, 2010). *QoL* is people's "emotional, social and physical well-being and their ability to function in the ordinary tasks of living" (Odili et al., 2010). The difference between QoL and HRQoL is the element of satisfaction with health care treatment and interventions from both the medical and therapeutic realms.

The referral of a client with diabetes to occupational therapy comes from a physician, although the reasons for referrals may occur on either a primary (dealing with diabetes symptom and medication management, self-care, or skin issues) or secondary (dealing with diminished sensation in the upper or lower extremities that impedes activity, safety, and movement; low vision; or amputation issues) basis in order to determine occupational needs.

The impact of a successful medical or therapeutic intervention can be reflected to the degree that the treatment or intervention has had a positive influence on the client's immediate or future well-being (Polotsky, 2000). The therapist can address sexual problems by using telling questionnaires, the BMI if obesity is present, and the structured PLISSIT model (Annon, 1976) of care.

Occupational therapists are experts in analyzing the performance skills and patterns that occur in daily life. Through the therapists' education and training interventions, clients with diabetes can achieve the 7 Self-Care Behaviors Promoted by AADE (2010) that include (1) healthy eating, (2) being active, (3) monitoring (e.g., physical symptoms, blood glucose testing, weight, blood pressure), (4) taking medications, (5) problem solving, (6) healthy coping, and (7) risk reduction (e.g., smoking cessation, foot inspections, maintaining health records, attending medical appointments). Sexual activity, an ADL according to the *Occupational Therapy Practice Framework: Domain and Process* (AOTA, 2008), appropriately falls under the 7 Self-Care Behaviors (AADE, 2010) as an issue dealt with in problem solving ("How can I have intercourse?" "When do I have more energy?") and healthy coping ("I am desirable," "I can live my life as a sexual being").

In occupational therapy, all aspects of an individual's life are reflected in the assessment and intervention process. This process should include both necessary and desired topics that are documented as goals. To affect positive influences on the client's QoL and his or her satisfaction with his or her personal health, providing holistic and client-centered interventions, including sexuality and sexual activity, should be considered an essential and consistent part of evaluation and intervention.

To address sexuality and sexual activity, a clear understanding of the client's status and personal goals for care must be secured. This can be achieved in the assessment process by including a thorough questionnaire such as the Stanford Patient Education Research Center's Diabetes Questionnaire (Stanford Patient Education Research Center, 2010). The Stanford questionnaire does not explicitly ask questions about sexual activity, but it questions life and relationship satisfaction, which are components of sexual activity and intimacy. Securing personal and intimate information using a questionnaire promotes client privacy and might also provide the opportunity to begin to talk about sexuality and sexual activity concerns with the client, if sexual activity is identified by the client as an area of concern or interest. If the PLISSIT Model (Annon, 1976) is adhered to, the questionnaire represents the "P" (permission to discuss) for "Permission on the basis of questionnaire answers."

Making the transition from an occupational therapy evaluation to dealing with the topic of sexual activity may seem daunting, but it does not have to be difficult. The use of a self-administered questionnaire (which should be optional for the client to complete) provides a bridge to the topic of sexual activity.

The Diabetes–39 (Boyer & Earp, 1997) is a tool that reviews different aspects of the client's life, including energy and mobility, diabetes control, anxiety and worry, social burden, sexual functioning, and diabetes medications. Over time, the Diabetes–39 questionnaire has proven to have good validity and reliability (Garratt, Schmidt, & Fitzpatrick, 2002). This questionnaire covers various subject areas, including sexual functioning. The questions are equally weighted and stated in a consistent manner so those concerning sexual functioning do not appear different or disjointed from questions relating to other areas of function.

Sexuality Problems Related to Diabetes

Diabetes is a disease that can potentially affect almost every system in the body. The constellation of problems associated with diabetes is great; therefore, sexual dysfunction, hormone imbalance, compromised circulation, cardiac problems, nerve and blood vessel damage, and many other issues are common among men and women. The ANS helps to control the digestion of food and to circulate blood, body functions that we do not have to think about consciously. The sexual response to stimuli is also involuntary and is governed by autonomic nerve signals that increase blood flow to the genitals and cause smooth muscles to relax. Damage to these autonomic nerves can hinder sexual function and responses (Vinik & Erbas, 2001).

Males

Erectile dysfunction

The most common sexual problem in males with diabetes is ED (National Diabetes Information Clearinghouse [NDIC], 2011). *ED* is the consistent inability to get an erection or to have an erection firm enough or that can be sustained long enough for sexual intercourse.

Men who have diabetes are 2–3 times more likely to experience ED than are men without diabetes (NCDI, 2011). Additionally, some males with diabetes are overweight or obese; therefore, the risk of ED in males is 1.5–3.0 times greater for men who are obese than men who are normal weight. The likelihood of ED increases with a greater BMI (Chitaley, Kupelian, Subak, & Wessells, 2009).

Research suggested that ED might be an early marker of diabetes, particularly in men ages 45 years or younger. In men with diabetes, ED begins earlier than in the general population (Chitaley et al., 2010). Although diabetes is a major cause of ED, other major causes include high blood pressure, alcohol abuse, and peripheral blood vessel disease. The side effects of medications, psychological factors, smoking, and hormonal deficiencies also contribute to ED. ED in men with diabetes is caused by nerve damage, high blood pressure, or peripheral artery disease; therefore, treatments vary greatly. Treatments might include taking oral medication, using a vacuum pump, placing a suppository pellet in the urethra, or having penile injections. Although treatments can produce considerable anxiety for clients, they are generally effective.

In the event that the client desires interventions by using medications for ED or by using the vacuum pump, pellet, or injections, the occupational therapist should secure training or education from a physician (urologist) or a certified sex therapist or should make a referral to a another health care professional. Additionally, a client and therapist of the same sex might make addressing this subject easier for all involved.

- *Oral medication.* Oral medications for the treatment of ED include commercially advertised and widely prescribed medication such as Viagara, Cialis, or Levitra. These drugs increase the effects of nitric oxide, a natural chemical in the body, which relaxes muscles in the penis. This action increases blood flow to the penis and results in an erection (Mayo Clinic, 2011a). The dosage level for these medications varies from man to man. Oral medications are effective for most males with diabetes if used properly.

- *Use of a vacuum pump.* With a vacuum cylinder device, the penis is placed in the cylinder with a pre-fit elastic band at the base of the device and penis. Air is pumped out of the device, creating a vacuum and drawing blood into the penis. An erection results from this action. Once the erection is attained, the cylinder device is removed from the penis, but the constricting band stays in place at the base of the penis to retain the erection (Delaware Urologic Associates,

2011). The vacuum pump is effective and might be used by men for whom oral medications are contraindicated.

- *Suppositories or pellets.* Known as "transdermal pharmacotherapy" or MUSE,® the male places Alprostadil, a vasodialator drug suppository or pellet, into the urethra using a plastic applicator. The vasodialator suppository drug dissolves, and this results in increased blood flow to the penis by relaxing and expanding the blood vessels (Cleveland Clinic, 2008). Suppository pellets are effective and might be used if other ED treatments are contraindicated.

- *Penile injections.* The penis base can be self-injected using a very fine needle with Alprostadil, a vasodialator (Cleveland Clinic, 2008). Pain resulting from this self-injection is minimal because of the small size of the needle used for injection. Although penile injections are effective for treating ED, this option is not widely used because of the self-injection action and the possibility of injection pain.

Retrograde ejaculation

Another sexual problem that affects males with diabetes is *retrograde ejaculation,* a condition in which part or all of a man's semen goes into the bladder instead of out the tip of the penis during ejaculation, resulting in a "dry ejaculation."

Semen enters the bladder and is expelled with no adverse consequences during urination. A man experiencing this problem might notice that little semen is emitted during ejaculation, or he might become aware of the condition if fertility problems arise. An analysis of the man's urine sample will reveal the presence of semen in the urine, and the urine might appear to be cloudy. Treatment for retrograde ejaculation caused by diabetes might be helped with medications that increase the sympathetic or decrease the parasympathetic tone of the bladder (Fedele, 2005).

Females

Women with diabetes experience sexual dysfunction differently than do men. In a research study by Fatemi and Taghavi (2009), women with diabetes experienced the following symptoms concerning sexuality and sexual activity:

- Decreased vaginal lubrication resulting in vaginal dryness

- Uncomfortable or painful intercourse because of vaginal dryness

- Decreased desire for sexual activity (lower libido)

- A decreased or absent sexual response, including the inability to become or remain aroused because of reduced sensation or no sensation in the genital area and the constant or occasional inability to reach orgasm.

The reasons that women with diabetes experience sexual problems are the same reasons experienced by men—the hormonal upheaval and the physiological and neurological implications of the disease. However, it is important for women to talk to their physicians and gynecologists about vaginal dryness, possible painful sexual intercourse (because of vaginal dryness), and urinary urgency or incontinence. Women with diabetes also experience frequent candida (yeast) infections that make the need for regular gynecological visits imperative. Candida is one component of the body's normal bacteria and organisms. When diabetes, infections, or antibiotics unbalance the body's acidity level, candida cells multiply, resulting in a yeast infection (Ross, 2008). If women with diabetes experience repeated candida infections, this might be a sign that the blood sugar level is high (Ross, 2008).

Treatments related to diabetes

The use of over-the-counter vaginal lubricants is suggested to decrease vaginal dryness and to increase comfort during intercourse. To increase comfort during intercourse, changing intercourse positions might be helpful. The traditional man-on-top position might not be the most comfortable position for the woman with diabetes. She should try side-lying, using pillows or bolsters (see Figures A.1 and A.5 in Appendix A), or stimulation during intercourse to increase comfort and responsiveness. Additionally, instruction in Kegel or pelvic exercises might help to strengthen the pelvic muscles that are inherent to sexual activity (Mayo Clinic, 2010), along with strengthening and toning muscles for urinary control. Muscles that are strong and toned provide more consistent support and strength integrity. Kegel exercises can tone the area, improve blood supply, and provide additional integrity for both sexual activity and muscles tone in general (see Exhibit 4.2).

Occupational therapy interventions should be comprised of thoughtful questioning regarding intimacy; sexual status; and potential problems, issues, or concerns. Talking about sexuality is such a personal subject; therefore, talking about it is usually accomplished with the least amount of distress or anxiety in a quiet area such as the patient's room or in an office.

The therapist should follow the PLISSIT Model (Annon, 1976) to insure that this subject is agreeable for the patient to discuss. Following the

Exhibit 4.2. Correctly Performing Kegel Exercises

Kegel or pelvic exercises can help to strengthen weak muscles, including the pelvic floor muscles, the sphincter muscles, the bladder muscles, and the urethra. These muscles can be weakened by childbirth, pregnancy, or being overweight, and they are affected by nerve damage that is associated with diabetes.

1. *Find the right muscles.* To perform pelvic exercises, you must be sure that you are exercising the correct muscles in the pelvic floor. Three "tests" ensure that you are strengthening the correct muscles: (a) try to stop the flow of urine while you are sitting on the toilet; if you can do this, you are using the correct muscles; (b) imagine that you are trying to stop passing gas and squeeze the muscles that you would use to stop this from happening—if you can do this, you are using the correct muscles; and (c) insert your finger into your vagina and squeeze as if you were trying to stop a flow of urine; if you feel a tightening around your finger, you are using the correct muscles.

2. *Relax.* When trying either to find the correct muscles or to perform the tightening exercises, remember not to squeeze your stomach or leg muscles. Do not hold your breath.

3. *Find a quiet place to perform your exercises.* A quiet location will help you focus on the exercises without distraction.

4. *Lie on your back (supine), preferably on the floor or a firm surface.* Pull in the pelvic muscles and hold for a count of 3 then relax for a count of 3. The goal is to work up to a total of 10–15 repetitions each time you exercise. Perform these exercises faithfully, 3 times each day for 5-minute sessions. Usually within a few weeks, you will notice improvement, and within 3–6 weeks, bladder control should improve.

Note. National Institutes of Health (2010).

PLISSIT Model (*P* = *Permission, LI* = *Limited Information, SS* = *Specific Suggestions, IT* = *Intensive Therapy*), the first step in this process should be to obtain permission to talk about sexuality and sexual activity. This should be done using compassion and courtesy, by asking the patient whether "we can talk about intimacy and sexual activity." Once assured that this subject is appropriate, the therapist should provide "limited information" about sexual activity being a normal part of daily life and about how diabetes (or any other problem or diagnosis) is known to affect sexuality and the sexual response. The therapist can also provide a handout if it is available. From the patient's responses, specific suggestions can be made (for women, perhaps reviewing pelvic exercises; for men, reviewing the ED medication guidelines). The "intensive therapy" component of the PLISSIT Model is generally considered to be outside the realm of occupational therapy. In cases in which intensive treatment interventions are required, a referral to a certified sex therapist should occur (Wallace, 2008).

Summary

Diabetes numbers are increasing in the United States. The frequent causes identified for the increase in this disease are poor nutritional intake and the lack of exercise, which results in obesity. Although the signs and symptoms are consistent regardless of the age or situation, diabetes can affect any individual throughout the lifespan. Sexuality and sexual activity are areas that are frequently identified as problematic for those who are diagnosed with diabetes. The occupational therapist can make significant interventions in addressing sexuality and sexual activity with patients with diabetes by providing compassion, an open mind, and useful tools to enhance daily activity. By using assessment questionnaires, open communication about the subject, and practicing practical skills and exercises, sexual activity and sexuality can be professionally and adeptly addressed in occupational therapy (see Case Example 4.1).

Case Example 4.1. Mrs. Smith: Type 2 Diabetes

Mrs. Smith, a 62-year-old woman with Type 2 diabetes, is experiencing frequent urinary tract infections, poor bladder control, and a loss of sexual desire. Her husband is a retired government employee. She and her husband are the parents of 3 grown children. She reports, "I know my husband still loves me, but I am just not interested in sex anymore. Maybe I'm too old—I don't know." She also reports, "I keep getting urinary tract infections and have a lot of vaginal infections or yeast infections. I can't control when I need to urinate. I just feel sort of dirty all the time."

Mrs. Smith has been diagnosed with Type 2 diabetes for approximately 15 years. She has gained approximately 35 pounds over the past 10 years and

---

(Continued)

Case Example 4.1. Mrs. Smith: Type 2 Diabetes (*cont.*)

is less physically active. She reports, "I don't have any get up and go—I think it got up and went. Where? I don't know."

Her symptoms and control of her blood sugar level have become more difficult since she experienced menopause about 10 years ago. She currently appears to be experiencing depression and frequently states, "I just don't feel attractive or desirable anymore. I've gained weight, I can't control when I need to void, and I just want to be left alone. I just don't feel like much of a woman anymore."

Questions to Consider

1. What are some of the usual signs of Type 2 diabetes?

2. What type of occupational therapy interventions could be made to address her issue of "feeling dirty" because of incontinence?

3. What type of therapeutic intervention could you introduce to help Mrs. Smith regain control of her pelvic muscles and her incontinence?

4. How would you begin and then follow through on dealing with her lack of interest in sexual activity?

5. What recommendations could you make concerning intimacy and sexual activity?

6. Can you make any suggestions about increasing her energy level and in helping her control her weight?

References

American Association of Diabetes Educators. (2010). *AADE 7 self-care behaviors*. Retrieved July 10, 2011, from http://diabeteseducator.org/ProfessionalResources/AADE7/index.html

American Congress of Obstetricians and Gynecologists. (2011). Committee opinion No. 504: Screening and diagnosis of gestational diabetes mellitus. *Obstetrics and Gynecology, 118*(3), 751–753.

American Diabetes Association. (2011a). *Diabetes basics: Symptoms*. Retrieved August 17, 2011, from http://www.diabetes.org/diabetes-basics/symptoms/

American Diabetes Association. (2011b). Standards of medical care in diabetes—2011. *Diabetes Care, 34*(Suppl. 1), S11–S61.

American Diabetes Association. (2011c). *Living with diabetes: Depression*. Retrieved September 9, 2011, from http://www.diabetes.org/living-with-diabetes/complications/mental-health/depression.html

American Diabetes Association. (2012). *What is gestational diabetes?* Retrieved February 13, 2012, from http://www.diabetes.org/diabetes-basics/gestational/what-is-gestational-diabetes.html

American Occupational Therapy Association. (2007). Obesity and occupational therapy [Position paper]. *American Journal of Occupational Therapy, 61,* 701–703. doi:10.5014/ajot.61.6.701

American Occupational Therapy Association. (2008). Occupational therapy practice framework: Domain and process (2nd ed.). *American Journal of Occupational Therapy, 62,* 625–683. doi:10.5014/ajot.62.6.625

American Occupational Therapy Association. (2011). *OT Fact Sheet—Occupational therapy's role in diabetes self-management.* Retrieved July 19, 2010, from http:www.aota.org/consumers/professionals/whatisOT/HW/facts/Diabetes.aspx?FT=pdf

Annon, J. S. (1976). The PLISSIT model: A proposed conceptual scheme for the behavioral treatment of sexual problems. *Journal of Sex Education and Therapy, 2,* 1–15.

Boyer, J. G., & Earp, J. A. (1997). *Diabetes–39.* Retrieved December 14, 2011, from http://www.musc.edu/dfm/RCMAR/D39.html

Centers for Disease Control and Prevention. (2011a). *Healthy weight: Assessing your weight.* Retrieved August 17, 2011, from http://www.cdc.gov/healthyweight/assessing/index.html

Centers for Disease Control and Prevention. (2011b). *National diabetes fact sheet: 2011.* Retrieved August 17, 2011, from http://www.cdc.gov/diabetes/pubs/pdf/ndfs_2011.pdf

Centers for Disease Control and Prevention. (n.d.). *SEARCH for diabetes in youth: Fact sheet.* Retrieved January 12, 2012, from http://www.cdc.gov/diabetes/pubs/pdf/search.pdf

Chapman, D. P., Perry, G. S., & Strine, T. W. (2005). *The vital link between chronic disease and depressive disorders.* Retrieved July 29, 2011, from www.cdc.gov/pcd/issues/2005/jan/04_0066.htm

Chitaley, K., Kupelian, V., Subak, L., & Wessells, H. (2009). Diabetes, obesity, and erectile dysfunction: Field overview and research priorities. *Journal of Urology, 182*(Suppl. 6), S45–S50.

Cleveland Clinic. (2008). *Erectile dysfunction treatment.* Retrieved August 2, 2011, from http://health.usnews.com/health-conditions/sexual-health/erectile-dysfunction/treatment

Delaware Urologic Associates. (2011). *Erectile dysfunction.* Retrieved August 2, 2011, from http://www.delawareurologic.com/erectile_dysfunction/

Fatemi, S. S., & Taghavi, S. M. (2009). Evaluation of sexual function in women with Type 2 diabetes mellitus. *Diabetes Vascular Disease Research, 6*(1), 38–39.

Fedele, D. (2005). Therapy Insight—Sexual and bladder dysfunction associated with diabetes mellitus. *Nature Clinical Practice Urology, 2*(6), 282–290.

Flegal, K. M., Carroll, M. O., Ogden, C. L., & Curtin, L. R. (2010). Prevalence and trends in obesity among U.S. adults, 1999–2008. *JAMA, 303*(3), 235–241.

Garratt, A. M., Schmidt, I., & Fitzpatrick, R. (2002). Patient-assessed health outcome measures for diabetes: A structured review. *Diabetes Medicine, 19,* 1–11.

Leontis, L. M., & Walker, K. A. (2011). *Type 2 diabetes complications.* Retrieved June 30, 2011, from http://www.endocrineweb.com/conditions/type-2-diabetes-complications

Mayo Clinic. (2010). *Kegel exercises: A how-to guide for women.* Retrieved August 31, 2010, from http://www.mayoclinic.com/health/kegel-exercises/WO00119

Mayo Clinic. (2011a). *Diabetic neuropathy.* Retrieved July 31, 2011, from http://www.mayoclinic.com/diabetic-neuropathy/OS01045

Mayo Clinic. (2011b). *Diabetes prevention: 5 Tips for taking control.* Retrieved January 1, 2011, from http://www.mayoclinic.com/health/diabetes-prevention/DA00127

MedlinePlus. (2011). *Type 1 diabetes.* Retrieved January 13, 2012, from http://www.nlm.nih.gov/medlineplus/ency/article/000305.htm

National Diabetes Education Program. (n.d.). *Diabetes is preventable.* Retrieved August 17, 2011, from http://ndep.nih.gov/am-i-at-risk/DiabetesIsPreventable.aspx

National Diabetes Information Clearinghouse. (2011). *Sexual and urologic problems of diabetes.* Retrieved August 2, 2011, from http://www.diabetes.niddk.nih.gov/dm/pubs/sup/index.aspx

National Institutes of Health. (2010). *Kegel exercises: Self-care.* Retrieved August 17, 2011, from http://www.nlm.nih.gov/medlineplus/ency/patientinstructions/000141.htm

Nauert, R. (2010). *Psychological, physical factors complicate care for chronic illness.* Retrieved July 19, 2011, from http://psychcentral.com/news/2010/10/12/psychological-physical-factors-complicate-care-for-chronic-illness/19512.html

Odili, V. U., Ugboka, L. U., & Oparah, A. C. (2010). *Quality of life with diabetes in Benin City as measured with WHOQOL–BREF.* Retrieved August 6, 2010, from http://www.ispub.com/journal/the-internet-journal-of-law-health-care-and-ethics/volume-6-number2/quality-of-life-of-people-with-diabetes-in-benin-city-as-measured-with-whoqol-bref.html

Polotsky, A. J. (2011). Obesity and sexuality in men and women: Myths, misconceptions, and the data. *Sexuality, Reproduction, and Menopause, 8*(2), 7–10.

Polotsky, W. H. (2000). Understanding and assessing diabetes-specific quality of life. *Diabetes Spectrum, 13,* 36–41.

Ross, H. M. (2008). *Yeast infections with diabetes.* Retrieved July 30, 2011, from http://diabetes.about.com/od/preventingcomplications/a/yeast.htm

Sattley, M. (2008). *The history of diabetes.* Retrieved April 2, 2012, from http://www.diabeteshealth.com/read/2008/12/17/715/the-history-of-diabetes

Stanford Patient Education Research Center. (2010). *Sample questionnaire: Diabetes.* Retrieved August 5, 2010, from http://patienteducation.stanford.edu/research/diabquest.pdf

U.S. Department of Health and Human Services. (2010). *Diabetes*. Retrieved August 2, 2010, from http://www.healthypeople.gov/2020/topicsobjectives2020/over view.as?topicid=8

Vinik, A. I., & Erbas, T. (2001). Recognizing and treating diabetic autonomic neuropathy. *Cleveland Clinic Journal of Medicine, 68*(11), 928–944.

Vinik, A. I., Maser, R. E., Mitchell, B. D., & Freeman, R. (2003). *Diabetic autonomic neuropathy*. Retrieved July 31, 2011, from http://www.diabetesjournals.org/content/26/5/1553.full

Wallace, M. (2008). Assessment of sexual health in older adults. *American Journal of Nursing, 108*(7), 52–60.

5

Spinal Cord Injury and Sexuality

Bernadette Hattjar, DrOT, MEd, OTR/L, CWCE

Key Terms and Concepts

- Apoptosis
- Autonomic dysreflexia
- Bowel and bladder program
- Excitotoxicity
- Psychogenic arousal
- Reflexogenic arousal
- Sexual persona
- Spinal shock.

Upon completion of this chapter, readers will be able to

- Distinguish between a complete and incomplete spinal cord injury;
- Identify the difference in how spinal cord injury affects the sexual function of males and females;
- State bowel and bladder programming differences for men and women with spinal cord injuries; and
- Identify positions, indicators, and contra-indicators for sexual activity for males and females with spinal cord injuries.

Introduction

Spinal cord injury (SCI) refers to either a complete or an incomplete injury of the spinal cord. An estimated 23% of individuals in the United States who experience paralysis attribute it to an SCI (Christopher and Dana Reeve Foundation, 2010). SCI was considered a "severe and untreatable condition" throughout most of scientific history until the early 1980s (Christopher and Dana Reeve Foundation, 2010). In the 1980s, regeneration capabilities, including axonal regrowth and retraining neural circuits to restore body functions, refuted this scientific belief (National Institute of Neurological Disorders and Stroke [NINDS], 2011).

In the 1990s, research suggested that axon growth could occur and growth-suppressing molecules could be blocked, thereby increasing the likelihood of recovery or partial recovery from an SCI. Experiments showed success in rebuilding injured neurons that also led to partial recovery of spinal cord function in some cases (Mayo Clinic, 2011). It was determined that treatment of injured neurons fostered improved neuronal function in uninjured areas, and this research may be especially helpful to individuals with incomplete SCIs.

In the case of an incomplete SCI, the individual may retain uninjured nerves below the site of the injury. The uninjured nerves could potentially be "coaxed into taking over the function for injured nerves" (Christopher and Dana Reeve Foundation, 2012). Current research supports past research endeavors, directs rehabilitation and exercise techniques that are more rigorous, and targets future genetic arenas for in-depth investigation. NINDS (2011) encourages research in the following areas to secure a better understanding of potential spinal cord repair:

- Protecting surviving nerve cells from future damage
- Replacing damaged nerve cells
- Stimulating regrowth of axons and targeting their connections
- Retraining neural circuits to restore body functions.

Such research facts casts hope on what was once considered to be a hopeless and irreversible diagnosis.

Demographics

Generally, SCIs are more common in younger individuals. More SCIs occur in young males, and more than 80% of clients with an SCI are men (NINDS, 2011). The average age of onset is 37.8 years, and 52% of these injuries occur between ages 16 to 30 years (Atkins, 2008). Almost 1.3 million individuals living in the United States have an SCI (NINDS, 2011). Because of the early onset of the injury, the sexual self is challenged by an SCI.

The most common causes for SCI (*n* = 1,275,000) in the United States are due to

- *Work-related accidents:* 28%, or 362,000 people

- *Motor vehicle accidents:* 24%, or 311,000 people. (This number includes automobile and motorcycle accidents.)

- *Sporting and recreation accidents:* 16%, or 206,000 people. (These injuries are usually the result of contact or impact sports or diving accidents.)

- *Falls:* 9%, or 112,000 people. (Falls that result in SCI are more common in the older population.)

- *Victims of violence:* 4%, or 57,000 people. (Violence relates to injuries sustained from a gunshot or knife wound.)

- *Congenital disabilities:* 3%, or 34,000 people

- *Natural disasters:* 1%, or 8,000 people

- *Unknown:* 9%, or 109,000 people

- *Other:* 6%, or 76,000 people. (Christopher and Dana Reeve Foundation, 2010)

Additionally, alcohol use, either by a perpetrator (in which alcohol might aggravate anger or poor judgment) or the victim (in which alcohol might increase risk-taking behaviors) is a factor in 1 of 4 SCIs (Mayo Clinic, 2011; NINDS, 2011). Although accidents and trauma are usually attributed as causes of SCI or spinal cord trauma, physiologic diseases such as osteoporosis, cancer, arthritis, and spinal cord inflammation can also be factors (Mayo Clinic, 2011).

SCI Signs and Symptoms

The preeminent sign of SCI is paralysis below the area of injury. In general, the higher the injury, the greater the extent of the paralysis (see Figure 5.1). Immediately following an SCI, *spinal shock* occurs, in which bone fragments and disc material or ligaments bruise or tear into spinal cord tissue after a sudden traumatic blow to the spinal cord. After the injury, axons are cut off or damaged beyond repair, and neural cell membranes are broken. Blood vessels may rupture and cause heavy bleeding in the central grey matter, which can spread to other areas of the spinal cord over the next few hours. The

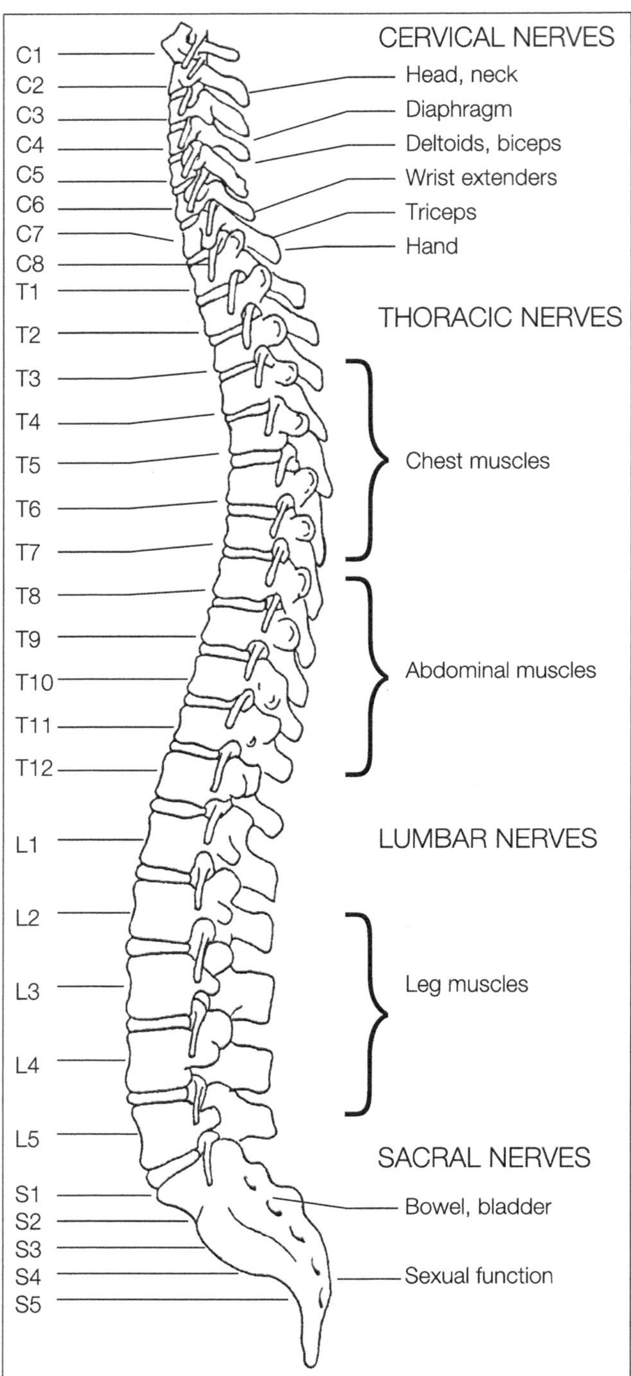

Figure 5.1. Spinal nerves and vertebrae.

Note. Copyright © 2011, by Delilah Cohn, The Medical Illustration Studio. Used under license.

spinal cord swells to fill the entire cavity of the spinal canal at the injury level. This swelling cuts off blood flow and oxygen to spinal cord tissue. Blood pressure drops, and the body loses its ability to self-regulate automatically. As blood pressure continues to lower, electrical activity of the neurons and axons becomes impaired.

Spinal shock takes place in approximately half of all SCIs and directly relates to the size and severity of the injury (NINDS, 2011). During spinal shock, deterioration occurs and even undamaged portions of the spinal cord become temporarily disabled, interfering with normal communication to the brain. Complete paralysis may develop, including the motor and sensory capacities.

The initial physical trauma continues and sets off biochemical and cellular events where inflammation reigns, neuronal death occurs, and the myelin sheath insulation is stripped off the nerves. Blood flow changes may spread to adjacent areas, causing further damage and nerve and tissue destruction. Additionally, an excessive release of neurotransmitters occurs, especially glutamate, an excitatory neurotransmitter, which disrupts normal processes, kills neurons, and sets off a destructive process called *excitotoxicity*. This disrupts normal processes and kills neurons and axon-protective *oligodendrocytes*, the insulators of axons in the central nervous system (CNS). Without the protective myelination provided by the oligodenrocytes, nerve impulses are slowed down, disrupted, or eliminated.

Inflammation of the spinal cord occurs when the blood–brain barrier is broken due to blood vessel bursting (Whetstone, Hsu, Eisenberg, Werb, & Noble-Haeusslein, 2003). Fluid accumulation and an influx of immune cells predominates this situation. Nerve cells also begin to self-destruct. *Apoptosis,* which occurs when the protective and insulating myelin sheath is stripped from intact axons in ascending and descending pathways, kills off oligodentrocytes in the damaged area of the spinal cord, further damaging the spinal cord and interfering with its ability to communicate with the brain. In essence, communication between the brain and spinal cord short-circuits.

The elements of secondary damage—inflammation, restricted or compromised blood flow, excitotoxicity, and free radical release and apoptosis—increase the area of damage in the spinal cord. Damaged axons become dysfunctional because they are stripped of their myelin sheath or because they are disconnected from communication with the brain. *Glial cells,* which are cells in the CNS that support and insulate the nerves, cluster to accelerate scar formation. The formation of scarring impedes communication between the brain and spinal cord and produces an impenetrable barrier. A few axons might be spared, but not enough intact axons remain to convey any meaningful information to the brain (NINDS, 2011). Exhibit 5.1 describes other terminology important to understanding SCI.

Exhibit 5.1. SCI Terminology

The following terms must be understood to comprehend the severity of an SCI:

- *Spinal shock* is related to the severity and location of an SCI. It occurs in about 50% of all SCIs and is characterized by deterioration of the integrity of the cord because of the injury. Blood flow, electrical impulses, and structural changes occur at the injury site, around the cord, and might extend to undamaged portions of the cord. Inflammation, which further compromises CNS communication, is also present. Spinal shock occurs immediately following the injury and might last from hours to weeks.

- *Tetraplegia (quadriplegia)* is an impairment in motor or sensory function in the cervical area of the spinal cord (American Spinal Injury Association [ASIA], 2010).

- *Paraplegia* is a motor and sensory impairment at the thoracic, lumbar, or sacral areas of the spinal cord. Depending on the location of the injury, upper-extremity function will be spared, but the trunk, pelvis, and lower extremity will be impaired.

- *Neurological level* is the lowest level at which key muscles grade 3/5 and sensation is intact according to the *dermatomes* (the areas on the skin supplied by sensory fibers from spinal nerves).

- *Functional level* refers to the lowest segments where key muscles are 3+/5 and sensation is intact.

- *Complete injury* is the absence of motor or sensory function at the lowest sacral segments.

- *Incomplete injury* is referred to only when there is partial preservation of sensory or motor function below the neurological level of the injury and at the sacral level.

- *Partial preservation* is referred to in clients with complete SCI who have partial innervation in dermatomes below the site of the SCI (ASIA, 2010).

Sexuality Issues Related to SCI

Rehabilitating Body and Mind

Upon review of SCI demographics and signs and symptoms, it is understandable that sexuality and sexual activity might encompass a significant aspect of rehabilitation because of the acute and sometimes traumatic status of the injury. After the client's medical status stabilizes, rehabilitation focuses on physiological stabilization; motor and sensory interventions; adaptive equipment use; assistive technology use; and the beginning of the return to the client's previous lifestyle, including sexual activity.

Sexuality has a particularly predictive correlation with how clients come to terms with their disability. As Novak and Mitchell (1988) succinctly stated, "Sexuality appears to play an important role in individuals' ability to cope with their disability" (p. 105). They cite Weiss and Diamond's work (1966), which found a positive correlation between patients' avoiding a realistic consideration of their sexuality and avoiding a realistic acceptance of their disability. The SCI presents a strong external "picture" of disability and probably an even stronger internal "script" of the personal and private ramifications of the disability. The individual's *sexual persona* (who that person is as a sexual being) is a part of a person's identity. Thus, the body and the mind must be simultaneously rehabilitated.

Research studies for both males and females have been conducted to determine the effect the SCI has on sexual activity (Alexander, Sipski, & Findley, 1993; Sipski & Alexander, 1993), both pre- and post-SCI. Four categories of sexual activity were used for the two studies cited and include (1) sexual activities and preferences; (2) sexual abilities; (3) sexual desire, arousal, and satisfaction; and (4) sexual adjustment.

For women with SCI, sex occurred more frequently prior to the injury. The act of having sexual intercourse was rated about 25% less important to women after they had sustained an SCI (Kettl et al., 1991) because of sensory losses related to the SCI. Sensory input was identified by females with an SCI as being pleasure producing. Post-injury sexual activity related more to kissing, hugging, and touching. Post-injury SCI issues difficulty achieving lubrication sufficient to have sexual intercourse and difficulty achieving or experiencing orgasm (McCluer, 1992).

For men with an SCI, a decreased frequency of sexual intercourse can correlate with an increased interest in alternative sexual activities post-injury. Only 38% of the complete SCI males reported being able to achieve an erection and orgasm after the SCI (Alexander et al., 1993). For both men and women, clients' perceptions of themselves and their partners as sexual beings decreased after the SCI. Additionally, sexual satisfaction decreased after the SCI. Sexual satisfaction was positively correlated with the patients' and their partners' interest in penile–vaginal intercourse (considered to be the "usual" type of sexual intercourse). Overall, the lower degree of sexual satisfaction and challenging sexual adjustment was reported by many of the male and female research participants.

Relationships

An SCI changes the client's life and can result in personal, physical, psychological, and relationship difficulties. Sexual problems can often be compounded by such difficulties, especially in relationships. However, it is important to highlight that these issues create interpersonal problems in any relationship, not just a disabled–nondisabled relationship. The SCI often magnifies problems in relationships, including the area of sexuality and sexual activity.

However, men and women who have experienced an SCI can sustain intimate relationships, develop new relationships, marry, and have children. Men can father children, and women can bear children. However, the actual act of intercourse will be different in its inception and execution.

An intimate relationship is more than having sex. Individuals in intimate relationships must be able to express their feelings and direct their partners to have fulfilling sexual activity. It is contingent on communication, touching, respect, and being psychologically turned on by the other individual. An SCI does not necessarily change any of these factors. However, the individual might feel frustrated, angry, or have a lower sex drive, and these things can affect any relationship. For men and women, intimacy is more likely to be compromised by sexual arousal problems that are directly related to the injury (U. S. National Library of Medicine, 2011).

Although the focus of this text is on the effect of chronic disability on the client, it is also important to consider the role of the caregiver. The spouse is the key support person for many individuals with an SCI. If a marriage, committed relationship, or caregiving relationship is positive, the caregiving experience is more likely to be positive for the care provider. The opposite is also true. Due to a significant role shift, caregiver stress is common. Caregiver stress, in regard to care of a loved one who has experienced an SCI, might be manifested by the caregiver as (1) *role overload* (juggling many roles to meet demands of the situation), (2) *loss of self* (needing to place the needs of another person first, thereby diminishing self needs), (3) *needing to deal and function within new personal and social relationships* (e.g., dealing with health care professionals, developing relationships or friendships with others who care for with SCIs), and (4) *dealing with financial constraints* (e.g., the individual with an SCI cannot work or has to seek alternative employment other than the pre-SCI work; Post, Bloemen, & Witte, 2005). The burden of care might be described as a *sense of responsibility* (a positive or neutral sense) or a *weight* (a more negative connotation) directed to the individual who has experienced the SCI. The burden aspect is reflected by the needs of the individual with an SCI being met by the caregiver.

Occupational Therapy Assessment and Evaluation

When used in conjunction with an occupational therapy evaluation, a sexuality questionnaire can provide information concerning sexual activity in general, psychosocial status, physical abilities and limitations, personal values, and communication abilities, as all of these areas comprise the constellation of sexual activity and sexuality. In the case of the use of a questionnaire, this should be considered supplemental to the more traditional occupational therapy evaluation, not in lieu of the occupational therapy evaluation. In the case of securing information on sexual activity with client with an SCI, use of the questionnaire format is common. In fact, most of the research studies available use the questionnaire format for securing information from this and many other diagnosis groups of clients.

Questionnaire formats are used for many reasons. They retain subject anonymity; secure personal attitudes, values, and perceptions; and permit thoughtfully considered answers done at the respondents' convenience (Portney & Watkins, 2000). This data-gathering tool can also be used with a larger group of subjects and with a sensitive and personal subject like sexual activity; a questionnaire might allow the subject to answer more honestly and thoroughly than a face-to-face interview would permit.

Two questionnaires that can be used in conjunction with the occupational therapy assessment or evaluation include

- Multidimensional Sexuality Questionnaire (MSQ; Snell, Fisher, & Walters, 1993) and

- Trueblood Sexual Attitudes Questionnaire (TSAQ; Trueblood, Hannon, & Hall, 1998).

These questionnaires cover a greater information landscape in relation to sexual activity and sexuality than would be included in a more typical assessment. The information gleaned in a questionnaire can be used to augment the regular assessment and thereby enrich and substantiate a client's treatment plan and goals concerning sexual activity and sexuality.

Multidimensional Sexuality Questionnaire

The MSQ (Snell et al., 1993) was developed to secure information about the psychological, individual tendencies associated with human sexuality through a multidimensional measure. To fully substantiate this questionnaire, the MSQ was subject to a thorough literature review conducted to highlight those tendencies that seem to have the greatest likelihood of affecting the sexual aspects of an individual's life. These areas are identified in the MSQ as follows:

- *Sexual esteem* is a generalized tendency to evaluate positively one's capacity to relate sexually with another person.
- *Sexual preoccupation* is the tendency to become absorbed in, obsessed with, and engrossed with thoughts about the sexual aspects of life.
- *Internal sexual control* is the belief that sexual aspects of one's life are determined by one's own personal control.
- *Sexual consciousness* is the tendency to think about and reflect about one's sexuality.
- *Sexual motivation* is the desire to be involved in a sexual relationship.
- *Sexual anxiety* is the tendency to feel tension, discomfort, and anxiety about the sexual aspects of one's life.
- *Sexual assertiveness* is being able to assert oneself about the sexual aspects of life.
- *Sexual depression* is the tendency to feel depressed about the sexual aspects of one's life.
- *External sexual control* is the belief that human sexuality is determined by influences like chance, good luck, bad luck, serendipity, being in the right place at the right time, or being in the wrong place at the wrong time.
- *Sexual monitoring* is the awareness of the public image that one's sexuality makes on others.
- *Fear of sex* is a fear of engaging in sexual relations with another individual.
- *Sexual satisfaction* is the tendency to be highly satisfied with the sexual aspects of one's life.

The MSQ has 61 questions with an alphabetized Likert-response scale with responses ranging from A (*not at all characteristic of me*) to E (*very characteristic of me*). The client can complete the questions, or the therapist or another individual can indicate the responses.

Trueblood Sexual Attitudes Questionnaire

The TSAQ (Trueblood et al., 1998) was developed to measure attitude change regarding the most common topics covered in a human sexuality college course. The questions mimic questions that are more typically related to sexual activity and sexuality; therefore, the author considered the inclusion of this item to be appropriate and relevant. The TSAQ questionnaire items were developed after a thorough review of human sexuality textbook topics. The questionnaire's 80 questions are placed on one of five major subscale topics: (1) *autoeroticism,* (2) *heterosexuality,* (3) *homosexuality,* (4) *sexual variations,* and (5) *commercial sex.* Each question is answered on a 9-point Likert scale ranging from 1 (*I completely disagree*) to 9 (*I completely agree*).

Sexual Activity After SCI

The ability to engage in sexual activity is considered to be an activity of daily living (ADL) in the *Occupational Therapy Practice Framework: Domain and Process* (American Occupational Therapy Association, 2008), along with the more typical ADLs such as dressing, bathing, grooming, and mobility activities. In the case of clients with SCIs, the typical ADLs are addressed with regularity in the rehabilitation setting, but sexual activity might not receive the same weight or time allotment in the clients' rehabilitation schedules. Appendix 5.A. describes occupational therapy interventions with SCI.

Arousal

Psychogenic arousal begins in the mind and might begin after thinking about sex, reading something romantic, and so on. Such arousal is caused by nerves in the T12 to L2 levels of the spinal cord (Mayo Clinic, 2009). *Reflexogenic arousal* occurs from physical touch to the labia, clitoris, penis, or other parts of the genital area and is caused by nerves in the S2 to S4 levels of the spinal cord.

Arousal results in an erection in the male and in lubrication in females. With an SCI, the male might experience erection difficulties. Males with complete SCI and upper-motor neuron injuries affecting the sacral segment of the cord lose the ability to have a psychogenic erection (visual and auditory sensory input), while reflex erectile function remains intact (arousal by touch or tactile sensory input). Males with incomplete upper-motor neuron injuries retain the reflexive erective function, and some might retain the psychogenic erectile function. Of males with lower-motor neuron injuries affecting the sacral area, 25% will retain the psychogenic erectile function, and none retains the reflex erectile function. With incomplete lower-motor neuron injuries, over 90% of males will be able to have some type of erectile function (Sipski, 2011). A woman might experience a loss of sensitivity in the genital region that could result in decreased vaginal lubrication that equates to uncomfortable or painful intercourse (Ferreiro-Velasco et al., 2005).

Men and women with SCIs are able to experience orgasm, although the orgasm sensation will be perceived differently after the SCI. Orgasm is frequently described as "a mind thing" or a "psychological response" (Rowles, 2010), as opposed to a physical response.

Addressing Sexuality

Sexuality and sexual activity issues present differently for males and females who have sustained SCIs. In a 1996 research study by McAlonan comprised of a convenience sample of 12 clients with SCI, 50% reported "dissatisfaction" with the manner in which sexual activity was addressed within the rehabilitation setting, 17% responded in a neutral manner, and 33% reported positive feelings about the manner in which sexuality and sexual activity was addressed in their treatment. The individuals involved in this study were sexually active before the SCI (11 of 12 participants). SCI client dissatisfaction was reported because of frustration about and disappointment in the manner in which sexuality was addressed and a sense of avoidance in health care professionals broaching the subject with them. Some study participants (17%) felt uncomfortable talking about sexual activity in a group venue and preferred a one-to-one situation that was not available. The quality of information presented in sexual rehabilitation sessions was identified as being helpful, but only 25% of the participants rated the content quality as "satisfactory." In general, the amount and quality of information was not perceived as being adequate. However, participants felt that open, direct communication; comfort with subject matter; and a willingness to listen and answer any questions were desirable traits in health care professionals when the issue of sexuality was addressed (McAlonan, 1996).

Magnan and Reynolds (2006) conducted an extensive research study related to barriers that inhibit sexual activity from being addressed in five nursing specialty areas (oncology, medical, surgical, obstetrics/gynecology, and rehabilitation). The results of this research indicate that nurses do not expect clients to ask about their sexuality concerns, and this result is consistent with other research studies. Magnan and Reynolds summarized their research results by stating,

> It may be that the nurses are correct in their assumption that patients do not expect nurses to address their sexuality concerns . . . [but] patients may not expect holistic nursing care that includes addressing one's sexuality concerns simply because they have never experienced it. (p. 286)

Gender Differences in Activity

There are significant differences in how a SCI affects sexual activity among males and females. The effect, of course, is determined by the level of the injury, the client's age, the presence of any other medical conditions or complications, culture, marital status, perceived importance, and innumerable other factors.

Males

In males, the two areas in the spinal cord that are most related to sexual function are T11–L2 and S2–S4 (McCluer, 1992; Rowles, 2010). The T11–L2 levels control *psychogenic erections* (erections stimulated in the brain when fantasizing), and the S2–S4 levels control *reflexogenic erections* (erections stimulated by tactile sensation and ejaculation). Male fertility is also often affected by an SCI. The male's ability to ejaculate will depend on the injury location. The ability to ejaculate is controlled by nerves that originate in the lowest part of the spinal cord, including T12–L2 and sacral Levels 2, 3, and 4 (RehabTeamSite, 2009; see Figure 5.1). If a man with an SCI is found to have viable sperm but cannot ejaculate, he may choose to undergo an electro-ejaculation procedure in which his sperm would be collected. This procedure would be followed by the insemination of his partner.

Male and female clients with SCIs might experience the sensation of orgasm differently. Orgasm might be experienced as more of a "tingle" sensation or as a psychological experience (Rowles, 2010), which might be more associated with internal feelings, sensory stimulation, and fantasy than with the actual act of intercourse. Or, orgasm might manifest as muscle contractions, muscle spasms, or a sensation of flushing above the injury site.

Females

Women experience a decrease or loss of lubrication and sensory loss following an SCI. It is also common for many females to experience *amenorrhea,* the absence of the menstrual cycle, following an SCI because of the physical and psychological stress the injury provides. The average time reported for resuming the menstrual cycle was 4.3 months, with a range from 1 week to 24 months, but the normal menses usually returns within 12 months

(McCluer, 1992). Monthly cycles are governed by hormonal, not neurological, factors, and a physician may prescribe hormones to stimulate the monthly cycle. Amenorrhea can occur in any woman when she experience stress, either physical or emotional (McCluer, 1992), and a female client with an SCI can have both physical and emotional stress associated with the situation. However, it is important to note that, even if a menstrual period is not evident because of the absence of blood flow, it does not mean that a woman is infertile. In most cases, female fertility is not permanently affected by an SCI.

Research concerning women with SCIs relates primarily to the physiologic and reproductive capacities as opposed to the emotional and psychological ramifications (Richards, Tepper, Whipple, & Komisaruk, 1997). It is additionally important to understand that more retrospective research has been conducted on the effects of an SCI on males than females.

Women are able to become pregnant after an SCI, but there are additional precautions that must be noted, including

- *Transferring difficulty.* Consider the movement problems that pregnant women have, and multiply that many times over for a pregnant woman with an SCI.

- *Increased chance of urinary tract infections (UTIs) and bladder management problems.* Urinary and bladder problems are common in a normal pregnancy. The likelihood of a UTI or bladder problems is greatly increased because of catheterization, impaired mobility in the hands, and the lack of sensory feedback from the urethra and anus (decreased cleanliness might be a prominent factor in the contribution to UTIs). Urinary and bladder health is compromised to a greater degree in a pregnant woman with an SCI. Even if the woman maintains a consistent bowel and bladder program, will she be able to reach her genital area with the increased abdominal girth associated with pregnancy?

- *Higher risk of autonomic dysreflexia,* an extreme spike in blood pressure or a persistent headache that might be life threatening. It is caused by an unopposed sympathetic response to stimuli in women with a T6 or higher injury (Atkins, 2008).

Bowel and Bladder Programs

Occupational therapy practitioners routinely work with clients with SCIs on bowel and bladder programs, yet they do not routinely address sexual activity problems. Sensation is compromised with an SCI, and bowel and bladder issues and catheterization are common with SCIs. A structured bowel and bladder program is a daily scheduled task for clients with SCIs. The bowel and bladder catheterization and a structured, timed schedule can create a multitude of problems concerning sexual activity, intimacy, and the act of intercourse. Sexual spontaneity might be thwarted because of the time structure of a bowel and bladder program. Any intimate act will need to be planned around the bowel and bladder time schedule. Additionally, the fact that voiding and defecation are no longer voluntarily controlled might create "messes" that can hinder intimacy.

Bowel and bladder function is controlled in the S2–S5 spinal segment, so any SCI at this level or above will lose voluntary bowel and bladder control. Voiding becomes reflexive and not consciously controllable. Therefore, catheterization and a bowel and bladder program become imperative. Bladder drainage is achieved using indwelling catheters, intermittent catheterizations, suprapubic catheters, condom sheath catheters, or a combination of any of these methods (Benevento & Sipski, 2002). Pharmacologic management of bladder problems might be required.

Bowel dysfunction presents a more serious problem and can easily affect the client's quality of life and self-esteem. A *neurogenic bowel problem* occurs when neurological control is lacking or limited because of the SCI. The two main types of neurogenic bowel problems are (1) lower-motor neuron bowel syndrome, or *areflexic bowel syndrome,* and (2) upper-motor neuron bowel syndrome, or *reflexive bowel syndrome.*

Lower-motor neuron bowel dysfunction is characterized by slow stool propulsion and a dry, round stool, which results in constipation and a risk of incontinence. *Upper-motor neuron bowel syndrome* is characterized by increased colon wall and anal muscle tone. There is stool propulsion and reflexive coordination of fecal matter through the intestine, but incontinence is common. Reflexive bowel syndrome is controlled by using an anal suppository, upright or right or left lateral positioning (partial sidelying), and digital stimulation of the anus until voiding occurs. In all bowel programs, prolonged bed rest and inactivity make the situation worse because the lack of movement impedes the digestion of food and the propulsion of this matter into the intestines. It is advisable for the client to ingest healthy, higher-fiber foods, especially fruits and vegetables, along with liquids, as these foods and any liquid facilitate a more normal and regular bowel movement.

For clients with paraplegia, the bowel program usually begins with taking an oral medication to facilitate defecation and establishing a regular schedule for toileting. This includes transferring to the toilet, clothing removal, insertion of an anal suppository (in addition to oral medications) to increase the ease of defecation, waiting for the medication and suppository to take effect, and inserting the finger into the anus for digital stimulation. This stimulation causes reflexive defecation. The use of a mirror and a light source sometimes aids in the step-by-step and safe completion of this process.

For clients who have low tetraplegia, this process is complicated by poor trunk control and finger paralysis. In this case, the use of a digital stimulator stick transposes for the use of a finger for anal reflexive defecation. The use of a mirror will also provide visual feedback and will help to accomplish this routine task correctly and safely.

The bladder program usually consists of catheterization. *Indwelling catheters* stay in the urethra and are periodically changed. They are usually used soon after an SCI occurs, but alternative methods of bladder control are reviewed as rehabilitation progresses. However, some clients will always use an indwelling catheter. Intermittent catheterization involves the insertion of the catheter approximately every 4–6 hours. This time schedule constitutes the bladder program. Reflex voiding occurs in males with the use of a condom catheter and a leg collection bag, whereas women must wear a diaper because of intermittent urine leakage. Reflex voiding occurs when the bladder is full, and urine must be expelled.

Overall, bladder management is more of a problem with females than males. Women have a shorter urethra and the opening for catheterization is located between the folds of the labia. This makes catheter insertion much more difficult and leakage of urine more likely; therefore, the use of a diaper is common. Skin irritation and breakdown is also more common in women because it is difficult to keep the area dry and clean.

In bowel and bladder programs for both men and women with an SCI, the major goal is to attain and sustain the voiding of urine and feces on a regular, scheduled basis to maintain optimal health and safety. If bowel and bladder programs are closely adhered to, as far as both the schedule and safety or cleanliness are concerned, there is less chance that sexual activity will be affected by problems related to bowel and bladder issues.

Respiration

Respiration is often compromised in clients with cervical SCIs. In the first year after an SCI, pneumonia is cited as the most common cause of death. In high cervical injuries, the phrenic nerve is partially or completely paralyzed, which results in paralysis of the diaphragm. In these cases, ventilator support is necessary and in some cases of unilateral phrenic nerve paralysis, combined intercostal and diaphragm pacing can be used for respiratory support (Di-Marco, Takaoka, & Kowalski, 2005).

Impaired respiration is also experienced in lower cervical and thoracic injuries where other muscles necessary for breathing are compromised. One of the integral components of sexual activity is the increased level of respiration; therefore, the client might experience fear and anxiety or may distrust his or her ability to sustain sexual activity. If respiration is severely compromised, sexual activity might need to be slowly and gently conducted with touching, hugging, and kissing. If respiration is less involved, sexual activity should be conducted in a slow and flowing manner. In this case, the client should be the judge of the level of involvement and excitement.

Pain

Pain, both acute and chronic, is a problem for many clients who have sustained an SCI. A study at the University of Washington found that 84% of clients with SCIs reported experiencing pain (Jensen, Kuehn, Amtmann, & Cardenas, 2007). Pain presents an additional impediment in rehabilitation and ADLs. Pain reports are related to the nature and context of the injury. Most SCIs result from a hard impact; therefore, the resulting pain reports are usually justified. Siddall and Loeser (2001) reported that individuals with tetraplegia are more likely to offer pain reports than patients with paraplegia. Atkins (2008) detailed the types of pain clients with SCIs might experience:

- *Mechanical pain* relates to soft-tissue injury at the site of the injury. Pain in the shoulders is a frequently reported location of pain in clients with tetraplegia.

- *Radicular pain* follows the segmental distribution of a nerve.

- *Neuropathic pain* originates in the spinal cord and is thought to be the result of misdirected neural sprouting after the injury.

If one considers the multitude of problems that are present with an SCI and that pain is also a component, sexual activity might become an ADL to which the health care provider might not give much importance or credence. Other areas are likely deemed to be more important to the rehabilitation of the patient.

Pain reports should never be disregarded and should be addressed with a physician. However, sexual activity might inadvertently reduce pain reports because of the engagement in a pleasurable activity that redirects focus and attention. Conversely, sexual activity might exacerbate pain because of positioning, the weight of another person, or the need to maintain one position for a long time.

Contraception

Men

Males with SCIs can father children, and females with SCIs can become pregnant. Contraception for males who engage in sexual intercourse and want to prevent both unwanted pregnancy and sexually transmitted disease should use a condom (McCluer, 1992).

Women

Contraception for female clients with SCIs involves using the following methods with indicators and contraindications for their use.

Oral contraceptives

Use of oral contraceptives can increase the risk of *thrombophlebitis,* or blood clots (van Hylckama Vileg, Helmerhorst, Vandenbroucke, Doggen, & Rosendaal, 2009). Women in wheelchairs are at greater risk for developing blood clots because of inactivity. Smoking also increases the risk of blood clots, especially in women ages 35 years or older. If a woman has a history of thrombophlebitis, she should avoid using oral contraceptives.

Hormonal implants

Although the implant of hormones under the skin might be more reliable in preventing pregnancy due to a reduction in the client forgetting to take an oral contraceptive, there is not enough long-term research on this form of contraception to determine potential risks.

Barrier methods

Barrier methods include the mechanical prevention of pregnancy by inserting a "barrier" or diaphragm coated with spermicide into the vagina to its placement on the cervix. The risks for this type of contraception relate to correct use of the spermicide, correct insertion, and appropriate placement of the coated barrier into the vagina and onto the surface of the cervix. Either the woman or her partner can insert the barrier into the vagina to cover the cervix.

Intrauterine devices

An *intrauterine device (IUD)* is a small, T-shaped device that is inserted into a woman's uterus by a physician. It prevents pregnancy by blocking sperm from meeting an egg and by altering the uterine lining. Some rare serious complications of IUD use (e.g., ectopic pregnancy) are recognized by pain or cramping. If sensation is not intact for a woman with an SCI, these complications might go unnoticed, with negative results (McCluer, 1992).

Rhythm method

The rhythm method relies on avoidance of sexual activity during the peak fertility period, based on the woman's monthly cycle and body temperature. If menstrual periods or body temperature are irregular, as is often the case for women with SCIs, the use of this form of contraception is questionable in its reliability to prevent pregnancy (Baylor College of Medicine, 2011).

Sexual Activity Recommendations for SCI

With some adaptation, clients with SCIs can engage in sexual activity.

Lubrication

Women can use an over-the-counter water- or silicone-based lubricating gel to combat vaginal dryness. Water-based lubricants tend to be easier to apply and clean up than creamy or oil-based lubricants. Male partners might consider the use of a lubricated condom.

Communication

Communication is essential. Letting a partner know your limitations and functional ability, sensation level, and desires will promote good communication and good sex. Communication between partners also fosters intimacy and closeness, which can enhance the sexual experience. Clients should consider the following:

- Express personal needs, wants, and desires.
- Be honest concerning your abilities and interests, and state these things to your partner; make assertive requests or statements (e.g., "I like it when you touch me there," "It is more comfortable in this position," "I like to be close to you, but this hurts").
- The partner should communicate where he or she is touching the client if the area is insensate.

Bowel and Bladder Management

The occupational therapy practitioner must take bowel and bladder issues into consideration. Advise clients to schedule sexual activity not to interfere with bowel and bladder programs. For many clients with SCIs, taking care of bowel and bladder activities right before sexual activity makes sex more comfortable and reduces the likelihood that urination or defecation will occur during the act itself.

For men with external catheters, two solutions are available. The occupational therapy practitioner might suggest either securing the catheter tubing (a sheath that fits over the penis, similar to a condom) to the shaft of the penis and engaging in sexual activities, or if the man knows when he has to urinate, remove the catheter for a short period after urination and engage in sexual activity at that time. If intermittent catheterization is used, the time for sexual activity can be adjusted to meet the catheterization schedule. If a woman has an indwelling catheter, the catheter tube can be taped to the abdomen, and the urine collection bag can be positioned away from the body. It is safe to engage in sexual activity while the tube is in place.

Stimulation

Males and females with tetraplegia or paraplegia can use a vibrator or other type of assistive device strapped to the hand for stimulation (if hand dexterity is a problem). If a reflexogenic erection is possible for males, it can be achieved by manual stimulation of the testicles, penis, and surrounding area. If an erection is not possible, the following should be considered:

- Engaging in sexual activities other than intercourse.
- Use of a vibrator (either hand-held or strapped on to the hand) to attain stimulation.
- Use of a vacuum device that facilitates a short-term erection.* Devices create a vacuum around the penis. Blood is drawn into the area, and a ring is placed at the base of the penis to sustain an erection. This device demands dexterity for use and should not be left in place longer than 30 minutes because the skin might break down (Ducharme, 2000).
- Obtain surgical implants that can mimic an erection or partial erection.* Implants are considered only if other methods have not been successful or if penile vascularity is poor. Penile implants range in complexity from a malleable prosthesis to a prosthesis with hydraulic components (Ducharme, 2000).
- Exploring pharmacological agents that can cause an erection.*

____

Note. *Consult a urologist.

Richards et al. (1997) conducted a research study related to relationship satisfaction and sexuality for women with complete SCIs. For this group of women with SCIs, "stimulation of nongenital areas, primarily breast and hypersensitive areas at or above the level of injury" (p. 277) promoted sexual arousal, pleasurable sensations, and some instances of self-reported orgasm. This study also indicates that one research subject achieved post-injury orgasm by imagery.

Positioning

Clients can explore alternative positions for sexual activity, such as

- *Being "on the bottom"* (i.e., "man-on-top" position; see Figure A.4 in Appendix A). This position allows a woman with an SCI to be in a traditional position for having sex. The position allows for genital stimulation, but the partner must be mindful not to place full weight on the woman's chest, as her breathing might become compromised. A male with tetraplegia will not be able to assume the "on-top" position because of muscle paralysis or weakness in the upper body. Sex positions for the male with tetraplegia and paraplegia male are described below.

- *Sitting supported.* Sitting with support from pillows or bolsters on a bed, or being supported with pillows and bolsters positioned by the headboard for clients with paraplegia increases stability and the ability to look at the partner during sexual activity (see Figure A.5 in Appendix A).

- *Sitting in the wheelchair.* For the male client with an SCI, the partner can straddle him while he is positioned in the wheelchair. For the female, her partner can caress, hug, and kiss her and can provide tactile or oral stimulation to sensate areas of her body (see Figure A.6 in Appendix A).

- *Laying on one's side.* Laying on one's side permits the client to be positioned by the partner when the partner assumes a more directive role in positioning of the client. The partner would have positioning control of the individual with an SCI. This type of position would work better with a client with paraplegia because of the amount of sensate body mass that is present (see Figures A.1 and A.2 in Appendix A).

Occupational therapy practitioners can encourage clients to explore new erogenous zones that correspond with the sensate areas at and above the site of the injury. In the case of most clients with SCIs, erogenous zones involved go to the level of the last surface area of sensation. In the case of incomplete SCI, sensate areas might vary from person to person in relation to the injury.

Summary

SCIs cover a wide range of functional limitations, including physiological, social, and emotional. The extent of these limitations is usually directly the result of the site of the SCI. Usually, the higher the injury, the greater the functional limitations will be to the individual. SCI is more common in younger individuals; therefore, the likelihood that sexual activity will factor prominently as a confounding limitation is great.

The occupational therapy practitioner can contribute to the rehabilitation of both male and female clients with SCIs. Teaching, educating, and informing the client of options for ADLs, including sexual activity, is of paramount importance. The occupational therapist can initially broach the subject of sexual activity using a questionnaire. The results of the questionnaire can be discussed with the client, and the educational and teaching component of the therapeutic intervention can begin. By educating the client on sexual activity options, position options, adaptive equipment to enhance sexual activity, and meaningful suggestions, the therapist can assist the client in reassuming his or her role as a sexual being in spite of an SCI (see Case Example 5.1).

Case Example 5.1. Mark: Thoracic SCI

Mark is a 24-year-old single male. He sustained a thoracic SCI 8 months ago. The injury occurred during a boating accident where he was thrown from his boat into shallow water during a storm.

Mark graduated with his master's degree in education prior to his boating accident. He plans to look for a teaching position within the next month. Mark resides in a first-floor, wheelchair-accessible apartment and drives a car equipped with hand controls.

Mark has a longtime girlfriend, but he remains unsure of the status of this relationship based upon physical limitations caused by his SCI. He says, "She's fine with me the way I am. I'm not." Mark and his girlfriend have attempted intercourse numerous times, but he reports, "If I can't do it like I used to. . . . with the man on the top, well, I don't want to try any fancy stuff."

Mark adheres to a strict bowel and bladder program, and this compounds his aversion to sexual activity. Mark uses a condom-type external catheter. He states, "It's a mess. I feel dirty." Although Mark occasionally appears to be motivated to explore his concerns regarding sexuality and sexual activity, he

---

(Continued)

Case Example 5.1. Mark: Thoracic SCI (*cont.*)

becomes very closed off when the subject is broached with him in therapy sessions at an outpatient facility. Mark presents with a bright and positive demeanor, but this façade wears thin when the subject of his relationship with his girlfriend is brought up.

Questions to Consider

1. Using the PLISSIT model (see Chapter 1), how can the occupational therapy practitioner secure permission to broach the subject of sexuality?

2. If Mark strongly resists dealing with his sexuality, what should the occupational therapist do?

3. How could Mark's girlfriend become involved in therapy sessions in relation to the ADL of sexual activity? Is it an appropriate intervention to secure the girlfriend's involvement with this issue?

4. If Mark's permission is gained by the occupational therapy practitioner, what type of limited information might be helpful to present to him?

5. If limited information sharing is a success, what specific suggestions could be made to assist Mark in the area of his involvement in sexual activity?

References

Alexander, C., Sipski, M., & Findley, T. (1993). Sexual activities, desire, and satisfaction in males pre- and post-spinal cord injury. *Archives of Sexual Behavior, 22*(3), 217–228.

American Occupational Therapy Association. (2008). Occupational therapy practice framework: Domain and process (2nd ed.). *American Journal of Occupational Therapy, 62,* 625–683. doi: 10.5014/ajot.62.6.625

American Spinal Injury Association. (2010). *International standards for neurological classification of spinal injury patients.* Chicago: Author.

Atkins, M. (2008). Spinal cord injury. In M. V. Radomski & C. A. T. Latham (Eds.), *Occupational therapy for physical dysfunction* (6th ed., pp. 1171–1213). Philadelphia: Wolters Kluwer/Lippincott, Williams & Wilkins.

Baylor College of Medicine. (2011). *Sexuality and reproductive health: Contraception.* Retrieved June 8, 2011, from http://www.bcm.edu/crowd/?pmid=1439

Benevento, B. T., & Sipski, M. L. (2002). Spinal Cord Injury Series Special—Neurogenic bladder, neurogenic bowel, and sexual dysfunction in people with spinal cord injury. *Physical Therapy, 82*(6), 601–612.

Christopher and Dana Reeve Foundation. (2010). *One degree of separation: Spinal cord injury in the United States.* Retrieved April 10, 2010, from http://www.christopherreeve.org/site/c.mtKZKgMWKwG

Christopher and Dana Reeve Foundation. (2012). *Accomplishments in spinal cord research.* Retrieved February 9, 2012, from http://www.christopherreeve.org/site/c.ddJFKRNoFiG/b.4434393/k.290F/History_of_spinal_cord_research.htm

DiMarco, A. F., Takaoka, Y., & Kowalski, K. E. (2005). Combined intercostal and diaphragm pacing provide artificial ventilation in patients with tetraplegia. *Archives of Physical Medicine and Rehabilitation, 86*(6), 1200–1207.

Ducharme, S. (2000). *Sexuality and spinal cord injury.* Retrieved June 6, 2011, from http://www.stanleyducharme.com/resources/sex_spinalcord_injury.htm

Ferreiro-Velasco, M. E., Barca-Buyo, A., de la Barrera, S. S., Montoto-Marques, A., Vazquez, X. M., & Rodriguez-Sotillo, A. (2005). Sexual issues in a sample of women with spinal cord injury. *Spinal Cord, 43*(1), 51–55.

Jensen, M. P., Kuehn, C. M., Amtmann, D., & Cardenas, D. D. (2007). Symptom burden in persons with spinal cord injury. *Archives of Physical Medicine and Rehabilitation, 88*(5), 638–645.

Kettl, P., Zarefoss, S., Jacoby, K., Garman, C., Hulse, C., Rowley, F., et al. (1991). Female sexuality after spinal cord injury. *Sexuality and Disability, 9,* 287–295.

Magnan, M. A., & Reynolds, K. (2006). Barriers to addressing patient sexuality concerns across five areas of specialization. *Clinical Nurse Specialist, 20*(6), 285–292.

Mayo Clinic. (2009). *Mayo Clinic guide to living with spinal cord injury: Moving ahead with your life.* New York: Demos Medical Publishing.

Mayo Clinic. (2011). *Spinal cord injury: Causes.* Retrieved August 8, 2011, from http://www.mayoclinic.com/health/spinal-cord-injury/DS00460/DSECTION=causes

McAlonan, S. (1996). Improving sexual rehabilitation services: The patient's perspective. *American Journal of Occupational Therapy, 50,* 826–834. doi:10.5014/ajot/.50.10.826

McCluer, S. (1992). *Female sexuality and spinal cord injury: Fact sheet 8.* Retrieved April 10, 2010, from http://www.spinalcord.uab.edu/show.asp?durki=21490.

National Institute of Neurological Disorders and Stroke. (2011). *Spinal cord injury: Hope through research.* Retrieved June 17, 2011, from http://www.ninds.nih.gov/disorders/sci/detail_sci.htm

Novak, P. P., & Mitchell, M. M. (1988). Professional involvement in sexuality counseling for patients with spinal cord injuries. *American Journal of Occupational Therapy, 42*(2), 105–112. doi:10.5014/ajot.42.2.105

Portney, L. S., & Watkins, M. P. (2000). *Foundations of clinical research: Applications to practice* (2nd ed.). Upper Saddle River, NJ: Prentice-Hall.

Post, M. W., Bloemen, J., & de Witte, L. P. (2005). Burden of support for partners of persons with spinal cord injuries. *Spinal Cord, 43,* 311–319.

RehabTeamSite. (2009). *Sexuality in spinal cord injury: The spinal cord injured male: Ejaculation, orgasm, and coitus.* Retrieved June 2, 2011, from http://calder.med.miami.edu/pointis/ejaculation.html

Richards, E., Tepper, M., Whipple, B., & Komisaruk, B. (1997). Women with complete spinal cord injury: A phenomenological study of sexuality and relationship experiences. *Sexuality and Disability, 15*(4), 271–283.

Rowles, D. (2010). *Spinal cord injury: Sexuality.* Retrieved April 6, 2010, from http://lifecenter.ric.org/index.php?tray=CONTENTPrint&tid=top163&cid=2560

Siddall, P. J., & Loeser, J. D. (2001). Pain following spinal cord injury. *Spinal Cord, 39*(2), 63–73.

Sipski, M. (2011). *Sexuality and spinal cord injury.* Retrieved July 31, 2011, from http://www2.ed.gov/pubs/AmericanRehab/spring97/sp9707.html

Sipski, M., & Alexander, C. (1993). Sexual activities, response, and satisfaction in women pre- and post-spinal cord injury. *Archives of Physical Medicine and Rehabilitation, 74*(10), 1025–1029.

Snell, W. E., Fisher, T. D., & Walters, A. S. (1993). The Multidimensional Sexuality Questionnaire: An objective self-report measure of psychological tendencies associated with human sexuality. *Annals of Sex Research, 6,* 27–55.

Trueblood, K., Hannon, R., & Hall, D. S. (1998). *Development and validation of a measure of sexual attitudes.* Paper presented at the meeting of the Society for the Scientific Study of Sexuality's Western Region Annual Conference, Honolulu.

U. S. National Library of Medicine. (2011). *Sexual problems overview.* Retrieved June 12, 2011, from http://www.nlm.nih.gov/medlineplus/ency/article/001951.htm

van Hylckama Vileg, A., Helmerhorst, F. M., Vandenbroucke, J. P., Doggen, C. J., & Rosendaal, F. R. (2009). The venous thrombotic risk of oral contraceptives, effects of oestrogen dose and progestogen type: Results of the MEGA case-control study. *British Medical Journal, 339.* doi:10.1136/bmj.b2921

Weiss, A. J., & Diamond, M. D. (1966). Sexual adjustment, identification, and attitudes of patients with myelopathy. *Archives of Physical Medicine and Rehabilitation, 47*(4), 245–250.

Whetstone, W. D., Hsu, J.-Y., Eisenberg, M., Werb, Z., & Noble-Haeusslein, L. J. (2003). Blood–spinal cord barrier after spinal cord injury: Relation to revascularization and wound healing. *Journal of Neuroscience Research, 74*(2), 227–239.

Appendix 5.A. Occupational Therapy Interventions With SCI

According to the American Occupational Therapy Association (2002), the occupational therapist can perform the following interventions with clients with an SCI:

- Evaluate a person's ability and level of functioning in his or her home, at work, and while engaging in leisure activities and hobbies.

- Determine how motivated a person is to participate in activities that he or she participated in prior to the injury.

- Identify any changes in roles a person may experience because of SCI.

- Provide individualized therapy to retrain people to perform daily living skills using adaptive techniques.

- Facilitate coping skills that could help a person overcome the effects of an SCI.

- Implement exercises and routines that strengthen muscles that might have been affected that are necessary in daily activities.

- Determine the type of assistive devices that could help a person become more independent with daily living skills.

The areas identified relate to all aspects of a person's life, including sexual activity involvement, although not explicitly mentioned. The initial occupational therapy evaluation should be functional in scope, with consideration given to the client's interests, needs, strengths, and limitations.

The client's level of motivation should be determined, as motivation and perseverance are necessary to overcome the effects of an SCI. These same characteristics are crucial for a client who wishes to resume involvement in sexual activity as well. A strong desire to resume life roles and responsibilities can make all the difference in the rehabilitation process and bolster client motivation. Therapy interventions should directly relate to function, with the ultimate goal to be performance in daily activities with the greatest level of independence possible.

Occupational therapy interventions cover a wide scope of tasks, including but not limited to dressing, bathing, grooming, transferring, strengthening, compensatory techniques for daily activities, use of assistive technologies, splinting, bowel and bladder programming, endurance building, and mobility training. The essence of sexual activity reengagement is easily laced into these intervention areas. Consider, for example, mobility and transfer skills that can

(Continued)

Appendix 5.A. Occupational Therapy Interventions With SCI (*cont.*)

be generalized into positioning for sexual activity or bathing and grooming activities that can be transferred into self-esteem-elevating "primping" and beauty rituals to heighten one's physical appearance and promote an increased feeling of sexual attractiveness. Through the implementation of exercises and task routines, and using assistive devices, ADL performance, including engagement in sexual activity, can be enhanced.

Reference

American Occupational Therapy Association. (2002). *Tips for living: Living with spinal cord injury.* Retrieved July 1, 2010, from http://www.aota.org/consumers/consumers/Health-and-Wellness/SCI/35140.aspx?FT=.pdf

6

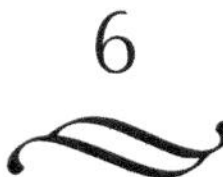

Cardiovascular Disease and Sexuality

Bernadette Hattjar, DrOT, MEd, OTR/L, CWCE

Key Terms and Concepts

- Activity configuration
- Atherosclerosis
- Cardiovascular disease
- Cardiac rehabilitation
- Congestive heart failure
- Coronary artery disease
- Energy conservation
- Erectile dysfunction
- Metabolic equivalent of task
- Myocardial infarction
- Stress reduction techniques
- Stroke.

At the end of this chapter, readers will be able to

- Understand the factors that contribute to cardiovascular disease,
- Identify the signs of myocardial infarction (heart attack),
- Identify appropriate assessment tools for this population,
- Identify appropriate interventions for addressing sexuality and sexual activity,
- Implement stress reduction techniques,

- Implement a configuration of daily activity to enable involvement in sexual activity,

- Identify communication impediments such as aggressive and passive behavior modes,

- Identify caregiver support styles and how these styles can affect the patient with cardiovascular disease,

- Recognize the myths and realities of cardiovascular disease symptoms, and

- Understand the diagnosis of erectile dysfunction and medications used to correct it.

Introduction

Cardiovascular disease (CVD) includes conditions that affect the structures or function of the heart, including diseases of the coronary arteries and blood vessels (Figure 6.1). CVD accounts for 1 in every 3 deaths in the United States (American Heart Association [AHA], 2011) and is considered the top killer in the country. The estimated cost for medical care for CVD was $316 billion in 2010 (Centers for Disease Control and Prevention [CDC], 2010).

Medical progress has improved heart care; therefore, CVD does not necessarily mean a death sentence for an individual. Advances in surgery, rehabilitation, and pharmaceuticals have also improved care; therefore, an individual with diagnosed CVD has an improved and extended life expectancy. With the improved quality of life (QoL) from medical interventions,

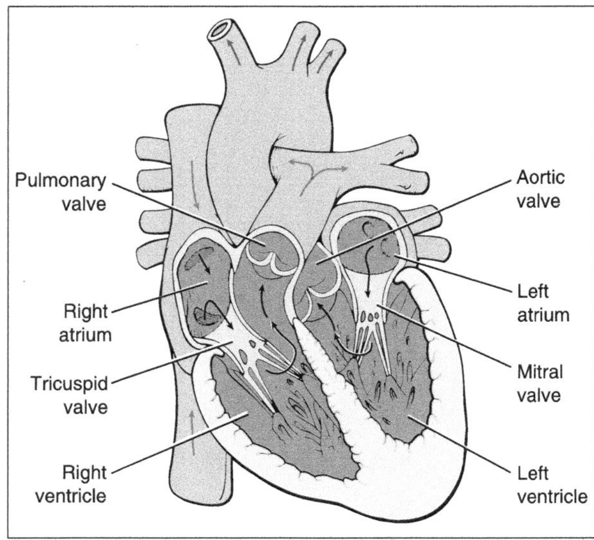

Figure 6.1. Chambers and valves of the heart.

Source. Richard Fritzler, Medical Illustrator, Roswell, GA. Used under license.

health care providers, especially occupational therapy practitioners, patients, and medical practitioners must consider daily activities that are common, usual, and reoccurring, including sexual activity.

CVD is comprised of the following components:

- *High blood pressure* is the excessive force of blood pumping through the blood vessels. It affects 1 in 4 Americans. High blood pressure can contribute to stroke and heart failure (AHA, 2011).

- *Coronary artery disease (CAD)* occurs when the arteries that supply the heart muscle with blood become occluded or blocked by athero-sclerotic plaque. CAD can lead to a myocardial infarction (MI), or heart attack, or to chest pain (Care to Act North Carolina, 2011).

- *Stroke* or *cerebrovascular accident* occurs when blood flow to the brain is interrupted *(ischemic stroke)* or when a blood vessel in the brain ruptures *(hemorrhagic stroke)*. High blood pressure increases the likelihood of a stroke (AHA, 2010a).

- *Heart failure* or *congestive heart failure (CHF)* occurs when the heart cannot pump enough blood to meet the needs of internal organs and tissues. The inefficient pumping of the heart leads to fatigue, fluid retention, and shortness of breath because of fluid collection (AHA, 2010a).

The most common type of CVD is coronary heart disease. Coronary heart disease is caused by *atherosclerosis,* the narrowing of the coronary arteries from a fatty plaque buildup. This is likely to cause chest pain or a heart attack (AHA, 2010a).

Exhibit 6.1. CVD Risk Factors

The following represents the percentage of adults in the United States with CVD risk factors in 2005–2006 (CDC, 2006):

- Inactivity, 39.5%
- Obesity, 33.9%
- High blood pressure, 30.5%
- Cigarette smoking, 20.8%
- High cholesterol, 15.6%
- Diabetes, 10.1%.

Note. About 37% of American adults have 2 or more of the risk factors listed above, which accounts for the high number of Americans with CVD.

Risk factors for CVD are well known and well documented, but the percentage of Americans with such risk factors is startling. Exhibit 6.1 lists the primary risk factors and their corresponding percentages.

The two measures commonly cited in history and literature that combat or prevent heart disease are exercise and diet. History shows that CVD is more prevalent in industrialized societies. In ancient and preindustrialized societies, the incidents of CVD were significantly lower; this was most likely because the people then ate diets that were low in fat and carbohydrates and higher in lean protein, vegetables, and legumes. Physical activity and work requirements were also greater in preindustrialized or agrarian societies, and this physical activity supports healthy heart function.

Demographics

The CDC (2006) reported that over 631,000 Americans died from cardiovascular complications. This number equals about 26%, or 1 in every 4, deaths in the United States.

Heart disease is the leading cause of death in both men and women. Although in decades prior to 2006 cardiovascular deaths were more common in men, in 2006 approximately 50% such deaths occurred in women (CDC, 2006). This increase in cardiovascular death in women is sometimes attributed to smoking and obesity. The death rate from CVD also varies by ethnicity, as is shown in Exhibit 6.2.

Signs and Symptoms

CVD presents with signs and symptoms, some of which are easily detectable by the individual or the physician. Other signs and symptoms might go unnoticed and undetected until a major cardiac event occurs.

The typical MI, or heart attack, presents with detectable signs. It is important to understand the five major signs of an MI:

Exhibit 6.2. CVD Deaths by Ethnicity

The percentage of deaths from CVD in the United States in 2004 (CDC, 2010) include

- Whites, 27.5%
- African Americans, 25.8%
- Asians or Pacific Islanders, 24.6%
- Hispanics, 22.7%
- American Indians or Alaska Natives, 19.8%.

1. Pain or discomfort in the jaw, neck, or back

2. Feeling weak, light-headed, or faint

3. Chest pain, discomfort, or tightness

4. Pain or discomfort in the arms or shoulders

5. Shortness of breath without exertion (CDC, 2010).

Other aspects of CVD are, more or less, silent in their development. CAD occurs when *plaque* (cholesterol deposits) builds up and partially or totally occludes arteries that supply blood to the heart muscle, causing atherosclerosis. Over time, atherosclerosis can weaken the heart muscle; it must work harder and is less efficient in pumping blood because it is overworking. This might eventually lead to *CHF,* in which the heart muscle cannot pump enough blood to meet the needs of the internal organs and tissue (Figure 6.2), or it might lead to an irregular heartbeat *(arrhythmia)*. For some individuals, a heart attack is the first observable sign that heart disease is present.

CVD signs and symptoms are often unnoticed or disregarded; therefore, regular physical check-ups are important. Typical tests used by physicians to detect the presence of heart disease include

- *Electrocardiogram (EKG).* Measures the electrical activity, rate, and regularity of the heartbeat.

- *Echocardiogram.* Uses ultrasound to create a picture of the heart.

- *Exercise stress test.* Measures the heart rate while the client walks on a treadmill. This test helps to determine how well the heart is working when it has to pump more blood.

- *Chest x-ray.* Creates a picture of the heart, lungs, and other organs in the chest.

- *Cardiac catheterization.* Checks the inside of arteries for blockage by threading thin, flexible tube through an artery in the groin, arm, or neck to reach the coronary artery. Can measure blood pressure and flow in the heart's chambers, collect blood samples from the heart, or inject dye into the coronary arteries.

- *Coronary angiogram.* Monitors blockage and flow of blood through the heart. Uses x-rays to detect dye flow injected via cardiac catheterization (CDC, 2010).

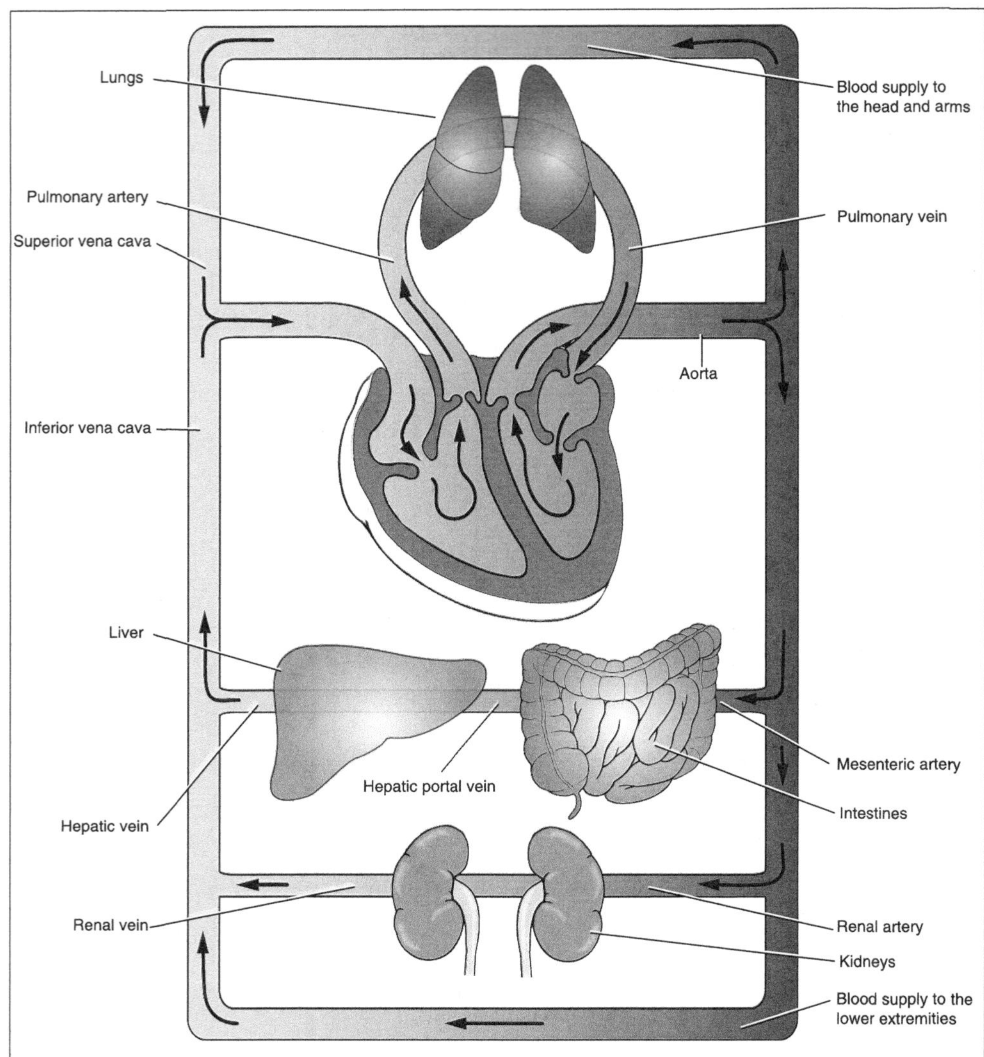

Figure 6.2. Circulatory system.

Source. Richard Fritzler, Medical Illustrator, Roswell, GA. Used under license.

Myths Related to Sexuality and Cardiac Dysfunction

Many myths persist about sexual activity and CVD:

- *Myth 1.* Sex is no longer permissible after a cardiac event such as an MI.

- *Myth 2.* Any person diagnosed with heart disease will experience chest pain during sexual activity.

- *Myth 3.* For older adults, sex is no longer important (Katz, 2007).

The media perpetuate these myths; hearing of someone dying of a heart attack during the act of sex is not rare. Consider a scene from the fictional film *Something's Gotta Give* (Block & Meyers, 2003), in which a man in his 60s experiences an MI during sex and has subsequent panic attacks (mimicking a heart attack) after his initial cardiac event. However, the actual likelihood of experiencing an MI during sexual activity is rare; therefore, showing such a death in a popular movie tends to fuel the myth that sexual activity is prohibitive for cardiac patients and older individuals.

Facts About Resuming Sexual Activity

Sex is not an easy subject for many individuals to broach with a health care provider. Sexual activity is also a subject that health care providers might not expect a patient or client to raise (Magnan & Reynolds, 2006). In short, the provider often does not address sexual activity, nor does the recipient question it. This commonly sets the stage for a "don't ask; don't tell" scenario that benefits neither the patient nor the health care provider.

This situation is first reinforced by the need for the health care provider to be highly productive and second by the short patient length of stay following a cardiac episode or cardiac surgery. Adding some probing questions to an initial assessment might grant permission to address the subject of sexual activity, but time constraints might not warrant discussion in an inpatient setting.

The therapist and patient should ask questions about sexual activity, as it will promote further discussion at the next level of care (e.g., cardiac rehabilitation, home care). Possible questions for beginning the discussion are listed in the "Occupational Therapy Assessment and Intervention" section later in this chapter.

Patients with CVD are usually adults (ages 18 years or older) with professional and personal responsibilities and roles. The CVD or heart attack experience frequently forces the patient to look at his or her life and the roles and responsibilities he or she encounters. This personal review of one's life might account for positive lifestyle changes such as exercise, diet, medication, or stress reduction, or it might precipitate negative lifestyle changes such as anxiety, depression, vigilance, withdrawal from life roles, or isolation. The positive and negative aspects of CVD also affect the caregiver, the spouse, or significant other. The method in which the caregiver provides care accounts for the caregiver's and patient's lived experience of CVD and the psychological and physical effects of CVD.

Providing Support

Healthy spouses or partners typically provide support for their ill partners in several ways:

- *Active engagement* includes constructive problem solving between the caregiver and the patient. This concept reflects open communication and dialogue exchange between individuals.

- *Protective buffering* consists of both parties hiding concerns and denying worries from the other. This *modus operandi* is assumed when the well and ill partner pretend that nothing is wrong, covers concerns with a smile, or dismisses any expressed concern ("Don't worry, you're fine").

- *Overprotection* refers to the caregiver's or the patient's underestimation of the patient's capabilities (Vilchinsky et al., 2010). This method of interacting places undefined limits and low expectations on the ill person and might place excessive burdens on the well person. Overdoing activity for the ill person and placing him or her in the traditional sick or patient role occurs.

Using an active engagement method of providing care promotes an open and honest exchange between the caregiver and the patient. Recovery from any disability or illness is best accomplished in a calm and stress-free environment. By maintaining an open dialogue and honest sharing of feelings and concerns, which occurs with the active engagement approach, stress is lowered externally with a calmer and more peaceful environment and internally because there is nothing to hide from or withhold.

According to the Person–Environment Fit Model, as identified by French, Rodgers, and Cobb in 1974, psychological adjustment (to anything) is a function of the degree of "fit" between the social or physical environment and the individual's traits (Vilchinsky et al., 2010). The social environment would be comprised of the caregiver's way of providing support, and the individual's traits would relate to the manner in which support is construed by the patient. If there is a lack of congruity between the manner of caregiver support and the way in which the patient experiences support, problems will be more likely to surface.

For example, if a patient with CVD is anxious and fearful of his or her status and caregiving is provided in an overprotecting manner, the caregiver and the patient might never realize his or her actual abilities. The patient might believe that he or she is more severely impaired than he or she actually is. On the other hand, if the caregiver does not assertively express concerns about the patient's status and covers up his or her feelings with a smile and laissez-faire attitude, and if the patient never vocalizes his or her personal concerns because he or she thinks everything is all right or all wrong, the dyadic relationship will be riddled with confusion, ambiguity, and lack of clarity. Therefore, a "match" between caregiving and the acceptance of caregiving is crucial to the relationship in all areas of occupation, including sexuality, sexual activity, and the resumption of an intimate relationship.

Discussing Sexual Activity

Sexuality and sexual activity are integral components of life satisfaction and are pleasurable and intimate aspects of being human. Yet, it is understandable that, after a cardiac event, a patient might feel that sexual activity is risky or an activity to be avoided.

Sexual activity and sexuality are not topics that are openly or freely discussed in the medical model of health care because the minimization and absence of symptoms is the primary focus of patient care—that is, the primary focus is on whether the patient is "symptom-free." To research and investigate the sexual activity aspect of patients after a cardiac event, the TRIUMPH (*T*ransitional *R*esearch *I*nvestigating *U*nderlying Disparities in Recovery from Acute *MI*: *P*atient's *H*ealth Status; Emory University, 2011) study reviewed participants' physical limitations, angina frequency, QoL, physical components (problems), and mental components (problems).

In the TRIUMPH registry (Emory University, 2011), which is comprised of 1,184 men and 576 women, nearly half the men and about one-third of the women reported receiving discharge instructions on resuming sexual activity. Even fewer men (40%) and women (20%) talked about sex with their physicians in the year following their heart attack. One year after the heart attack, more than 66% of the men and about 40% of the women reported some sexual activity.

Although the consensus of physicians indicates that it is safe to resume sexual activity after a heart attack once the patient feels better, physicians and other health care professionals do not always address patient questions about when it is safe to resume sexual activity:

> Sexuality is an important part of life throughout life, and most heart attack patients are sexually active. For the most part, physicians just aren't discussing this topic with their patients after a heart attack. . . . not raising the question (with patients) leaves the door closed. (AHA, 2010b)

Determining Risk

Objective guidelines for having sexual activity after MI were conceived and developed to provide clinical management of sexual dysfunction in patients with CVD (DeBusk et al., 2000). A stratified classification system includes high-, medium-, and low-risk categories of sexual activity and cardiac risk and provides a systematic set of guidelines concerning the patient's resumption of sexual activity after a cardiac event (Exhibit 6.3).

Objectively, the cardiovascular risk for sexual activity is similar to mild-to-moderate daily nonsexual activity. Only a small risk of MI is associated with sexual activity. The baseline for absolute risk of an MI during normal daily life is low: 1 chance in a million per hour for a healthy adult, and 10 chances in a million per hour for a patient with documented CVD. In other words, people may think that sex will precipitate another heart attack or will compromise their cardiac status in some way, but it offers no more of a threat to the heart than other daily activities. However, this assumption causes many patients with CVD to shy away from sexual activity.

The cardiovascular response to sexual activity, including sexual intercourse, is similar to mild-to-moderate activity effort (Jackson, 2009; see Table 6.1). In various cardiac research studies on the effect of sexual intercourse or sexual activity on heart rate and blood pressure, no significant or prohibitive effect was identified in relation to sexual activity or intercourse for clients with CVD, who were post heart attack, or with stable angina (Bohlen, Held, Sanderson, & Patterson, 1984; Garcia-Barreto, Sin-Chen, Rivas-Estany, Nieto, & Hemondez-Catiero, 1986; Jackson, 1981; Nemec, Mansfield, & Kennedy, 1964; Sainz, Amaya, & Garcia, 2004).

In fact, sexual intercourse or any type of sexual activity demands no more metabolic energy or exertion than walking 1 mile on a level, stable surface (Jackson, 2009) or walking 2–3 miles per hour (Katz, 2009; see Table 6.1). To understand more fully energy expenditure in activity, the metabolic equivalent of task (MET) is used. *MET* is the

> amount of energy expended when a person is engaged in activity. In a semireclined position with the extremities supported, the amount of energy expended is 2.5 milliliters of oxygen per minute per kilogram of body weight. This equals 1 MET of energy expenditure. (Latham, 2008, p. 359)

The actual energy expenditure and cardiac and pulmonary task requirements of sexual activity is not substantially different from daily, common activities. However, the patient's personal perception of engaging or re-engaging in

---

Exhibit 6.3. Classification for Sexual Activity Levels for Patients With CVDs

Low risk includes a large majority of patients. Identifiers include

- Controlled hypertension
- Mild, stable angina
- Successful coronary revascularization
- History of uncomplicated MI
- Mild valve disease
- No symptoms and <3 cardiovascular risk factors.

These patients can be safely encouraged to initiate or resume sexual activity or to receive treatment for sexual dysfunction.

Medium risk identifiers include

- Moderate angina
- Recent heart attack (<6 weeks ago)
- Left-ventricle dysfunction or Class II CHF
- Nonsustained low arrhythmias
- >3 risk factors for CAD.

Further evaluation by a cardiologist is suggested.

High risk identifiers include

- Unstable or refractory angina
- Uncontrolled hypertension
- CHF (Class III or IV)
- Very recent heart attack (<2 weeks ago)
- High-risk arrhythmias
- Obstructive cardiomyopathy
- Moderate-to-severe valve disease.

Patients in this category should be medically stabilized before resuming sexual activity.

Note. From DeBusk et al. (2000). Copyright © 2000 by the American College of Cardiology. Used with permission.

CAD = coronary artery disease; CHF = congestive heart failure.

Table 6.1. Metabolic Equivalent of Task Units in a Guide to Relating Daily Activity to Sexual Activity

Daily Activity	METs
*Lower-range or normal sexual activity	2–3
*Lower-range orgasm	3–4
*Upper-range activity (vigorous)	5–6
Lifting or carrying objects of 10–20 lbs.	4–5
Walking 1 mile on level surface for 20 min	3–4
Golf	4–5
Gardening or digging	3–5
Wall-papering or house do-it yourself work	4–5
Light housework	2–4
Heavy housework	3–6

Note. From "Sexual Response in Disease," by G. Jackson, 2009, *Journal of Sex Research*, Vol. 46, pp. 233–236. Copyright © 2009, by Taylor & Francis. Used with permission.

METs = metabolic equivalent of task units.

*Sexual intercourse with an established partner. Sexual intercourse or activity executed in a more casual manner or with a new or less familiar partner might involve a greater cardiac workload. This might be accounted for by an age difference between the partners, partner unfamiliarity, anxiety presented by a new or different sexual situation, increased sexual excitement about a new or different partner, and lack of knowledge about partner likes or dislikes regarding sexual activity.

sexual activity places undue stress or anxiety on the intimate relationship. This contributes to tension and, perhaps, to racing thoughts about the outcome of a sexual experience: Will I survive the actual act of having sex and orgasm?

Factors to Consider Prior to Resuming Sexual Activity

Nevertheless, patients with CVD should consider some physical, pain, and psychological factors when they and their partner resume sexual activity. General physical barriers that have been identified with the resumption of sexual activity in patients with CVD include heart *palpitations* (beating too fast or a sensation of heart fluttering), *arrhythmia* (beating too fast, too slow, or beating in an irregular manner), ongoing heart problems related to heart failure, heart muscle problems, or heart valve problems (these might include shortness of breath, irregular heartbeat, or chest pain; National Heart, Lung, & Blood Institute, 2011).

Psychological barriers that have been identified with the resumption of sexual activity in patients with CVD include fear (of having another cardiac event during the act itself), anxiety (related to the ability to physically perform the sex act), and self-esteem issues (Am I still attractive or desirable since having this cardiac problem?). When both the psychological and physical barriers coexist, lack of interest in sexual activity—for whatever reason—is a common symptom in patients with CVD.

Pain

The two most common types of pain that occur during sex for patients with CVD are (1) chest pain and (2) pain related to an incision site. Chest pain is frequently a fear-producing physiological fact for a few patients with CVD (remember that chest pain is not the norm!). If chest pain is experienced during usual daily activity, it will probably be experienced during sex.

This issue should be addressed with a physician before ongoing, regular sexual activity is resumed. Physicians frequently prescribe nitroglycerine for chest pain that occurs with activity, which serves to decrease chest pain caused by ischemia or decreased blood flow. *Nitroglycerine* is a small pill that is placed under the tongue and allowed to dissolve if or when chest pain occurs. The tissue in the mouth promotes fast absorption into the blood stream. As the medication is absorbed into the blood stream, chest pain should decrease. (After taking nitroglycerine, if chest pain does not subside within 15 minutes, medical care should be secured.)

If bypass surgery has occurred, tightness or pulling at the chest incision site or sternum is common. As the healing process takes place and physical status is improved, pulling and a sensation of tightness at the surgical incision decrease. Additionally, the patient should protect or buffer the sternum area after bypass surgery until healing occurs. (Frequently, small pillows are given to the patient to provide protection and "padding" over the incision site.) To accommodate both pain and healing, consider the use of pillows or positioning aids like bolsters to position the upper extremities and to avoid excessive pulling at the incision (see Figure A.5 in Appendix A).

It was once considered prudent for an individual with cardiac problems to avoid the traditional position and chest incision pulling or tightness because of the upper-extremity support that is assumed by some individuals during intercourse (Katz, 2009). Conversely, it is also sometimes suggested that he or she not lay supine during sexual activity because of increased pulmonary demands and the tendency for fluid to "pool" in the chest area while in this position. Actually, the couple should feel free to use whatever position is the most comfortable and familiar for sexual activity (Jackson,

2009). Sexual activity abstinence is not considered a typically occurring limitation of CVD.

That said, it is recommended that anal intercourse be avoided for patients with CVD. The position for anal intercourse can provide stimulation to the vagus nerve, one of the longest nerves in the body. This nerve stimulation can slow down heart rate and might contribute to chest pain (Katz, 2009). If the partners favor this position, they should explore and agree upon alternative positions for intercourse.

Lack of Libido

Lack of libido (decreased interest in sexual activity) might be the external presentation of depression or anxiety and might warrant medication or at least sharing this information with a health care provider. Some individuals might find that they or their partners are fearful of initiating sexual activity; they feel that sexual activity might cause additional cardiac compromises, precipitate a heart attack, or even result in death. These types of feelings should be openly discussed and shared with both the partner and the health care providers.

Erectile Dysfunction

Erectile dysfunction (ED) might be an early sign of cardiac problems in males as young as 45 years of age and might represent an early warning sign for CVD (Bankhead, 2009). *ED* relates to the male's inability to attain or sustain an erection sufficient in firmness to engage in sexual intercourse. In clients with CVD, ED often occurs as the result of medications or poor circulation. ED usually is exacerbated by the psychological symptoms of fear, anxiety, and low or diminished self-esteem.

ED is also correlated with CVD. One component of the Massachusetts Male Aging Study (Araujo et al., 2009) identified that ED and CVD often occur together; however, the risk of mortality from CVD or other causes has not been clearly established (Bankhead, 2009). One study (Thompson et al., 2005) analyzed more than 4,000 men without symptoms of CVD or ED and found that men who subsequently experienced ED were nearly 50% more likely to experience a cardiovascular event within 7 years than men who did not experience ED. Although this is only one study, the link between ED and CVD is well documented (Sainz et al., 2004). Approximately 40% of men experience ED after having a heart attack or a cardiac event such as an increase of CHF symptoms (e.g., shortness of breath, fluid retention, excessive fatigue; Russell, Khandheria, & Nehra, 2004).

Although the most common treatments for ED are oral medications such as sildenafil (Viagra), tadalafil (Cialis), or vardenafil (Levitra), these medications dilate the blood vessels and should be used with extreme caution and only under a physician's care. Additionally, nonprescription, herbal, or homeopathic medications for the treatment of ED are not regulated by the Federal Drug Administration and should not be used. Any medication used for ED should be used only with the knowledge of a licensed physician (Katz, 2009).

Resuming Sexual Activity

After a cardiac event, deferring sexual activity for 7–10 days is recommended (Katz, 2009) for individuals with lower risk, although many individuals usually wait longer before resuming any sexual activity because of fear or fatigue. For individuals at high risk or with unstable symptoms, it is usually advisable to obtain an exercise stress test prescribed by a physician before resuming sexual activity (DeBusk et al., 2000).

Usually, by 6 months after a cardiac event, most couples return to some form of sexual activity. It is usual for *cardiac rehabilitation,* a structured, monitored program of exercise in increasing intensity levels, to occur after physiological stabilization of the cardiac condition or event. A physician prescribes cardiac rehabilitation, and the rehabilitation team usually includes the referring physician or cardiologist, nurse, occupational therapist, physical therapist, exercise physiologist, social worker, and psychologist. Within the cardiac rehabilitation program, activity and exercise intensity gradually increase. It provides safety and substantiation for the resumption of more rigorous activities such as sexual activity. During cardiac rehabilitation, the occupational therapist can make interventions that relate to sexual activity resumption using the "PLISSIT" model (Annon, 1976; see Chapter 1). Cardiac rehabilitation (along with home care or outpatient settings) provides the time to establish a working relationship with the patient, thereby making the discussion of sexual activity more appropriate and, most likely, comfortable for both the patient and the therapist.

Occupational Therapy Assessment and Intervention

Assessment

Occupational therapists are adept in assessing the client's activity of daily living (ADL) performance and in making valid suggestions for activity modification and accommodations. After a cardiac event, the patient's occupational roles and responsibilities might be radically changed, and the patient might need to adapt to his or her current level of function. The occupational therapist can recommend energy conservation and work simplification techniques to enable the patient to be as independent and safe as possible in his or her execution of daily activities and tasks. *Energy conservation* means saving or storing energy to accomplish the activities one wants to accomplish; it does *not* mean doing nothing. In relation to sexual activity, a patient might not embark on a long-term, fatiguing activity if he or she plans to have sex on a particular day. Generally, assessment does not include addressing intimacy or sexual activity, but there is no reason why it cannot.

When intervening in any personal and intimate area of a patient's life, the occupational therapist must possess the paramount traits of compassion, sensitivity, and understanding. To address sexuality, consider asking the following type of questions:

1. How do you feel about your current physical status with regard to attractiveness and being desirable to your partner?

2. Do you believe that your intimate relationship has changed or will change because of your diagnosis?

3. How much physical or intimate contact have you had with your partner since the time of your diagnosis?

4. Do you have concerns about resuming your intimate relationship with your partner? Do you believe that you are still desirable or attractive to your partner? Has your intimate relationship changed? Have you engaged in touching, kissing, or hugging with your partner since the time of your diagnosis? If you have had a cardiac event, have you engaged in touching, kissing, or hugging with your partner since the time of your heart attack or heart surgery?

5. Do you have other concerns about intimacy that you would like to share? (Hattjar, Parker, & Lappa, 2008, p. CE6)

Asking questions in this manner will secure information but will not be intrusive or overtly sexual in nature.

Intervention

Occupational therapy practitioners can provide interventions to address sexual activity for clients with CVD. Stress reduction and energy conservation are the two primary interventions that can be generalized to sexual activity and nonsexual activities.

Stress reduction

Entertaining the thought of resuming sexual activity can add stress to the patient who fears another cardiac incident or heart attack and might question his or her ability to execute the act of having sexual activity. Anxiety about the ability to initiate, execute, and sustain sexual activity might be prominent in the patient's mind and add fuel to the level of stress. The patient might even deny his or her desire and assume that he or she cannot "fail" if he or she does not try. To alleviate stress and to help the patient address feelings of anxiety, stress reduction techniques might be included as a component of occupational therapy intervention.

Stress affects most people at some time and in some way. Although the causes of stress vary from person to person, the effects of stress are almost universal in their manifestations. Physically, stress is characterized by increased heartbeat, elevated blood pressure, pupil dilation, a sense of urgency, a sense of a loss of control, and mood changes. Stress can be beneficial in times of crises or emergency, but ongoing stress can cause physical and negative changes. Psychological effects of stress such as worrying, anticipation, and agitation can elevate cortisol levels and result in detrimental physiological effects. Generally, long-term stressors are the result of work problems, relationship problems, financial issues, loneliness, and worry or obsessions about physical health issues (Smith, Segal, & Segal, 2011). However, the effects of stress on patients with CVD can affect their physical status in many dangerous ways:

- Increasing the pumping action of the heart muscle
- Causing arrhythmia
- Thickening the blood (an automatic response to danger)
- Impeding fat molecules from clearing from throughout the body
- Causing the body to release inflammatory markers in the bloodstream, which might increase the likelihood of a heart attack or stroke (American Institute of Stress, n.d.).

To decrease the likelihood of detrimental stress effects, stress reduction techniques can be incorporated into the treatment interventions. Common stress reduction techniques include, but are not limited to,

- *Using a stress ball.* Squeezing the stress ball with one or both hands can help the patient to focus on the task and less on stress-producing issues.

- *Visual imagery.* Calming and pleasant visual imagery can be attained by having the patient close his or her eyes and imagine a calm, tranquil, peaceful place or memory.

- *Progressive or guided relaxation techniques.* When using a progressive relaxation activity, the therapist speaks in a soft, slow manner. The patient can be seated or in a supine position. Ask the patient to think about areas in his or her body where he or she retains stress, such as sites of muscle tightness or joint discomfort. Ask the patient to imagine that the stress-prone area is filled with sand, and as he or she relaxes, the sand will flow out of that area, thereby decreasing stress or pain.

- *Involvement in a tabletop creative activity.* Drawing, painting, making a collage, knitting or crocheting, or constructing a puzzle can divert attention away from stress.

- *Yoga.* If permitted by the physician, patients can try yoga. Use and stretching of muscles, along with focused breath, can lead to relaxation. For the patient with CVD, yoga should be done only with a certified yoga instructor, and the instructor must be made aware of the client's cardiac status.

- *Simple stretch-and-relax techniques.* Include isometric tense-and-relax techniques (in which the client tries to squeeze the shoulder blades together for a slow count of 3, and then relaxes) and slow isotonic muscle stretching (the type of stretching one might do upon awakening from sleep).

Stress-reducing activities can be incorporated into treatment sessions and might be useful for the client to do outside of the therapy session. Any of the above-mentioned stress reduction techniques could be effective for a variety of patients. The commonalities of these techniques are that (1) the activities divert the conscious attention to something other than the stress-producing situation or thought; (2) the focused use of muscles, followed by a period of relaxation of the muscles, produces a relaxation response to stress; (3) if the mind is encouraged to think and thereby divert and change stressful thoughts, relaxation is more likely to occur; and (4) all of these activities provide time to think, plan, assess, and talk about the perceived stressor of sexual activity.

Energy conservation

Another inroad to addressing intimacy and sexuality can be attained by addressing energy conservation techniques (Exhibit 6.4).

Exhibit 6.4. Basic Energy Conservation Techniques for Daily Activities

Energy conservation techniques maximize the patient's ability to become engaged in activities without compromising his or her physical or physiological status. Basic guidelines for energy conservation include, but are not limited to, the following recommendations:

1. *Activity planning.* Decide which tasks are most important to you or that you desire most to become involved in. Do these tasks occur many times throughout the day, once a day, a few times each week, weekly, or monthly?

2. *Activity ranking.* What activities are the most crucial to daily success or well-being?

3. *Energy awareness.* Determine at what time or times during the day that energy levels are higher or lower.

4. *Activity adaptation.* In what manner is the task usually accomplished? Can this be modified to create a "storage bank of energy"? For example, if an activity is usually done standing, can it be performed in a sitting position? If you cook or clean the house, can the tasks be modified so that you can avoid expending large amounts of energy while still accomplishing the task? For example, can items you wish to dust or clean be slid on a flat surface rather than lifted or moved? Does every room need to be vacuumed daily, or can one room be vacuumed each day? Is energy saved by creating a less-aggressive method of performing common tasks?

5. *Activity simplification.* Can tasks be performed in a simpler manner with similar results?

6. *Opt for meaningful tasks.* Do not waste energy unnecessarily on tasks that are not important. Save energy for tasks that are meaningful (Canadian Association of Occupational Therapists, 2012).

Although energy conservation might seem to be such a basic construct that it does not warrant therapist attention, many patients do not have a clear idea of how they actually spend their time and energy on a day-by-day basis. To highlight how time and energy are spent, it is appropriate that the patient begin therapeutic interventions by completing an activity configuration.

An *activity configuration* is a simple, charted review of how time is spent by the individual. Provide a basic chart with a general activity category legend (see Appendix 6.A). The patient can complete the form over a period of a few days or a week, and the completed form will provide an objective and visible review of how time is spent.

The activity configuration can help both the therapist and the patient determine when energy and the desire to become engaged in any activity is high and when interest and energy are low. Thus, this can help both individuals determine when higher energy-expending activities should occur.

Regarding sexual activity, patients should consider having sexual activity at alternative times from "what was usual" before the cardiac event. Perhaps the patient has more energy in the early evening and not as much energy before sleep. Perhaps the patient has more energy on weekend days or weekdays, depending on his or her life schedule. Timing should be considered to increase the likelihood that enjoyable sexual activity can occur. These things need to be considered before further discussion on sexual activity can or should occur. Additionally, by including sexual activity as an ADL, the patient gives the therapist permission for (or an inroad into) further discussion and intervention of this very personal subject.

The energy levels of most patients are usually low following the cardiac event. Rest and rehabilitation are tasks that a patient should undertake following a cardiac event and when the physician feels that the patient is ready for cardiac rehabilitation. The patient's ability to address feelings and stressors is also a crucial aspect of re-engaging with life and occupational roles. When the patient gains confidence and energy, and when interest levels increase, then dealing with the conservation of energy for tasks that the patient wants to become engaged in becomes important so that the patient can re-establish life roles. Sexual activity is a crucial component for any patient in returning to the premorbid life.

Summary

CVD is extremely prevalent in American society. The symptoms of CAD and cardiac dysfunction might remain silent until a cardiac event occurs, or they might be discovered only when the patient is monitoring, along with his or her physician, high-risk signs or symptoms to prevent a major cardiac event from occurring.

The occupational therapist can be an essential member in the cardiac interdisciplinary team. Occupational therapy can evaluate for function and can assess and intervene in occupational role re-engagement, including intervening in the patient's role of being an intimate partner and in helping the patient address stress.

Compassion and sensitivity are essential for addressing sexual activity with patients with CVD. This subject can be initially introduced by not only asking questions related to the patient's perception of his or her attractiveness and esteem but also by addressing energy conservation and having the client identify daily high- and low-energy levels. This component of intervention might be accomplished through an activity configuration to secure client input. This type of intervention can be performed in the inpatient setting if time (length of stay) permits; however, it is probably more aptly performed in the rehabilitation, home care, or outpatient settings because of increased time and the ability to establish a working relationship with the client. Nevertheless, it is essential that the patient grant the therapist permission to broach the subject of sexual activity.

Through providing a realistic, meaningful, and purposeful assessment and intervention, the occupational therapist can enhance patients' ability to become re-engaged in all aspects of life, including sexual activity.

Case Example 6.1. Ben: MI

Ben is a 58-year-old married man who had an MI about 4 months earlier. He resides with his wife of 20 years. They live in a one-story ranch home.

Ben is employed as a supervisor at a local electronics plant.

Since the time of his MI, Ben has stopped smoking and drinking and walks approximately 1 mile each day. His wife adheres to preparing low-fat, low-cholesterol food, and Ben frequently helps with food preparation. Ben's major avocational activity is cooking and baking. His wife states, "He is a much better cook than I ever could hope to be. I'm glad to have his help."

Ben has lost 15 pounds since the MI and reports, "Overall, I feel better, but I am still afraid that I'm going to have 'the big one.' It makes me feel funny. I've never been afraid of or shied away from anything until now." In essence, Ben has resumed his life and is doing well at work and in leisure and social tasks and is getting adequate rest. He has also incorporated stress reduction techniques (e.g., visual imagery, Wii™ bowling and tennis games, walking, low-cholesterol recipe adaptation for baking) into his daily routine.

However, he has not initiated any sexual activity with his wife since his MI. His wife reports, "He doesn't seem to be interested, and I don't press him for sex. I am just glad that he's okay. He's my best friend, and I don't want to lose him."

(Continued)

Case Example 6.1. Ben: MI *(cont.)*

About sex, Ben reports, "I'm afraid that I either won't be able to have sex or that I'll have another heart attack if I do have sex with my wife. I'm also not sure if I can, you know, get an erection. That bothers me. I never had a problem before, but I don't know about now."

Ben is symptom-free at this point and has recently brought up the topic of ED with his therapist but not with his physician. He is unclear about bringing up the topic of sexual activity with his doctor, and he has begun to address this subject in a limited manner with the occupational therapist.

Questions to Consider

1. Is Ben likely to have another MI if he engages in sexual activity? If so, why? If not, why not?

2. What type of caregiving style are both Ben and his wife adopting?

3. In what ways would an activity configuration assist Ben with sexual activity engagement? Remember that he is working and exercising.

4. What types of energy conservation techniques might allow Ben to develop an energy reserve?

5. Provide 2 ideas for stress reduction techniques that would be beneficial to Ben.

6. How would you recommend that Ben bring up the subject of resuming sexual activity engagement with his physician?

7. Because intimacy is more than engaging in sexual activity, how can Ben retain intimacy? Or, are Ben and his wife retaining a level of intimacy in their relationship?

8. How could you explain the concept of METs to Ben as a means of assuaging his concern about resuming sexual activity?

References

American Heart Association. (2010a). *Diseases and condition that put your heart at risk*. Retrieved May 28, 2010, from http://www.americanheart.org/presenter.jhtml?identifier=1200002

American Heart Association. (2010b). *Sexual activity declines for heart attack patients not getting doctors' advice, study finds*. Retrieved May 28, 2011, from http://www.sciencedaily.com/releases/2010/05/100521092424.htm

American Heart Association. (2011). *Heart disease and stroke statistics 2011 update: A report from the American Heart Association.* Retrieved June 29, 2011, from http://circ.ahajournals.org/cgi/reprint/CIR.0b013e3182009701

American Institute of Stress. (n.d.). *Stress and heart disease.* Retrieved June 29, 2011, from http://www.stress.org/topic-heart.htm?AIS=999f4996782edda398f6aa87f29344a0

Annon, J. (1976). The PLISSIT model: A proposed conceptual scheme for the behavioral treatment of sexual problems. *Journal of Sex Education Therapy, 2,* 1–15.

Araujo, A. B., Travison, T. G., Ganz, P., Chiu, G. R., Kupelian, V., Rosen, R. C., et al. (2009). Erectile dysfunction and mortality. *Journal of Sex Medicine, 6*(9), 2445–2454.

Bankhead, C. (2009). ED linked with 43% higher risk of CVD-related death. *Urology Times, 37*(12), 18.

Block, B. (Producer), & Meyers, N. (Writer/Director). (2003). *Something's gotta give* [Motion picture]. United States: Columbia Pictures & Warner Brothers Pictures.

Bohlen, J., Held, J., Sanderson, O., & Patterson, R. (1984). Heart rate, rate-pressure product, and oxygen uptake during four sexual activities. *Archives of Internal Medicine, 144,* 1745–1748.

Canadian Association of Occupational Therapists. (2012). *Energy for everyday living.* Retrieved April 2, 2012, from http://caot.ca/default.asp?pageid=3689

Care to Act North Carolina. (2011). *Types of cardiovascular disease.* Retrieved June 14, 2011, from http://caretoactnc.com/CardiovascularTypes.assx

Centers for Disease Control and Prevention. (2006). *America's heart disease burden.* Retrieved May 19, 2010, from http://www.cdc.gov/heartdisease/facts.htm

Centers for Disease Control and Prevention. (2010). *Coronary artery disease.* Retrieved June 1, 2010, from http://www.cdc.gov/heartdisease/coronary_ad.htm

DeBusk, R., Drory, Y., Goldstein, I., Jackson, G., Kaul, S., Kimmel, S., et al. (2000). Management of sexual dysfunction in patients with cardiovascular disease: Recommendations of The Princeton Consensus Panel. *American Journal of Cardiology, 86*(2), 175–181.

Emory University. (2011). *TRIUMPH registry.* Retrieved June 13, 2011, from http://www.medicine.emory.edu/divisions/cardiology/_epicore/research/registries/triumph.cfm

French, J. R. P., Rodgers, W., & Cobb, S. (1974). Adjustment as person–environment fit. In G. V. Coelho, D. A. Hamburg, & J. E. Adams (Eds.), *Coping and adaption* (pp. 316–333). New York: Basic Books.

Garcia-Barreto, D., Sin-Chen, C., Rivas-Estany, E., Nieto, R., & Hemondez-Catiero, A. (1986). Sexual intercourse in patients who have had a myocardial infarction. *Journal of Cardiopulmonary Rehabilitation, 6,* 324–328.

Hattjar, B., Parker, J. A., & Lappa, C. L. (2008). Addressing sexuality with adult clients with chronic disabilities: Occupational therapy's role. *OT Practice, 13*(11), CE1–CE8.

Jackson, G. (1981). Sexual intercourse and angina pectoris. *International Rehabilitative Medicine, 3*, 35–37.

Jackson, G. (2009). Sexual response in cardiovascular disease. *Journal of Sex Research, 46*(2/3), 233–236.

Katz, A. (2007). Sexuality and myocardial infarction: *American Journal of Nursing, 107*(3), 49–52.

Katz, A. (2009). *Sex after heart attack.* Retrieved September 2, 2010, from http://www.health4women.org/e/sex_after_heart_attack_159

Latham, C. (2008). Occupation as therapy: Selection, gradation, analysis, and adaptation. In M. Radomski & C. Latham (Eds.), *Occupational therapy for physical dysfunction* (6th ed., pp. 358–381). Philadelphia: Wolters Kluwer/Lippincott Williams & Wilkins.

Magnan, M., & Reynolds, K. (2006). Barriers to addressing patient sexuality concerns across five areas of specialization. *Clinical Nurse Specialist, 20*(6), 285–292.

National Heart, Lung, and Blood Institute. (2011). *What causes palpitations?* Retrieved June 28, 2011, from http://www.nhlbi.nih.gov/health-topics/hpl/causes.html

Nemec, E., Mansfield, L., & Kennedy, J. (1964). Heart rate and blood pressure responses during sexual activity in normal males. *American Heart Journal, 92*, 274–277.

Russell, S., Khandheria, B., & Nehra, A. (2004). Erectile dysfunction and cardiovascular disease. *Mayo Clinic Proceedings, 79*, 782–794.

Sainz, I., Amaya, J., & Garcia, M. (2004). Erectile dysfunction in heart disease patients. *International Journal of Impotence Research, 16*, S13–S17.

Smith, M., Segal, R., & Segal, J. (2011). *Understanding stress: Symptoms, signs, causes, and effects.* Retrieved June 13, 2011, from http://www.helpguide.org/mental/stress_signs.htm

Thompson, I., Tangen, C., Goodman, P., Probstfield, J., Moinpour, C., & Coltman, C. (2005). Erectile dysfunction and subsequent cardiovascular disease. *JAMA, 294*(23), 2996–3002.

Vilchinsky, N., Haze-Filderman, L., Leibowitz, M., Reges, O., Khaskia, A., & Mosseri, M., (2010). Spousal support and cardiac patients' distress: The moderating role of attachment orientation. *Journal of Family Psychology, 24*(4), 508–512.

Appendix 6.A. Activity Configuration Chart

Indicate each activity as L = leisure time; W = work as compensated, volunteer, child care, housework; ADLs = dressing, bathing grooming or hygiene, sexual activity, instrumental activities of daily living (including shopping, finances, driving); R = rest, naps, sleep time, relaxation time.

Date Time	Sunday	Monday	Tuesday	Wednesday	Thursday	Friday	Saturday
Midnight–1:00 a.m.							
1:00–2:00							
2:00–3:00							
3:00–4:00							
4:00–5:00							
5:00–6:00							
6:00–7:00							
7:00–8:00							
8:00–9:00							
9:00–10:00							
10:00–11:00							
11:00–Noon							
Noon–1:00 p.m.							
1:00–2:00							
2:00–3:00							
3:00–4:00							
4:00–5:00							
5:00–6:00							
6:00–7:00							
7:00–8:00							
8:00–9:00							
9:00–10:00							
10:00–11:00							
11:00–midnight							

Note. Courtesy of Bernadette Hattjar. Used with permission.

7

Traumatic Brain Injury and Sexuality

Vicki Pritchard, OTR/L; Tammy L. Kordes, PhD; and
Ashley Hofmann, MA

Key Terms and Concepts

- Erectile dysfunction

- Hypersexuality

- Hyposexuality

- Ranchos Los Amigos Scale of Cognitive Functioning

- Sexually inappropriate behaviors

- Socially appropriate interactions

- Target behaviors

- Traumatic brain injury

- Vaginismus.

Upon completion of this chapter, readers will be able to

- Recognize common symptoms associated with traumatic brain injury;

- Identify modalities that decrease symptoms of traumatic brain injuries;

- Select appropriate screen or assessment tools to enhance treatment planning, client satisfaction, and outcomes for goal development; and

- Develop appropriate treatment interventions on the basis of evaluation results.

Introduction

The Brain Injury Association of America (2011) defined a *traumatic brain injury (TBI)* as the disruption of cerebral functioning because of a blow to the head. Such injuries can result in physical, cognitive, and behavioral alterations. People with TBI might experience short-term memory loss, have difficulty concentrating, become easily disoriented, experience headaches or migraines, have slurred speech, experience seizures, become depressed or easily agitated, and experience increased anxiety or impulsive behaviors (American Occupational Therapy Association [AOTA], 2002).

TBI can also affect sexual response and sexuality (Aloni & Katz, 1999; Blanchard et al., 2003; Langevin, 2006; Ponsford, 2003; Simpson, McCann, & Lowy, 2003), and occupational therapy practitioners should be sensitized to the potential impact of TBI on intimacy and prepared to integrate sexual issues into rehabilitation (Gill, Sander, Robins, Mazzei, & Struchen, 2011). However, sexuality is typically an uncomfortable topic of discussion for clients, family members, and clinicians (Hattjar, Parker, & Lappa, 2008). It does not often elicit much attention during the rehabilitation process, unless seen as a barrier to treatment, such as a client's inappropriate sexual behavior toward the practitioner. At this point, sexuality and sexual behavior might be treated in a haphazard manner that inadvertently reinforces negative behavior.

Despite its lack of attention, sexual activity is a domain of occupational therapy and considered to an activity of daily living (ADL; AOTA, 2008). Clients who have sustained a TBI often have physical and cognitive challenges that require occupational therapy. Because of the wide range of impairments and severities, occupational therapy practitioners who work with this population "utilize every intervention strategy learned in their educational preparation—biomechanical, neurological, and psychosocial, often combining restorative and compensatory intervention approaches to address clients' valued activities and occupations" (Golisz, 2009, p. 10). Occupational therapy practitioners working with clients who have sustained a TBI can address sexuality for those clients who desire to participate in sexual activity.

Demographics

The incidence of TBI in the United States is staggering. The Centers for Disease Control and Prevention (CDC; 2010) estimates that approximately 1.7 million people sustain a TBI of varying degrees each year. More than 124,000 individuals are estimated to have long-lasting effects with some degree of permanent disability (CDC, 2011).

According to the CDC (2010), children ages 0–4 years, older adolescents ages 15–19 years, and adults ages 65 years or older comprise the groups most likely to sustain a TBI, and among all groups, males have a higher incidence of TBI. Leading causes of TBI include falls (35.2%), motor-vehicle accidents (17.3%), the head striking or being struck against (16.5%), assault (10%), and unknown or other causes (21%).

A meta-analysis on the incidence of TBI by Bruns and Hauser (2003) found that the highest occurrence of TBI is during teenage and young adult years. Although the risk seems to decrease through middle adulthood, it elevates quite dramatically in the elderly population because of the increased incidence of falls.

Veterans With TBIs

Another source of many TBIs has occurred in veterans returning from Operation Enduring Freedom (OEF) and Operation Iraqi Freedom (OIF). Approximately 20% of OEF/OIF veterans are estimated to have sustained a TBI (Corby-Edwards, 2009). Blast injury is the most common cause of war injury (Warden, 2006), but unlike blows to the head that might occur in an accident or sport, blast injuries emit energy waves that add a unique dimension to these types of TBIs (Alvarez, 2008). Little research has focused on blast TBIs, so in 2005 the Pentagon opened the Defense Centers of Excellence for Psychological Health and Traumatic Brain Injury, a clearinghouse for treatment, education, prevention, and research (Alvarez, 2008; Capehart & Bass, 2011).

Symptoms of posttraumatic stress disorder (PTSD) can overlap with those of TBI (U.S. Department of Veterans Affairs [VA], 2011). With an estimated 19% of returning veterans reporting signs of PTSD (AOTA, 2009; Tanielian & Jaycox, 2008), TBI rehabilitation coinciding with the psychological effects of PTSD is very real. Occupational therapy practitioners must take into consideration physical, cognitive, and psychosocial effects of veterans' combat-related PTSD to promote their health, participation, and well-being in military and family life (AOTA, 2009). Like TBI, PTSD can significantly affect sexuality among returning veterans (Cameron et al., 2011).

In 2006, the U.S. Army Surgeon General established the Traumatic Brain Injury Task Force to assess the current state of treatment for soldiers who receive a head injury ranging from a mild concussion to severe trauma. The task force found that soldiers who were wounded by blast injuries often did not show the external signs of a brain injury; therefore, they were not being identified as needing treatment (Corby-Edwards, 2009). Soldiers themselves might neglect mentioning difficulties, desiring to reconnect with family and friends and re-enter normal community life (Hofmann, 2008). However, with TBI being referred to as the "signature injury" of the war in Iraq (Abreu & Yancy, 2011, p. 380; Alvarez, 2008, p. A1), and complaints from soldiers and their advocates concerned by lack of recognition for complications resulting from TBIs, it is crucial for occupational therapy practitioners and other health care providers to accurately evaluate and address TBIs.

Classifying TBIs

The human brain is very fragile yet amazingly resilient, and is the most complex organ in the body (Figure 7.1). As a result, injury to the brain can result in a complex, wide range of symptoms and impairments. TBIs are classified as either *closed-penetrating* or *open-penetrating*, depending on whether the skull and brain matter are breached (Golisz, 2009). A closed-penetrating TBI occurs when the brain rapidly oscillates within the skull, perhaps with bruised or torn brain tissue or blood vessels. Falls, battlefield blasts, and motor-vehicle accidents typically cause this sort of TBI (Golisz, 2009). Open-penetrating injuries occur when there is direct continuity between scalp and brain tissue, in which the dura matter is torn and the brain substance is exposed (Golisz, 2009; Griffith & Lemberg, 1993).

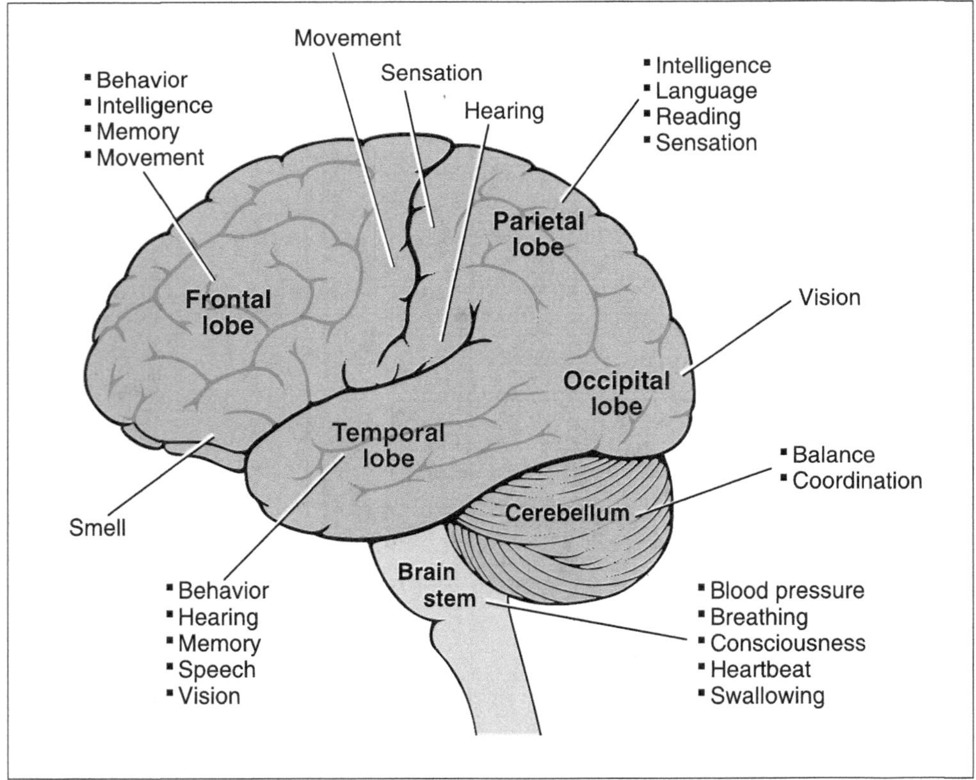

Figure 7.1. Functions of the major lobes of the brain.

Note. Copyright © 2011, by Richard Fritzler, Medical Illustrator, Roswell, GA. Used under license.

TBIs are also classified as primary or secondary, depending on whether the injury occurred at the time of the traumatic event or from secondary brain occurrences because of the initial neural injury (e.g., edema, anoxia, brain herniation). Depending on which areas of the brain sustain damage, persons with a TBI can present with ataxia; incoordination; apraxia; impairments in attention, memory, perception, and executive functioning; disinhibition; impulsivity; and emotional lability (Golisz, 2009).

Sexuality and TBI

Persons who have sustained a TBI have significantly higher reports of reduced sex drive, frequency of engaging in sexual activities, ability to give their partners sexual satisfaction, ability to perform sexual intercourse, ability to achieve orgasm, and enjoyment of sexual activity (Aloni & Katz, 2003; Katz & Aloni, 1999; Ponsford, 2003). TBI is also correlated with premature ejaculation (Simpson et al., 2003), impotence (Cohen, 2003), inappropriate sexual behavior (e.g., pedophilia, sexual offenses; Blanchard et al., 2003; Langevin, 2006), and hyposexuality and hypersexuality (Bianchi-Demicheli, Rollini, Lovblad, & Ortigue, 2010).

TBI can also significantly affect many important but perhaps less overt aspects of sexuality, such as social and relationship skills, self-esteem, and behavioral control (Katz & Aloni, 1999). The causes and effects of sexual functioning after TBI are highly confusing, and current literature does little to clarify it (see Exhibit 7.1; Aloni & Katz, 1999, 2003).

Physical Challenges

It is difficult to identify the physical causes that affect sexuality after TBI, as varying cultural, educational, psychological, anatomical, and physiological factors comprise human sexuality. A change to any of these can affect sexual behavior, and it is not always clear if damage to the brain directly causes a change in sexuality, or if the change is secondary (Cohen, 2003). For example, a study by Katz and Aloni (1999) found the greatest concern for single clients with a TBI was inappropriate social behavior, while married clients reported impotence as their greatest concern. Age, experience, and situational aspects among study participants varied, and the study illustrates how interconnected the factors of sexual life are and how challenging it is to separate out one aspect for cause and effect.

Pinpointing which anatomical areas of the neural systems are responsible for sexual response and functioning is difficult, but some patterns and conclusions can be made. Damage to the frontal lobes is a critical component to sexual behavior, as this area regulates the expression of cognitive

---

Exhibit 7.1. The Brain and Behavior: Current Understandings

The field of cognitive neuropsychology focuses on the functional consequences of disease and injury to the brain. Theories are rapidly evolving, but there is agreement that

- The brain has highly specialized areas of function for memory, reasoning, sensation, motor control, and emotion; thus, injuries exhibit unique characteristics depending on the areas of the brain affected.
- Multiple sensory pathways can be used to process information, so a lesion in one area can influence one function but not another.
- Human behavior is influenced not only by cognition but also by emotional (affective) and motivational states. These are influenced by environmental changes.
- Although tremendous advances are being made in neuroimaging, the complexity of the brain and the lack of valid predictive models do not yet permit reliable and precise mapping of functional cognition.
- Executive dysfunction after brain damage may be associated with decreased instrumental activities of daily living such as bathing, money management, community integration, and social skills.
- Brain functions extend beyond learning and memory and are necessary for producing the cortisol response to psychosocial stress.

Note. From "Everyday Living for Individuals With Cognitive Deficits After Alzheimer's Dementia and Traumatic Brain Injury," by B. C. Abreu and S. M. Yancy, 2011, *Ways of Living: Intervention Strategies to Enable Participation,* edited by C. H. Christiansen and K. M. Matuska, p. 381. Copyright © 2011, by the American Occupational Therapy Association. Reprinted with permission.

---

processes. The frontal lobes are particularly vulnerable to injury during head trauma and are seen as guiding impulse controls (Lezak, 2004). Damage to the frontal lobes is highly correlated with hypersexuality, exhibitionism, and impaired judgment and self-control (Olson, Plotzker, & Ezzat, 2007).

The brainstem contains many neurological centers and pathways important to sexuality; it is connected to the peripheral nervous system (PNS), the limbic system, and the hypothalamus and thalamus. All injuries to the brain stem could potentially affect sexuality (Cohen, 2003). The hypothalamus and pituitary are closely related, as the hypothalamus influences the release of hormones and the pituitary. The sensory, autonomic, and motor neurons of the PNS form the nerves of the genitalia.

Motor and praxis challenges related to sexual activity after TBI can affect posture, positioning, rhythmical movements, gentle or controlled touch, balance, use of upper limbs to hold, undressing, and use of contraceptives (Cohen, 2003; Griffith & Lemberg, 1993). Sensory challenges might include changes in perception of sensation (e.g., touch, pressure, pain, temperature) and visual, auditory, taste, and olfactory stimuli. Persons with a TBI might have difficulty processing such information within a sexual context (Cohen, 2003; Griffith & Lemberg, 1993).

Some sexual dysfunction in clients who have sustained a TBI can be attributed to medications. Some anticonvulsive drugs to prevent seizures (a common complication after TBI) can lead to impotence and decreased libido (Cohen, 2003). However, some common medications often used with clients who have sustained a TBI (e.g., anti-Parkinsonian drugs) are suggested to improve libido and erectile dysfunction (ED).

Cognitive Challenges

The impact of cognitive deficits after a TBI can be far reaching and can certainly affect sexual behavior (Aloni & Katz, 2003; Griffith & Lemberg, 1993). Memory impairments are the most common issue that occupational therapy practitioners see in TBI populations (Golisz, 2009). Changes in attention, concentration, planning ability, and abstract thinking can affect how well a client might recognize normal boundaries and lead to inappropriate sexual behavior (Aloni & Katz, 2003).

The Rancho Los Amigos Cognitive Scale (Hagen, 1998) is often used to describe cognitive and behavioral functioning (Golisz, 2009). Appendix 7.A describes each level in detail. Typically, sexually inappropriate behaviors begin at Level IV (confused/agitated), which might include exposure, fondling, self-stimulation, and the use of inappropriate language (Griffith & Lemberg, 1993). These behaviors might decrease during Level V (confused/inappropriate/nonagitated), and at Level VI they might disappear altogether as the client becomes more aware.

At cognitive levels in which the client can independently function to varying degrees (Level VII and above), those who have sustained a TBI may still have impaired judgment and abstract reasoning skills (Griffith & Lemberg, 1993; Katz & Aloni, 1999). Cognitive capacity in general may be limited, which could lead clients with a TBI to initiate inappropriate behaviors or become easy targets for designing individuals (Katz & Aloni, 1999).

TBIs can cause vision impairment by changing how visual information is relayed to the brain centers for processing as well as how the brain processes visual input (Warren, 2011). This can lead to misdirected reactions and movements as well as increased safety risk.

Finally, aphasia or dysphagia can occur after a TBI, especially in clients with damage to the dominant brain hemisphere. Such language and communication disorders can generate frustration that interferes with sexual desire (Cohen, 2003).

Emotional–Behavioral Challenges

Many factors are involved in the etiology of behavioral disturbance. They might include intellectual and cognitive changes (e.g., amnesia, agnosia, apraxia, aphasia, apathy), neurotransmitter dysfunction (e.g., dopamine, serotonin, cholinergic, adrenergic, GABA), and instinctual behaviors under stress (e.g., territoriality, defensiveness; Lezak, 2004).

In short, "the brain controls and mediates human emotions and is therefore the organ that regulates sexual function and behavior" (Aloni & Katz, 2003, p. 23). Sexual relationships (e.g., married couples) are highly vulnerable to the emotional aspects following a TBI, as changes in personality and roles can lead to lack of self-esteem and confidence and increased frustration, anxiety, depression, and communication difficulties (Aloni & Katz, 2003; Ponsford, 2003). However, it is important to note that such changes might be secondary to the TBI, not a direct result of it.

A problematic behavioral change involving challenges with sexual response after TBI might include *hyposexuality,* which presents as a significant decrease or total lack of sexual desire, or *hypersexuality,* which is significant increase in sexual preoccupation and sexually driven behaviors (Kaplan & Krueger, 2010).

The temporal poles are believed to be involved in socioemotional regulation, and injury to this area can result in hyposexuality (Olson et al., 2007). Miller, Cummings, McIntyre, Ebers, and Grode (1986) reported that it was difficult to pinpoint specific neuroanatomical structures involved in hyposexuality but found that lesions in the hypothalamus often resulted in decreased sexual desire.

Hyposexuality has long been associated with individuals who have temporal-lobe epilepsy or temporal lobectomies to control a seizure disorder

(Blumer & Walker, 1967; Morrell, 1991). The temporal lobes contain the emotional regulating structures of the limbic system, including the hippocampus and the amygdala. Injuries that involve these structures can cause changes in behavior and personality (McGee, 2004). Individuals who experience hyposexuality typically do not enjoy intimate contact with their partners, including touching, caressing, kissing, or intercourse, and the impact on relationships can feel devastating. Clients in a committed relationship might wonder, "What is wrong with me?" The client's partner might also entertain that question, not understanding the change in his or her loved one who was previously more sexually attracted to him or her. This lack of understanding of how the brain injury can affect sexual desire should be a focus of rehabilitative care and education.

In contrast to hyposexuality, individuals whose brain injuries have led to hypersexuality often demonstrate impulsive (and sometimes planned) acts of inappropriate touching of caregivers or strangers, socially and sexually inappropriate comments, and an increased need for sexual gratification (Eghwrudjakpor & Essien, 2008; Kaplan & Krueger, 2010). Persons with hypersexuality might experience a new or enhanced preoccupation with pornography, compulsive self-stimulation, phone sex, cybersex, and strip clubs (Kaplan & Krueger, 2010).

Although these behaviors significantly affect spousal relationships, other behaviors connected to hypersexuality (e.g., verbal dysinhibition, inappropriate touching, impulsivity) can also have a far-reaching impact on social and vocational situations. For example, an individual might publicly stare at a woman's breasts while her boyfriend notices, which could lead to a dangerous confrontation, or a female client could endanger herself by making inappropriate comments during a social event to a male she does not know. From a vocational perspective, an individual with hypersexuality secondary to TBI is particularly vulnerable to sexual harassment charges by superiors or coworkers.

The rather shocking nature of hypersexuality has garnered a greater level of attention by caregivers, medical staff, and occupational therapy practitioners, but it is actually less common than hyposexuality in patients with TBI (Kreutzer & Zasler, 1989).

Assessment

As part of a client's occupational therapy evaluation, two assessments that give good insight into the client's challenges regarding sexuality include the Canadian Occupational Performance Measure (COPM; Law et al., 1998) and the Beck Depression Inventory, 2nd Edition (BDI–II; Beck, Steer, & Brown, 1996).

The COPM (Law et al., 1998) is designed to detect change in a client's self-perception and is a first step in addressing occupational performance areas. The BDI–II (Beck et al., 1996), a 21-item self-report measure of depression, has been found useful in identifying symptoms of depression in the early stages following TBI (Rowland, Lam, & Leahy, 2005), and depression is correlated with decreased sexual activity (Shabsigh, Zakaria, Anastasiadis, & Seidman, 2001). However, this type (i.e., self-report) of assessment might not produce a valid result because of the tendency for lack of self-awareness as a prevalent problem in brain injury.

Caregiver evaluation should be incorporated to fully understand the impact of injury on the client's life and is vital to accurate, successful intervention. Clients might demonstrate impaired awareness of deficits or be unable to cognitively understand assessment measures. Caregiver report will offer valuable insight into the clients' performance and adjustment related to sexuality.

Occupational Therapy Intervention

Occupational therapy practitioners addressing sexuality with clients do so within the context of a multifaceted, holistic approach to rehabilitation that includes physical, cognitive, and emotional–behavioral concerns. It is beyond the scope of this chapter to detail every possible approach in working with adults with a TBI, so the space devoted to each intervention is relatively small. The main thing for practitioners to remember is that sexuality should be addressed in a way that takes into account the complex interactions that can affect sexuality. Deficits in physical, cognitive, and emotional–behavioral areas can occur alone or together, but all can significantly affect a client's recovery.

Physical Interventions

Physical areas that might affect sexual activity include muscle tone and range of motion (ROM), sensation, coordination, balance, mobility, and presence of pain. These areas should be observed as they relate to the performance of ADLs. ROM exercises can increase mobility. Depending on a client's sensory evaluation, he or she might be a candidate for sensory and perceptual retraining with short-term, achievable goals that increase function despite the loss of sensation (Cooper & Abrams, 2006; Griffith & Lemberg, 1993).

For pain during sexual activity (e.g., muscular pain), possible interventions include alternative positioning (Figures A.1, A.2, and A.7 in Appendix A might be particularly more comfortable). Gentle stretching, application of heat, and pain medication prior to sexual activity might also be helpful. It is unlikely for painful intercourse to be directly caused by a TBI, but psychological factors related to the injury can certainly lead to physical pain (Griffith & Lemberg, 1993). Typically, adequate lubrication with a water- or silicone-based lubrication can address this issue. *Vaginismus,* a muscular constriction of the vagina, can make penetration by the penis difficult or very painful. In this case, the use of dilators can gradually desensitize the area.

ED can often be treated pharmacologically—either by changing current medications that cause ED or by the administration of medications intended to treat erectile issues. (Consult a physician.) In the case of premature ejaculation, applying a topical anesthetic can help (Simpson et al., 2003).

For those with hyposexuality, a physician can help determine if medications are contributing to loss of desire and possibly adjust them. A physician can also explore pharmaceutical and hormonal options with the client.

Cognitive Interventions

Cognitive evaluation should include areas of memory, problem solving, processing, communication, and judgment. Visual–perceptual deficits may also be present, such as visual field deficits, figure–ground perception, position in space, and diplopia. As with all other treatment interventions, observation of client performance of cognitive skills is the best method for determination of approach.

For memory deficits that interfere with sexuality, clients can use a ledger or audio recorder to track occurrences of sexual activity as well as a checklist of preparation activities (e.g., contraception, medications). Personal digital assistants or smart phones have particularly great potential to help individuals be more independent, as they can store and track limitless information.

Vision and perception can also affect sexuality, as the client might lack awareness around parts of his or her body or field of vision. It is common to incorrectly attribute changes in vision to changes in cognition in individuals who have sustained a TBI, causing vision difficulties to go undetected (Warren, 2011). Interventions aimed at compensating for visual–perceptual deficits are typically preferable to the intensive rehabilitation that restoring hemianopic visual field requires (Warren, 2011). Occupational therapy intervention for low vision would address compensation, adaptation, and other strategies for function, and those strategies can be applied to situations involving sexual activity. Educating the client is key, as he or she must learn—and believe—that he or she cannot trust the blind side's visual input. Next, to stay safe during sexual activities, clients must learn to quickly turn their heads and entirely search the blind area automatically when moving or changing positions.

Behavioral and Psychosocial Interventions

Professionals working with people who have sustained a TBI most often address sexuality through a behavioral approach (Katz & Aloni, 1999). Any behavior plan must be developed with special consideration for the patient's cognitive, emotional, and behavioral strengths and weaknesses as well as his or her presentation. Behavioral problems can be acute (sudden behavioral challenges) or chronic (persistent behavioral challenges) and often add to the burden of caring for a patient with a TBI. In addition, these challenges often lead to placement in a long-term-care facility (Neurologic Rehabilitation Institute at Brookhaven Hospital, 2011).

Inexperience

Many TBIs occur when individuals are teens or young adults, and they may have had limited experience with dating or sex prior to their injury. Depending on the nature of the TBI, this inexperience may be compounded by a decreased ability to read the emotional and social cues of others (Ylvisaker, Turkstra, & Coelho, 2005). In these instances, social skills training and role-playing can be useful. Clients might practice the following skills:

- How to appropriately converse with someone he or she is interested in
- How to invite someone on a date
- How to plan for and go on a date.

Additionally, the occupational therapist might facilitate opportunities for younger clients to practice basic social skills with their peers in natural environments.

Sexually inappropriate behaviors

Sexually inappropriate behaviors can be defined as the use of sexually explicit language, sexual advances, or actual touching of others in a sexual manner, as well as self-stimulation in public areas. In contrast, *socially appropriate interactions* are the absence of the above-stated target behaviors and the exhibiting of behaviors in keeping with age-appropriate standards.

Hypersexuality, for example, can be quite disruptive to the therapeutic environment and potentially dangerous. Clear and concise behavioral strategies are needed. A behavior plan must be established that takes into account the client's level of cognition (e.g., ability to learn, recall, awareness, insight into the implications of the behavior), the behavior that is being targeted to extinguish, and the antecedents to that behavior and patient's response to past and current interventions.

For clients recovering from a TBI, the behavioral interventions must be as individualized as any other part of a treatment plan; any attempt to use a "cookie cutter" approach will miss the nuances of the injury and fall short in terms of success. The most important part of any successful behavior plan for clients with TBI is consistency of implementation (Feeney & Ylvisaker, 2011).

Changes in personality and behavior can require multiple interventions and might include both behavioral and pharmacological treatments (Bradford, 2000; Kaplan & Krueger, 2010). Behavioral problems often do not occur in isolation; occupational therapists must consider the entire situation when determining the most effective intervention. When determining what the most effective behavioral intervention may be, consider the following questions to orient yourself to the pattern and nature of the behavior:

- Is the behavior constant, regardless of stimuli?
- Does the behavior typically occur during a specific time of day?
- Does it occur only with caregiving activity?

In general, some basic guidelines can improve outcomes when working with clients recovering from a TBI:

- *Don't wait for a crisis.* Anticipate that sexually related disruptive behavior or social problems might arise because of the TBI. Intervene as early as possible.
- *Avoid change.* Set up and follow routines to compensate for decreased memory or cognitive skills and to provide the client with predictable structure.
- *Don't overstimulate.* Plan and prepare for or around events that might be overstimulating, keep noise to a minimum, allow only one person to speak at a time, and keep questions or conversation basic and direct.
- *Enhance orientation.* Help the client become gradually more aware of other people, environments, situations, and time of day.
- *Augment verbal communication.* Depending on the degree of injury and impairment, use body language, pictures, or communication boards.

- *Avoid changes in the environment.* Keep environments simple, clean, and well organized, and avoid introducing overly stimulating objects, sounds, or people.

- *Expect variability.* Clients with a TBI present with a wide range of symptoms, and even the individual client can behave or progress drastically differently from day to day.

- *Plan and anticipate.* Assist clients ready for sexual activity with planning it, and anticipate possible environmental or emotional barriers.

- *Attend to those behaviors you want increased.* Using approaches such as positive behavioral support or applied behavioral analysis to positively reinforce appropriate behavior.

- *Ignore those behaviors you want extinguished.* Do not encourage disruptive or inappropriate behavior by giving the client attention; doing so might increase his or her desire to continue it.

With hypersexuality, the goal is to decrease behaviors that preclude a successful return to premorbid levels of functioning while simultaneously increasing those that are serving in an adaptive manner. This means the occupational therapy practitioner must increase the client's capacity for appropriate self-control. Use of initial neurobehavioral interventions focus on increasing a patient's self-control while also gathering baseline data to be used for future behavioral interventions. Although establishing this baseline allows the practitioner to evaluate the effectiveness of an intervention, it also raises possible reinforcers for later use. Even the most astute occupational therapy practitioner cannot always predict which interventions will be most successful for different clients, and the knowledge of the meaningfulness of behavioral reinforcers comes with time spent with clients and their loved ones. For example, a practitioner should learn what activities, foods, objects, and so on are meaningful to the client, who perhaps previously enjoyed watching television. The practitioner might use television time as a reinforcer but discover that, following TBI, the patient no longer enjoys watching television and finds it overwhelming. The practitioner would then change the chosen reinforcement.

Determine *target behaviors,* which are those behaviors identified as problematic and "targeted" for change. Possibilities might include public self-stimulation, exposure, or explicit language. From a neurobehavioral perspective, it is important to operationally define the target behaviors (e.g., "John exposes himself during treatment sessions"). Different disciplines work with each client; therefore, a consistent definition of the target behavior reduces the likelihood of another health care professional inadvertently reinforcing a problem behavior.

When a sexually inappropriate behavior occurs, the clinician should ask himself or herself:

- Was the comment or touch sexual in nature?

- Was the comment or touch unwelcome?

- Was the comment or touch uninvited?

Sometimes, sexually inappropriate behaviors are used to garner attention are intended to shock, elicit sympathy, annoy, gain attention, or interrupt others. Usually, the best intervention for these types of behaviors is simply to ignore the behavior, as evidence shows that overtly reacting to the target behavior increases its frequency (Fyffe, Kahng, Fittro, & Russel, 2004). When the behavior occurs, immediately cease all interaction and ignore the patient until either of the following criteria is met:

- Interaction will resume following 5 consecutive seconds of silence.

- Interaction will resume immediately upon his or her resumption of normal speaking volume or appropriate comments or behaviors without the 5-second delay.

- While implementing this procedure, be sure to avoid eye contact.

Next, change the topic or distract the client. Debating behaviors or situations with an individual recovering from a TBI is typically futile. Avoid scolding, criticizing, or punishing. After all, even the most behaviorally disturbed client who has sustained a TBI is still human and should be treated in a way that maintains maximum privacy and personal dignity.

In the absence of sexually inappropriate behaviors, provide age-appropriate praise whenever the client exhibits socially acceptable behavior (e.g., conversation, quiet behavior). For example, the practitioner might say to a client, "It's so nice talking to you about football. I love football!"

The following guidelines can help ensure that occupational therapy practitioners conduct themselves in a way that best supports their intervention efforts:

- Always model appropriate behavior when in the presence of a client who has sustained a TBI.

- Be consistent, with timely follow-through.

- Do not discuss personal issues with the client.

- Present a cohesive and united front (among therapists, other professionals, family members) when providing treatment and during general social interactions.
- Never debate care issues or behavioral interventions with colleagues or family members in the presence of clients.

Keep in mind that memory deficits are very common in patients recovering from a TBI (AOTA, 2002; Golisz, 2009). A client's ability to recall an episode of frank behavioral dyscontrol or even simple social misjudgment an hour or more later might be questionable. Therefore, this question arises: If the client cannot recall an event after a period of time, how does he or she learn from a behavioral intervention? It takes time to change behavior and consistent interventions are the key. For the patient with a brain injury, consistency breeds predictability.

Finally, inform family members and caregivers (who might be extremely appalled or embarrassed by their loved one's sexually inappropriate behavior) that such behaviors are common after a TBI and will most likely decrease over time (Bezeau, Bogod, & Mateer, 2004).

Relationships

Clients with TBI must be able to negotiate their communities without sexually offending others or finding themselves in dangerous situations. Relationships are a key component of community integration (Fleming & Nalder, 2011). For people who have sustained a TBI, loss of role and social isolation are often results of unsuccessful attempts at community reintegration. Unfortunately, impairments in social skills might become evident only after discharge (Golisz, 2009).

Evidence shows that those clients who maintain meaningful relationships report better quality of life (Dijkers, 2004), and this can certainly include the sexual aspect of such relationships. Goal setting, role-playing, and videotaping social interactions can help clients address the social skills needed for the emotional connection between the client and his or her partner.

Hyposexuality in particular will most often need to be addressed within the relationship context. Psychological counseling or sex therapy can help couples determine what they want in a sexual relationship and to adapt any limitations the TBI may have caused.

Education

Education is a primary part of occupational therapy intervention, and it might include sex education concerning TBI, caregiver education, and contraception.

Sex education

Health care professionals generally agree that providing information to clients that explains the emotional, behavioral, and physical impairments that can result from a TBI, as discussed earlier in this chapter, reduces clients' anxiety, feelings of guilt, rejection by partners, and shame on the part of both the client and partner (Katz & Aloni, 1999). Candidly discussing these issues with clients and their partners might prevent extremely negative reactions to perceived sexual failures and the connected loss of self-esteem or self-confidence, all of which could result in further sex-related issues.

Caregiver education

During the provision of therapeutic and educational services, clinicians should strive to enhance empathy for patients while increasing a caregiver's tolerance for maladaptive behaviors. Occupational therapy practitioners can assist both clients and caregivers in establishing more realistic expectations and preparing for the future, including the following steps:

- Inform family members of typical sequelae of TBIs.

- Encourage caregivers to take care of themselves rather than neglect self-care, proper nutrition, exercise, and respites.

- Keep realistic expectations, and be prepared for irritability, apathy, and disorganization.

- Arrange for education and support. Brain injury support groups provide clients and their families with ongoing support, education, and real world problem-solving assistance (Golisz, 2009; VA, 2010).

Particularly in situations in which a spouse is the primary caregiver, changing from a partner to a more parental role can be extraordinarily stressful and significantly affect sexual intimacy (VA, 2010). Explaining to caregiving spouses or partners that decreased libido or personality changes are a result of the TBI, not anything the spouse or partner has or has not done, can greatly reduce their guilt and anxiety. In some cases, referral to marital or couples counseling is appropriate, if the client with a TBI has the cognitive functioning to gain from it (VA, 2010).

Contraception

It is critical for persons who have sustained a TBI and their partners to be thoroughly educated on protecting themselves from sexually transmitted diseases (STDs) and pregnancy. Options differ depending on the client's circumstances, and a physician should be consulted.

For women with a TBI, oral contraception (i.e., the pill), is not recommended, as it requires the client to remember to take it each day. Additionally, the hormones it contains could react with other medications or conditions related to the TBI that the client is currently experiencing. Intrauterine devices (IUDs) are a good option for women who are in monogamous relationships, especially if they already have a child (as the uterus has already amply stretched). A physician installs the IUD into the woman's uterus, and depending on the brand the client selects, it will prevent pregnancy for 5–7 years. It does not protect against STDs.

Condoms, cervical caps, and diaphragms prevent pregnancy, but memory deficits and general noncompliance on the part of the client with a TBI require that the client's partner supervise their use (Griffith & Lemberg, 1993). Permanent options, such as tubal ligations (cutting and tying the fallopian tubes) or a vasectomy (cutting and tying the vas derens part of the scrotum), might be considered. However, the client must be involved in all contraception decisions.

Summary

TBIs can affect sexuality in many ways—physically, emotionally, cognitively, and behaviorally. Educating clients and their partners on common TBI sequelae and its affect on sexuality can reduce guilt, anxiety, and frustration; increase patience and empathy; and mange expectations. Through the rehabilitation process and perhaps with adaptation, many clients can resume sexuality activity (see Case Example 7.1).

Case Example 7.1. Chloe: TBI

Chloe is a 34-year-old woman who sustained a severe brain injury as the result of a motor vehicle accident while traveling to work. Rehabilitation focused on remediation of deficits, including right visual field loss, right hemiparesis, impaired cognition, and decreased balance. Prior to her injury, Chloe had been employed as a trauma nurse and was living with her husband and toddler son.

During her recovery, Chloe demonstrated excellent progress and was functionally independent with her own care but continued to experience cognitive difficulties characteristic of a Ranchos Los Amigos Level VI. Her treatment shifted from the traditional hospital-based care and began to incorporate community and family after approximately 2 months.

During occupational therapy, Chloe voiced some anxiety regarding her ability to resume sexual activities with her husband. The occupational therapist shifted focus and informed both Chloe and her husband of the various

---

(Continued)

Case Example 7.1. Chloe: TBI *(cont.)*

ways a TBI could affect sexuality. She suggested that they set small, reachable goals, such as having an honest conversation about their anxieties and hopes for their sex life, a date night without the pressure of sex, kissing, and so on.

The occupational therapist brought up the subject of contraception, and Chloe and her husband indicated that, although they hoped to have another child some day, they did not want to become pregnant for the next couple of years. The occupational therapist informed them of various contraception options, particularly the IUD, as Chloe had cognitive deficits that made remembering to take an oral contraceptive quite risky, was in a monogamous relationship, and did not want a permanent contraceptive solution. The occupational therapist referred Chloe to a physician to further explore contraceptive options.

Chloe continued to rehabilitate, working toward increased muscle tone, strength, and balance. She also learned ways to compensate for her vision impairment. Eventually, Chloe and her husband felt ready for sexual intercourse, and in light of her muscle weaknesses and balance, the occupational therapist suggested they begin with the man-on-top position. The occupational therapist reminded Chloe's husband to remain within her field of vision so she wound not be caught by surprise at any point.

During a follow-up appointment with the occupational therapist, Chloe reported that she had felt very anxious but kept talking to her husband, who continually assured her that she was in control and he would back off at any point, if she wanted him to. They took their time, eventually achieving penetration. Although Chloe did not have an orgasm, she and her husband were surprised at how much they emotionally connected, and they felt they had taken a step to strengthen their relationship.

Questions to Consider

1. What sorts of things did the occupational therapist need to consider when addressing sexuality with Chloe?

2. How did the occupation of sexuality fit into Chloe's life?

3. How did the occupational therapist's caregiver education affect Chloe and her husband's intimacy?

References

Abreu, B. C., & Yancy, S. M. (2011). Everyday living for individuals with cognitive deficits after Alzheimer's disease and traumatic brain injury. In C. H. Christiansen & K. M. Matuska (Eds.), *Ways of living: Intervention strategies to enable participation* (4th ed.; pp. 379–404). Bethesda, MD: AOTA Press.

Aloni, R., & Katz, S. (1999). A review of the effect of traumatic brain injury on the human sexual response. *Brain Injury, 13*(4), 269–280.

Aloni, R., & Katz, S. (2003). *Sexual difficulties after traumatic brain injury and ways to deal with it.* Springfield, IL: Charles C Thomas.

Alvarez, L. (2008, August 26). War veterans' concussions are often overlooked. *The New York Times*, p. A1.

American Occupational Therapy Association. (2002). *Traumatic brain injury: Effects and intervention.* Retrieved October 12, 2011, from http://www.aota.org/Consumers/consumers/Health-and-Wellness/TBI/35199.aspx

American Occupational Therapy Association. (2008). Occupational therapy practice framework: Domain and process (2nd ed.). *American Journal of Occupational Therapy, 62*, 625–683. doi:10.5014/ajot.62.6.625

American Occupational Therapy Association. (2009). AOTA's societal statement on combat-related posttraumatic stress. *American Journal of Occupational Therapy, 63*, 845–846. doi:10.5014/ajot.63.6.845

Beck, A. T., Steer, R. A., & Brown, G. K. (1996). *Beck Depression Inventory* (2nd ed.). San Antonio, TX: Psychological Corporation.

Bezeau, S. C., Bogod, N. M., & Mateer, C. A. (2004). Sexually intrusive behavior following brain injury: Approaches to assessment and rehabilitation. *Brain Injury, 18*(3), 299–313.

Bianchi-Demicheli, F., Rollini, C., Lovblad, K., & Ortigue, S. (2010). "Sleeping Beauty paraphilia": Deviant desire in the context of bodily self-image disturbance in a patient with a fronto-parietal traumatic brain injury. *Medical Science Monitor, 16*, 15–17.

Blanchard, R., Kuban, M. E., Klassen, P., Dickey, R., Christensen, B. K., Cantor, J. M., et al. (2003). Self-reported head injuries before and after age 13 in pedophilic and nonpedophilic men referred for clinical assessment. *Archives of Sexual Behavior, 32*(6), 573–581.

Blumer, D., & Walker, A. E. (1967). Sexual behavior in temporal lobe epilepsy. *Archives of Neurology, 16*(1), 37–43.

Bradford, J. M. W. (2000). The treatment of sexual deviation using a pharmacological approach. *Journal of Sex Research, 37*(3), 248–257.

Brain Injury Association of America. (2011). *About brain injury.* Retrieved May 2, 2011, from http://www.biausa.org/index.htm

Bruns, J., & Hauser, W. A. (2003). The epidemiology of traumatic brain injury: A review. *Epilepsia, 44*(10), 2–10.

Cameron, R. P., Mona, L. R., Syme, M. L., Cordes, C. C., Fraley, S. S., Chen, S. S., et al. (2011). Sexuality among wounded veterans of Operation Enduring Freedom (OEF), Operation Iraqi Freedom (OIF), and Operation New Dawn (OND): Implications for rehabilitation psychologists. *Rehabilitation Psychology, 56*(4), 289–301.

Capehart, B., & Bass, D. (2011). Traumatic brain injury among veterans returning from Afghanistan and Iraq: Strategies for diagnosis and treatment. *Psychiatric Times, 28*(7), e1–e5.

Centers for Disease Control and Prevention. (2010). *Traumatic brain injury in the United States.* Retrieved October 12, 2011, from http://www.cdc.gov/traumaticbraininjury/pdf/blue_book.pdf

Centers for Disease Control and Prevention. (2011). *Traumatic brain injury in the U.S.* Retrieved November 9, 2011, from http://www.cdc.gov/features/dsTBI_BrainInjury/

Cohen, M. (2003). Physical and medical aspects of sexuality after traumatic brain injury. In R. Aloni & S. Katz (Eds.), *Sexual difficulties after traumatic brain injury and ways to deal with it* (pp. 42–54). Springfield, IL: Charles C Thomas.

Cooper, C., & Abrams, M. P. (2006). Evaluation of sensation and intervention for sensory dysfunction. In H. M. Pendleton & W. Schultz-Krohn (Eds.), *Pedretti's occupational therapy: Practice skills for physical dysfunction* (6th ed., pp. 513–531). St. Louis: Elsevier/Mosby.

Corby-Edwards, A. K. (2009). *Traumatic brain injury: Care and treatment of Operation Enduring Freedom and Operation Iraqi Freedom veterans.* Washington, DC: Congressional Research Service.

Dijkers, M. P. (2004). Quality of life after traumatic brain injury: A review of research approaches and findings. *Archives of Physical Medicine and Rehabilitation, 85*(Suppl. 2), S21–S35.

Eghwrudjakpor, P. O., & Essien, A. A. (2008). Hypersexual behavior following craniocerebral trauma: An experience with five cases. *Libyan Journal of Medicine, 3*(4), 192–194.

Feeney, T. J., & Ylvisaker, M. (2011). Positive behavioral interventions. In J. M. Silver, T. W. McAllister, & S. C. Yudofsky (Eds.), *Textbook of traumatic brain injury* (2nd ed., pp. 587–598). Arlington, VA: American Psychiatric Publishing.

Fleming, J., & Nalder, E. (2011). Transition to community integration for persons with acquired brain injury. In N. Katz (Ed.), *Cognition, occupation, and participation across the life span: Neuroscience, neurorehabilitation, and models of intervention in occupation therapy* (3rd ed., pp. 51–70). Bethesda, MD: AOTA Press.

Fyffe, C. E., Kahng, S., Fittro, E., & Russell, D. (2004). Functional analysis and treatment of inappropriate sexual behavior. *Journal of Applied Behavior Analysis, 37*(3), 401–404.

Gill, C. J., Sander, A. M., Robins, N., Mazzei, D. K., & Struchen, M. A. (2011). Exploring experiences of intimacy from the viewpoint of individuals with traumatic brain injury and their partners. *Journal of Head Trauma Rehabilitation, 26*(1), 56–68.

Golisz, K. (2009). *Occupational therapy practice guidelines for adults with traumatic brain injury.* Bethesda, MD: AOTA Press.

Griffith, E. R., & Lemberg, S. (1993). *Sexuality and the person with traumatic brain injury: A guide for families.* Philadelphia: F. A. Davis.

Hagen, C. (1998). *The Rancho Los Amigos Levels of Cognitive Functioning: The revised levels* (3rd ed.). Downey, CA: Los Amigos Research and Educational Institute.

Hattjar, B., Parker, J. A., & Lappa, C. L. (2008). Addressing sexuality with adult clients with chronic disabilities: Occupational therapy's role. *OT Practice, 13*(11), CE1–CE8.

Hofmann, A. O. (2008). Veterans Affairs. *OT Practice, 13*(16), 12–15.

Kaplan, M. S., & Krueger, R. B. (2010). Diagnosis, assessment, and treatment of hypersexuality. *Journal of Sex Research, 47*(2), 181–198.

Katz, S., & Aloni, R. (1999). Sexual dysfunction of persons after traumatic brain injury: Perceptions of professionals. *International Journal of Rehabilitation Research, 22*(1), 45–53.

Kreutzer, J. S., & Zasler, N. D. (1989). Psychosexual consequences of traumatic brain injury: Methodology and preliminary findings. *Brain Injury, 3*(2), 177–186.

Langevin, R. (2006). Sexual offenses and traumatic brain injury. *Brain and Cognition, 60*(2), 206–207.

Law, M., Baptiste, S., Carswell, A., McColl, M., Polatjko, H., & Pollock, N. (1998). *Canadian Occupational Performance Measure* (3rd ed.). Ottawa: CAOT Publications ACE.

Lezak, M. (2004). *Neuropsychological assessment* (4th ed.). New York: Oxford University Press.

McGee, J. (2004). Neuroanatomy of behavior after brain injury, or you don't like my behavior? You'll have to discuss that with my brain directly. *Outlook, 4*(2), 24–32.

Miller, B. L., Cummings, J. L., McIntyre, H., Ebers, G., & Grode, M. (1986). Hypersexuality or altered sexual preference following brain injury. *Journal of Neurology, Neurosurgery, and Psychiatry, 49,* 867–873.

Morrell, M. J. (1991). Sexual dysfunction and epilepsy. *Epilepsia, 32*(Suppl. S6), S38–S45.

Neurologic Rehabilitation Institute at Brookhaven Hospital. (2011). *Frequently asked questions about brain injury.* Retrieved November 3, 2011, from http://www.traumaticbraininjury.net/faqs/

Olson, I. R., Plotzker, A., & Ezzyat, Y. (2007). The enigmatic temporal pole: A review of findings on social and emotional processing. *Brain, 130*(7), 1718–1731.

Ponsford, J. (2003). Sexual changes associated with traumatic brain injury. *Neuropsychological Rehabilitation, 13*(1–2), 275–289.

Rowland, S. M., Lam, C. S., & Leahy, B. (2005). Use of the Beck Depression Inventory–II with persons with traumatic brain injury: Analysis of factorial structure. *Brain Injury, 19*(2), 77–83.

Shabsigh, R., Zakaria, L., Anastasiadis, A. G., & Seidman, S. N. (2001). Sexual dysfunction and depression: Etiology, prevalence, and treatment. *Current Urology Reports, 2*(6), 463–467.

Simpson, G., McCann, B., & Lowy, M. (2003). Treatment of premature ejaculation after traumatic brain injury. *Brain Injury, 17*(8), 723–729.

Tanielian, T. L., & Jaycox, L. H. (Eds.). (2008). *Invisible wounds of war: Psychological and cognitive injuries, their consequences, and services to assist recovery.* Santa Monica, CA: Rand.

U.S. Department of Veterans Affairs. (2010). *Traumatic brain injury.* Retrieved November 14, 2011, from http://www.publichealth.va.gov/docs/vhi/traumatic-brain-injury-vhi.pdf

U.S. Department of Veterans Affairs. (2011). *Traumatic brain injury and PTSD.* Retrieved January 25, 2012, from http://www.ptsd.va.gov/public/pages/traumatic_brain_injury_and_ptsd.asp

Warden, D. (2006). Military TBI during the Iraq and Afghanistan wars. *Journal of Head Trauma Rehabilitation, 21*(5), 398–402.

Warren, M. (2011). Intervention for adults with vision impairment from acquired brain injury. In M. Warren & E. A. Barstow (Eds.), *Occupational therapy interventions for adults with low vision* (pp. 403–448). Bethesda, MD: AOTA Press.

Ylvisaker, M., Turkstra, L., & Coelho, C. (2005). Behavioral and social interventions for individuals with traumatic brain injury: A summary of the research with clinical implications. *Seminars in Speech and Language, 26*(4), 256–267.

Appendix 7.A. Rancho Los Amigos Levels of Cognitive Functioning

Rancho Cognitive Level	Cognitive, Behavioral, Psychosocial, and Functional Characteristics
Level I: No Response *Total assistance*	• Complete absence of observable change in behavior when presented with visual, auditory, tactile, proprioceptive, vestibular, or painful stimuli
Level II: General-ized Response *Total assistance*	• Demonstrates generalized reflex response to painful stimuli • Responds to repeated auditory stimuli with increased or decreased activity • Responds to external stimuli with generalized physiological changes, gross body movement, or nonpurposeful vocalization • Responses noted above may be the same regardless of type and location of stimulation • Responses may be significantly delayed
Level III: Local-ized Response *Total assistance*	• Demonstrates withdrawal or vocalization to painful stimuli • Turns toward or away from auditory stimuli • Blinks when strong light crosses visual field • Visually follows moving object passed within visual field • Responds to discomfort by pulling tubes or restraints • Responds inconsistently to simple commands • Responses directly related to type of stimulus • May respond to some people (especially family and friends) but not to others
Level IV: Confused/ Agitated *Maximal assistance*	• Alert and in heightened state of activity • Purposeful attempts to crawl out of bed or remove restraints or tubes • May perform motor activities such as sitting, reaching, and walking, but without any apparent purpose or upon another's request • Very brief and usually nonpurposeful moments of sustained, alternating, and divided attention • Absent short-term memory • May cry or scream out of proportion to stimulus even after its removal • May exhibit aggressive or flight behavior • Mood may swing from euphoric to hostile with no apparent relationship to environmental events • Unable to cooperate with treatment efforts • Verbalizations frequently are incoherent or inappropriate to activity or environment

(Continued)

Appendix 7.A. Rancho Los Amigos Levels of Cognitive Functioning *(cont.)*

Level V: Confused, Inappropriate, Nonagitated *Maximal assistance*	• Alert, not agitated, but may wander randomly or with a vague intention of going home • May become agitated in response to external stimulation or lack of environmental structure • Not oriented to person, place, or time • Frequent, brief periods of nonpurposeful sustained attention • Severely impaired recent memory, with confusion of past and present in reaction to ongoing activity • Absent goal-directed, problem-solving, and self-monitoring behavior • Often demonstrates inappropriate use of objects without external direction • May be able to perform previously learned tasks when structure and cues are provided • Unable to learn new information
	• Able to respond appropriately to simple commands fairly consistently with external structures and cues • Responses to simple commands without external structure are random and nonpurposeful in relation to command • Able to converse on a social, automatic level for brief periods of time when provided external structure and cues • Verbalizations about present events become inappropriate and confabulatory when external structure and cues are not provided
Level VI: Confused, Appropriate *Moderate assistance*	• Inconsistently oriented to person, time, and place • Able to attend to highly familiar tasks in nondistracting environment for 30 minutes with moderate redirection • More depth and detail of remote memory than of recent memory • Vague recognition of some staff • Able to use assistive memory aid with maximum assistance • Emerging awareness of appropriate response to self, family, and basic needs • Moderate assistance needed to resolve barriers (problem solve) to task completion • Supervised for old learning (e.g., self-care) • Shows carry-over for relearned familiar tasks (e.g., self-care) • Maximum assistance for new learning with little or no carry-over • Unaware of impairments, disabilities, and safety risks • Consistently follows simple directions • Verbal expressions appropriate in highly familiar and structured situations

(Continued)

Appendix 7.A. Rancho Los Amigos Levels of Cognitive Functioning *(cont.)*

Level VII: Automatic-Appropriate *Minimal assistance for routine daily living skills*	• Consistently oriented to person and place within highly familiar environments; moderate assistance for orientation to time • Able to attend to highly familiar tasks in a nondistracting environment for at least 30 minutes with minimal assistance to complete tasks • Able to use assistive memory devices with minimal assistance • Minimal supervision for new learning; demonstrates carryover of new learning • Initiates and carries out steps to complete familiar personal and household routines, but has shallow recall of what he or she has been doing • Able to monitor accuracy and completeness of each step in routine personal and household activities of daily living (ADLs) and modify plan with minimal assistance
	• Superficial awareness of his or her condition but unaware of specific impairments and disabilities and the limits they place on his or her ability to safely, accurately, and completely carry out household, community, work, and leisure tasks • Unrealistic planning; unable to think about consequences of a decision or action • Overestimates abilities • Unaware of others' needs and feelings; unable to recognize inappropriate social interaction behavior • Oppositional or uncooperative
Level VIII: Purposeful and Appropriate *Standby assistance for routine daily living skills*	• Consistently oriented to person, place, and time • Independently attends to and completes familiar tasks for 1 hour in a distracting environment • Able to recall and integrate past and recent events • Uses assistive memory devices to recall daily schedule, create to-do lists, and record critical information for later use with standby assistance • Initiates and carries out steps to complete familiar personal, household, community, work, and leisure routines with standby assistance; can modify the plan when needed with minimal assistance • Requires no assistance once new tasks or activities are learned • Aware of and acknowledges impairments and disabilities when they interfere with task completion, but requires standby assistance to take appropriate corrective action • Thinks about consequences of a decision or action with minimal assistance • Overestimates or underestimates abilities

(Continued)

Appendix 7.A. Rancho Los Amigos Levels of Cognitive Functioning *(cont.)*

Level VIII: Purposeful and Appropriate *Standby assistance for routine daily living skills*	• Acknowledges others' needs and feelings and responds appropriately with minimal assistance • Depressed, irritable; low tolerance for frustration; easily angered and argumentative • Self-centered • Uncharacteristically dependent or independent • Able to recognize and acknowledge inappropriate social interaction behavior while it is occurring; takes corrective action with minimal assistance
Level IX: Purposeful and Appropriate *Standby assistance on request for daily living skills*	• Independently shifts back and forth between tasks and completes them accurately for at least 2 consecutive hours • Uses assistive memory devices to recall daily schedule, create to-do lists, and record critical information for later use with assistance when requested • When asked, initiates and carries out steps to complete familiar personal, household, work, and leisure tasks independently; completes unfamiliar personal, household, work, and leisure tasks with assistance • Aware of and acknowledges impairments and disabilities when they interfere with task completion and takes appropriate corrective action; requires standby assistance to anticipate a problem before it occurs and take action to avoid it • When asked, able to think about consequences of decisions or actions with assistance • Accurately estimates abilities but requires standby assistance to adjust to task demands • Acknowledges others' needs and feelings and responds appropriately with standby assistance • May continue to be depressed • May be easily irritable • May have low tolerance for frustration • Able to self-monitor appropriateness of social interaction with standby assistance

(Continued)

Appendix 7.A. Rancho Los Amigos Levels of Cognitive Functioning *(cont.)*

Level X: Purposeful and Appropriate *Modified independent*	• Able to handle multiple tasks simultaneously in all environments but may require periodic breaks • Able to independently procure, create, and maintain own assistive memory devices • Independently initiates and carries out steps to complete familiar and unfamiliar personal, household, community, work, and leisure tasks; may require more than the usual amount of time or compensatory strategies to complete them • Anticipates impact of impairments and disabilities on ability to complete ADLs and takes action to avoid problems before they occur; may require more than the usual amount of time or compensatory strategies • Able to think independently about consequences of decisions or actions but may require more than the usual amount of time or compensatory strategies to select the appropriate decision or action
	• Accurately estimates abilities and independently adjusts to task demands • Able to recognize the needs and feelings of others and automatically respond in an appropriate manner • May be periodically depressed • Irritability and low tolerance for frustration when sick, fatigued, or under emotional stress • Social interaction behavior is consistently appropriate

Note. Adapted from *Rancho Los Amigos Levels of Cognitive Functioning* (3rd ed.), by C. Hagen, 1998, Downey, CA: Los Amigos Research and Educational Institute. Copyright © 1998 by, the Los Amigos Research and Educational Institute. Adapted with permission.

8

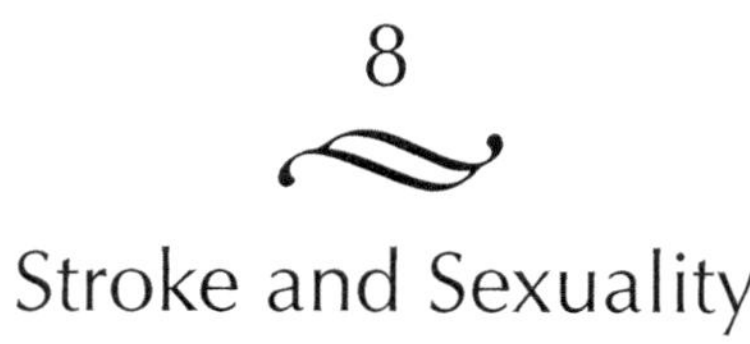

Stroke and Sexuality

Michelle Mioduszewski, MS, OTR/L

Key Terms and Concepts

- Aphasia
- Body mapping
- Disablement model
- Dysarthria
- Dysphagia
- Dyspraxia
- Hemiparesis
- Hemiplegia
- Hemorrhagic stroke
- Hypersensitivity
- Hypertonic and hypotonic muscle tone
- Ischemic stroke.

Learning Objectives

By the end of the chapter, readers will be able to

- Discuss the basic causes of stroke,
- Understand physical effects of stroke as they relate to hemiplegia and the change in sexuality role,

- Understand how communication can change after a stroke and how it affects the sexuality role,

- Describe mood changes after a stroke and how they affect sexuality,

- Understand the cognitive changes after a stroke and how they might affect sexuality,

- Describe the possible visual changes after a stroke and how they can affect sexuality,

- Understand bowel and bladder changes after a stroke and how they can affect sexuality,

- Describe complications that can occur with the caregiver relationship,

- Implement the components of the PLISSIT Model (Annon, 1976) into the therapeutic intervention to sexual activity, and

- Understand billing for services rendered as an occupational therapist for education on sexuality.

Understanding Stroke

In the United States, someone has a stroke every 45 seconds, which translates to 700,000 people experiencing this trauma every year, and 500,000 for the first time (Vega, 2010). Stroke is one of the leading causes of death in the United States and a major cause of serious, long-term, and chronic disability in adults (American Speech and Hearing Association, 2004). Approximately two-thirds of those who have a stroke will survive (Woodson, 2008). Strokes, or cerebral vascular accidents (CVAs), are divided into categories by the cause for damage to the brain. Sexuality starts in the brain, particularly in the amygdala, mesencheplalic tegmentum, and the septal nuclei (Rees, Fowler, & Maas, 2007); therefore, persons with this diagnosis require attention to sexual function.

The most common type of stroke is an *ischemic stroke*, in which a physical blockage occurs in the artery that supplies blood to the brain. The blockage of the artery then cuts off the supply of oxygen-rich blood to a particular area of the brain, causing damage. Some 87% of all strokes fall into this category (Vega, 2008). *Hemorrhagic stroke* occurs when a blood vessel ruptures *(aneurysm)* or leaks *(arteriovenous malformation)*. In this situation, pressure builds in the brain and causes the brain damage.

The most commonly described signs and symptoms of a stoke occurring include numbness, tingling, or weakness on one side of the body; confusion; difficulty with communication (receptive or expressive); problems with vision;

coordination difficulties (e.g., unbalanced, dropping things); or severe pain in the head (American Stroke Association [ASA], 2012).

Impact of Stroke

A stroke leaves a varying list of residual issues for the survivor. The most common issues that are seen include hemiplegia or hemiparesis, communication and oral–motor limitations, mood or personality changes, cognitive impairments, visual–perceptual impairments, bowel and bladder dysfunction, and an overall change in life roles. This chapter briefly discusses the areas that are affected by stroke and then discusses how these might potentially affect a stroke survivor's sexuality and how an occupational therapy practitioner might intervene.

To determine the effect of a CVA on occupational performance and role disruptions, the implementation of the disablement model (Ueda & Okawa, 2003) for therapy assessment and interventions is suggested. The *disablement model* is "an evaluation and intervention model based on specific impairment, functional loss, and attainable quality of life, rather than on a medical diagnosis" (*Mosby's Medical Dictionary,* 2008). For example, rather than stating "The client has a CVA," using the disablement model, the client would experience decreased balance, right-side weakness (hemiparesis), and possible vision limitations that will affect her ability to return to her job as an elementary school teacher, to drive independently, and to return to live independently in her two-story home. The client is concerned about the ability to remain gainfully employed, live independently, and resume her relationship with her significant other.

The use of the disablement model redirects the focus of assessment and intervention and provides client-centered and client-specific opportunities for interventions. As the therapist custom designs therapeutic interventions, the client's needs can be met by using this model of care. The disablement model allows the occupational therapy practitioner to focus less on the medical diagnosis and more on the client's impairment and the functional and role resumption level.

Hemiparesis and Hemiplegia

Hemiparesis is weakness on one side of the body, and *hemiplegia* is the loss of movement on one side of the body (*Mosby's Medical Dictionary,* 2008). After a stroke, a person's one-sided impairments can be minor or profound. Such impairments are related to the damage in the brain to the motor area on the parietal lobe. Not only can the muscles on the one side of the body be weak, but changes in tone can impair and limit function. Initially, a person experiences *hypotonic* (low or flaccid) muscle tone and usually progresses into a *hypertonic* (high or spastic) muscle tone situation. *Spasticity* is the hypertonic response after central nervous system trauma. On the basis of the progression from low tone to high tone, hypertonic muscle tone requires a greater need for intervention.

Hypertonic muscle tone can be very difficult to manage in daily life because a person cannot easily control it, and it often makes tasks more difficult to perform. The increase in tone and weakness often leads to limited use and reduced range of motion (ROM), along with the possibility of increased pain. The increased pain creates an environment of nonuse or limited use. With fewer opportunities for movement, a person's ROM and strength fades. With less movement, pain often increases and the cycle begins. Pain discourages movement and can cause tighter muscles and more pain that limit use of a joint, causing the loss of more strength and ROM. Pain can be a significant secondary stroke symptom, limiting function and roles.

Sensation

Sensation changes are another challenge experienced with hemiparesis and hemiplegia. Sensation changes can vary among people and even locations in one person's body. For example, a person's shoulder might be extremely hypersensitive to touch and movement, while he or she has no sensation in his or her hand. This type of impairment comes with multiple complications. When sensitivity is hyperactive, touch is often avoided and met with great fear. Clothing selection must be carefully chosen and movements completed with caution. When sensitivity is hypoactive, safety becomes a concern, as the person could be unaware of his or her position, might come in contact with potentially dangerous items (e.g., hot, sharp), drop items, and experience significant frustration with fine-motor tasks. When strength, tone, ROM, sensation changes, and pain impairments are experienced in all or parts of a person's body, mobility, movement, and function are affected.

With hemipareisis and hemiplegia, fatigue, endurance, and sensation changes can also affect a stroke survivor's physical barriers. Often they both present as barriers for many of an individual's daily routines. A person requires more focus and energy to move and complete each component of a task and, depending on the situation, might require assistance to complete the task. As clients with hemiparesis and hemiplegia have to complete physical activities with one side of the body and fluctuating muscle tone, the energy expenditure is greater than in the person without such impairments.

Communication and Oral–Motor Impairments

In addition to the possible physical deficits after a stoke, communication and oral–motor impairments might also be present. A common type of oral–motor impairment is *aphasia*, which is divided into three broad areas: (1) receptive aphasia, (2) expressive aphasia, and (3) global aphasia. *Receptive aphasia* occurs when the stroke survivor experiences difficulty understanding incoming language, such as the directions a therapist or caregiver says. *Expressive aphasia* occurs when the stroke survivor is unable to produce understandable communication. For example, he or she might answer "no" to every question, even open-ended questions. *Global aphasia* is the combination of receptive and expressive aphasia. In this case, the person is unable to understand incoming communication and unable to produce outgoing communication.

Other common communication deficits can include dysarthria and dyspraxia. *Dysarthria* is limited or poor articulation of verbal speech. *Dyspraxia* is characterized by a lack of motor planning and can be seen with verbal skills or the entire body. Dyspraxia presents like very uncoordinated movement.

Along with communication deficits, swallowing difficulties can occur. *Dysphagia* is the limited ability or inability to effectively consume nutrition. It includes the swallow as well as all aspects of eating. A possible additional symptom associated with dysphagia is oral leakage or drooling. This can significantly affect social roles in a stroke survivor's life.

Personality Changes

When a stroke affects a person's personality due to brain damage, relationships change. Common personality changes include impulsive actions, depressed mood, flat affect, and irritability (Gillen, 2006). Caregivers report apathy, increased frustration, decreased patience, and increased dissatisfaction in those recovering from stroke, and their perception of the client's personality change tends to correlate with their own distress in coping with the changes (Stone et al., 2004). The roles and relationship between spouses in particular can change dramatically after a stroke as one member of the relationship becomes a caregiver and support system and has additional responsibility. Although changes in personality might be an exacerbation of pre-stroke personality traits, they can affect the client's everyday life.

Cognitive and Executive Function Impairment

Cognitive processes occur in the brain, so they are frequently impaired after a stroke takes place. The range at which a person can be impaired is extremely variable, depending on the severity of the CVA, and might range from low-level skills (e.g., alertness, arousal, orientation) to higher-level skills (e.g., sequencing multiple steps, planning, problem solving, acquiring new learning; Gutman & Schonfeld, 2009). Thus, a stroke survivor's awareness of basic needs could be impaired, or he or she might have deficits only in executive functioning skills (e.g., planning, organizing, strategizing). No matter what the intensity or degree of cognitive impairment, it affects the client's function in daily life, especially in complex social situations. Cognitive impairments could prevent the client from holding employment or being left unsupervised.

Visual–Perceptual Impairment

As the brain is the control center for the visual and perceptual systems, one frequently sees vision and vision-related deficits after a stroke (Warren, 2011). There are very few reliable and consistent statistics on the frequency of visual deficits after a stroke because of the lack of consistent and reliable assessment in research. Vision deficits that can occur after a stroke could include field deficits or ocular–motor limitations. *Field deficits* are the loss of visual field caused from damage to the occipital lobe of the brain; this can occur in varying degrees. The most common is a *homonymous hemianopsia* (loss on the entire side of the visual field), but the loss could be in an isolated quadrant as well. Ocular–motor deficits create symptoms such as double vision, eye pain or strain, and headaches (Warren, 2011).

The challenge in vision rehabilitation with clients who have experienced a stroke is that signs of visual impairments—difficulty in completing vision-related activities of daily living (ADLs), reduced speed in information processing, or errors—can be erroneously attributed to cognitive impairments rather than to vision (Warren, 2011).

Bowel and Bladder Dysfunction

Bowel and bladder dysfunction are common after a stroke and are reported to be an issue for 15% of stroke survivors per year after the stroke, and these dysfunctions are a cause for not being discharged home after rehabilitation (National Stroke Association [NSA], 2007). Such impairments could include a complete lack of control, limited control, impaired sensation, or limitations in only one of the systems. Considering the nature and location of this dysfunction, it is not surprising that bowel and bladder dysfunction is a barrier in life and sexuality.

Sexual Activity as Occupation

In the *Occupational Therapy Practice Framework: Domain and Process* (*Framework;* American Occupational Therapy Association, 2008), sexual activity is considered an ADL and classified as an area of occupation. *Occupation* can be defined as

- "Daily activities that reflect cultural values [and] provide structure to living and meaning to individuals; these activities meet human needs for self-care, enjoyment, and participation in society" (Crepeau, Cohn, & Schell, 2003, p. 1031).

- "Activities that people engage in throughout their daily lives to fulfill their time and give life meaning. Occupations involve mental abilities and skills and might or might not have an observable physical dimension" (Hinojosa & Kramer, 1997, p. 865).

- "A dynamic relationship among an occupational form, a person with a unique developmental structure, subjective meanings and purpose, and the resulting occupational performance" (Nelson & Jepson-Thomas, 2003, p. 90).

When considering sexual activity within the context of occupation, it clearly falls under the scope of occupational therapy. The connection between sexual activity and ADLs makes occupational therapy practitioners the ideal allied health professionals to address this topic with a client. If the profession seeks to provide holistic interventions, addressing sexual activity becomes an integral part of this process.

Sexuality After Stroke

A stroke changes the role of being sexual for both the client and his or her partner (McVeigh, 2009). The changes at the impairment and disability levels previously discussed can lead to challenges in intimacy. Positions can be painful to achieve and maintain. Tone, weakness, and ROM limitation might completely eliminate some positions such as quadruped-based positions that require significant strength and balance to stabilize in a dynamic situation. Personality changes might affect how a partner emotionally reacts. Perceptual and cognitive changes might create a disorganized approach to the task.

The occupational therapy practitioner's role is to assist the client in returning to his or her prior roles and maximizing independence. Vaughan (2009) suggested that occupational therapy practitioners need to give clients permission to be sexual and discuss sex, although the biggest barrier is bringing up the subject. Occupational therapy practitioners frequently work with clients in some of their most vulnerable moments, such as balancing at the edge of the bed to put on pants, bathing in the shower, or using the toilet. Although occupational therapy practitioners are comfortable in these settings, taking the conversation to the topic of sex is not often done (Hattjar, 2007).

In many therapeutic settings, occupational therapy practitioners have the opportunity to address sexual activity with clients. In the acute care setting, when preparing a client with a stroke for discharge, especially if there is no plan for follow-up therapy, sexuality should be included in the discharge instruction education with a heavy focus on tools and resources, as the therapist might not be involved after this time.

In the neurorehabilitation setting, practitioners complete training on so many aspects of daily life. The need in the neurorehabilitation program must include tone management with sexual positions and possible practice on a home visit.

In the long-term-care (LTC) facility, the client's living environment has drastically changed, and finding the space and situation to engage in a sexual role is difficult. When someone is a resident in a LTC facility, he or she has usually experienced many changes leading to the move. Often, individuals in LTC facilities have lost a spouse, so sex roles may have already dramatically changed in the client's life. Additionally, in most cases, a medical event or loss of function has caused the client to require more care, and this change (physical or mental) can affect sexual interest and function. In a facility environment, privacy is restricted (e.g., roommates, nursing supervision, medical management). The client no longer has a secure home environment that restricts the access of others, obviously limiting the romantic relationship and sexual relationship, be it with a spouse or new partner.

Compounding issues in a LTC facility could be relationship policies in the facility and family concerns. In this situation, the role of the occupational therapy practitioner is to educate the client on facility restrictions while acting as a client advocate to the facility administration. An occupational therapy practitioner can facilitate a situation to give a client privacy and time with a partner, either at the facility or on a day pass at the client's home. This can be difficult, but when approached in an objective light and done in an organized and respectful format, maximal results can be achieved.

As the client leaves an inpatient setting to a lesser-care setting like the home health and outpatient settings, the client has the opportunity to experience the changes and implement information from therapy in relation to sexual activity. Here, reengagement in sex becomes tangible.

In the home health environment, the occupational therapy practitioner is personally involved in the client's home and routine. The outpatient setting is often the last opportunity for occupational therapists to approach the topic sex. The home health and outpatient settings offer a unique opportunity for sex training with the neurologic population. Practitioners can send a client home (or work with the client in the home) with trial interventions and get feedback upon future visits. The occupational therapy practitioner can then adjust the interventions.

Frequently, clients who have had a stroke move though many stages of therapy such as those just mentioned. Although the thought of one's sexuality role might not be a priority initially, it might become a more relevant topic at another stage in the recovery process. It is the responsibility of health care professionals who claim to be the specialist in role resumption and functional training to consider sexual activity and sexuality.

Addressing Sexuality in Stroke Survivors

In general, the role of an occupational therapist is to assist clients in returning to their pre-illness, injury, or disability roles and occupations. The most important issue in addressing sexuality is to do so with dignity. Sexual activity is a personal, intimate, and sometimes uncomfortable topic for both the therapist and client to broach. Vaughan (2009) suggested that occupational therapists need to obtain permission from the client to address the subject of sexual activity because of the intimate and personal nature of this ADL.

To address a topic such as sexual activity more comfortably, occupational therapists can use a structured and sequenced framework, like the PLISSIT Model (Annon, 1976; see Chapter 1 of this text). The PLISSIT Model is considered the "gold standard" for addressing sexual activity and sexuality intervention and counseling within the health care arena (Klein & Merritt, 2011; Linder, 2007). Although the PLISSIT model provides a structure and sequence for addressing sexual activity in a therapeutic setting, the practitioner must also acknowledge his or her own feelings about addressing sexual activity with a client and understand his or her own biases.

To address sexual activity with a client, the practitioner must clarify his or her own feelings about the topic. When presented with a chronic and debilitating medical diagnosis like stroke, the client might not know the impact of the diagnosis on sexual activity, although he or she will probably understand the need to take medication, acknowledge mobility limitations, and see the necessity of reconfiguring how he or she must approach daily activities. However, if a client does not understand what to expect concerning sexual activity, education by the occupational therapy practitioner is a very appropriate intervention.

Debunking Myths

Kaufman, Silverberg, and Odette (2007) listed two significant mistruths: People with disabilities are (1) not sexual and (2) not desirable. Kaufman et al. (2007) also pointed out the myth that sexual activity must be spontaneous and come naturally. This is as untrue for the individual with a disability as it is for a person with no disability. Planning is frequently a component of the task of sex.

Kaufman et al. (2007) also noted the misperception that people with a disability do not need education about sex. Sexuality is important to a person's quality of life, including those who have survived a stroke. After a stroke, there is a reduction in frequency of sexual activity and a decrease in partner sexual satisfaction (Rees et al., 2007). Research suggests that physical issues rarely cause true sexual dysfunction but that depression and psycho-social issues have a greater effect (Rees et al., 2007). Clients who have had a stroke need to understand how the stroke affects sexual activity as well as how psychological factors can influence sexual satisfaction.

Introducing the Topic of Sex

Sexual activity is a very sensitive subject, and respecting privacy is of par-amount importance. However, placing too much emphasis on an intimate conversation can place the client "on the spot." For example, completely changing the therapy session's routine and pattern to move into a quiet room and sit across from your client will inherently stress the therapeutic rela-tionship. Instead, an occupational therapist can carefully plan the treatment session to integrate time and space for this conversation. For example, in the rehabilitation facility setting, it could be suggested that practice be done getting in and out of a bed in a mock bedroom. While in the space that is separate from the main occupational therapy clinic space, the topic of sex can be gently addressed. Based on the client's response, the rest of treatment session can be transformed into an educational session, or positions could be practiced while on the bed. Although this is an optimal setting for addressing sexual activity, some clients may feel that talking about the subject while on a bed is too uncomfortable, so the setting may need to be modified.

Another example for an introduction is to allow the client to prepare for the conversation. The day or weekend before the topic is discussed in the treatment session, the therapist can inform the client about the upcoming topic and give him or her some flyers and information on the subject. The therapist can instruct the client to generally review the information and pre-pare with thoughts and questions for the next session.

Alternatively, the occupational therapist can introduce the topic during another intervention. For example, during a stretching routine, the therapist can inquire about the client's home and inform the client that sexuality can be very important and that there are things that can be done to return to prior function or improve limitations. Following the introduction of the topic of sex (in any way that is appropriate for the client), it is paramount that the occupational therapist or any other professional respect the client's wishes. If the client wants to discuss his or her sexuality, the therapist can assist in all ways; if he or she declines interest, the therapist can indicate a willingness to discuss it later but not force the issue. If seeing the client for a period of months, it might be relevant to introduce the topic again in a few months but again respect his or her decision to direct care and privacy.

Intervention

After beginning the conversation on sexuality, and assuming the conversation continues, suspend judgment and holistically approach the client and therapy. The conversation can continue to include customized education based on the client's concerns and deficits. It should also be noted that there are no "stroke sexual positions." There are many sexual positions, and some tend to be easier and better for some diagnoses, including stroke.

Physical Considerations

When discussing the physical component of sexual activity with the client after a stroke, the most common factors are passive ROM, active movements or strength, spasticity, sensation, and pain. Because a person who has had a stroke changes over time, he or she might need to alter the best position as his or her body changes. Consider beginning with man-on-top, woman-on-top, side-lying, and seated (with back supported) postures (see Figures A.1–A.5 in Appendix A).

A key factor when discussing appropriate positions with the client is to include the ability to stimulate (Kaufman et al., 2007). It would be awkward if a hemiparetic arm were on the bottom in a side-lying position. It would also be difficult for someone with one-sided weakness to hold himself or herself up in a prone prop or quadruped position. The client could be in the supine posture, which would allow him or her not to fight gravity. Pillows and other wedges can also be use to support body parts for more control.

Spasticity

Spasticity can be a significant challenge with sexual arousal, as any excitement usually increases the level of spasticity. Some suggestions to help manage spasticity include taking a bath in warm water before sexual activity to relax muscles and joints. Another option that can be discussed with the client's neurologist is taking additional medication before sexual activity to reduce the spasticity. Using pillows and props are extremely helpful with spasticity challenges.

Sensation Changes

When sensation changes are involved, it is very appropriate and highly recommended that couples engage in *body mapping* (Kaufman et al., 2007), in which partners slowly and specifically explore with light and heavy touch all over each others' bodies. (The primary option is for the partner to do this to the client, but the roles might also be reversed if desired.) Although this might be a healthy exercise for many couples, mapping the sensation system of the client can be even more enlightening for his or her partner. The body-mapping process is important, as it allows the partner to have a clearer understanding of the sensation limitations from the stroke.

Sex is heavily driven by sensation, so, with impairment to a person's sensation because of a stroke, sex will literally and figuratively "feel" different. During foreplay and intercourse, touch is a significant form of communication. Using body mapping, the touching partner slowly moves from place to place to allow for delays in processing the sensory information. Also, the touching partner should change the level of pressure to see whether different intensities change the way the sensory input is received. The person receiving the touch responds by describing how it feels. The descriptions should be clear so that the touching partner can learn what areas of the body are most sexually charged. This can also help with learning how and where to apply pressure if spasticity becomes problematic. The specific procedure would not be appropriate to conduct during therapy but should be given as an assignment to be done at home. As this task involves both partners, education might be done with both parties present, depending on the relationship and persons involved.

Pain

Pain must be respected with any activity, especially such an intimate one as sex. Pain often results in a reduced libido because it limits movement and comfort, both important precursors to sexual activity. If this is the situation, the first line of defense is to alleviate the pain. If pain reduces one's libido, it most likely affects other areas of one's life. If pain is a primary and intrusive symptom, it must be eliminated or decreased through position or medication prescribed by a physician.

Relief for pain often associated with stroke needs to be discussed with a neurologist, as there are medications that can help to alleviate neurological pain. Like many things with sex, finding the right and least painful position takes trial and error. This might require a significant amount of patience from both partners, but the time and effort are worth it in the end. The important skill to reinforce during education is communication between partners. It is not possible to explain and understand the full depth of the pain felt by a partner, but the partner should try to understand how the pain affects the sexual experience (Kaufman et al., 2007). Once these are understood, the communication mind frame can be nonjudgmental, open, and patient.

Hypersensitivity

Hypersensitivity is a touch that is misperceived. It is often described as sharp, as an irritant, or painful. When hypersensitivity is found in the genital region, orgasm creates the feeling that one has to urinate (Kaufman et al., 2007). Some strategies that could be implemented in therapy are desensitization to the hypersensitivity. This is traditionally done by starting with a very soft or innocuous stimulus to the sensitive area and slowly increasing the level of stimulation. For example, if the forearm were hypersensitive, the client might gently rub the skin with satin or silk. Then the treatment might progress to cotton, denim, and corduroy fabrics. When the genital areas are hypersensitive, the client's partner can "translate" therapy information to the sexual area. The occupational therapist can conduct the training with appropriate demonstrations (in non-genital areas) and monitor the training via interview with the client and his or her sexual partner.

Fatigue

The key to a client having sex when he or she is sensitive to fatigue is to remember that sex does not have to be a marathon of aggressive activity. Foreplay, flirting, and intercourse can be done in creative and planned ways that will manage energy expenditure. If ongoing fatigue is present, sexual activity could be scheduled for times when the client's energy and interest are high (Hattjar, 2011). Tantric sex, planning, energy conservation techniques, and choosing appropriate positions can help manage fatigue.

Tantric sex

One option in managing fatigue is tantric sex. The difference between traditional Western world sexual intercourse and tantra-based sex is that the Western view has a beginning (foreplay), middle (penetration), and finale (orgasm), and tantric sex is focused on the feeling and has no defined start, middle, or end (Kaufman et al., 2007). Fulbright (2009) described tantric sex as cultivating awareness, exploring sexual energy, dissolving the sense of self as contrasted with others and the rest of the world, and not focusing on an orgasm. The benefits of tantric sex include cultivating better communication and more empathic sexuality, relishing slow arousals, supporting the skill of becoming more focused in stimulating the erogenous zones, and inviting a prolonged sexual pleasure experience (Fulbright, 2009). Through tantric sex, one can increase his or her awareness, develop spiritual enlightenment, create richer and more meaningful sex, and realize his or her sexual potential (Fulbright, 2009; Kaufman et al., 2007).

Planning

Planning is another method of compensation for fatigue management. Educating a client in the skill of observing his or her routines and involvement in energy-expending activities is the key to such planning. When clients can assess themselves and know what periods of the day or week are particularly stressful and tiring, they can begin to determine when they have the most energy and when the ideal time for sexual activity would be.

Completing this self-assessment as a log or diary can also carry over into planning for other activities, besides sexual activity, that require more energy. The process can be very enlightening for a person to see his or her week at a glance and see the trends. Although such planning sacrifices some of the spontaneity of sex, it provides an opportunity for longer foreplay and intercourse.

Energy conservation

An energy conservation technique during sex (e.g., foreplay, oral sex, penetration) is a pacing method where the client pauses or changes the activity to a less-strenuous activity when he or she begins to feel tired. This might involve changing positions, changing the style of sexual experience, or pausing for a few minutes. The most energy conservative position is side-lying (both participants on their sides) and can be a fatigue management option when or if endurance is a barrier (Bosworth, 2012).

Positions

Intercourse positions that require the least amount of effort are the side-lying position or having the client on his or her back. Both of these positions are the least physically taxing. Oral sex can be accomplished by having the client lay in a supine position for receiving and giving. Having the stroke survivor seated at the edge of the bed, in a chair or wheelchair (Kaufman et al., 2007) is an energy-conserving position for receiving. An alternative position for giving is the side-lying position in which the entire body is supported.

Dysphagia

The primary areas of concern for a stroke survivor with dysphagia are kissing, oral sex, and aspiration during intimacy. Kissing can be challenging, as the muscles in the mouth are not as strong and equal (usually right to left) as they used to be. To further complicate kissing, clients are placing an increased demand on the coordination and strength of their tongue. This can cause drooling or saliva dripping while kissing, but this is easily remedied by having a tissue readily available. To minimize the risk of aspiration in prolonged kissing, having the client be in a higher position creates a natural chin tuck. This can be done by having the partner sitting or lying below him or her.

Similar challenges occur in oral sex. Oral–motor control, aspiration, and endurance issues should be monitored. Control of the tongue and mouth is being challenged, and the result is usually oral leakage, poor endurance, and the risk for aspiration. Encourage clients to have a tissue or washcloth handy for leakage, take breaks to monitor endurance, and monitor position.

Better positions for the client for giving oral sex is to have his or her partner seated in front of him or her (maintaining an upright posture and allowing for chin tucks when the neck is flexed to create a more effective and safer swallow) as needed, or having his or her partner in supine and the giver on their side (allows easier transition to a more upright posture). Finally, aspiration needs to be considered in any position during any activity. The head of the bed should be fixed at least at 30 degrees when holding a position for an extended period of time, and care should be given to consider the angle of the neck and relationship of the mouth. Extensive education for the client in this area can be shared by a speech–language pathologist.

Oral–motor impairment can affect communication during sexual activity. Not being able to communicate in a traditional fashion creates difficulty during sexual activity, but it does not preclude someone from being sexually active. The use of nonverbal communication is crucial with clients with oral–motor or communication impairments. Hand signs and taps (established before activity with both partners) are extremely helpful when used with an attentive partner. The development of clear signs for pain and discomfort should be well established. Verbal or nonverbal cues can be used to orient a partner that pain is being experienced and that a change is needed. Changes might be as minor as position or support, but they are critical in producing a pleasant experience. In addition to physical signs, a particular look can be given to a partner that indicates a particular desire.

Cognitive and Communication Impairments

In clients with cognitive impairment, a common barrier in exploring their sexuality is motivation and drive (Korpelainen, Nieminen, & Myllylä, 1999). For some individuals, organization and planning to engage in sexual activity might be too complex. In this situation, adding a pre-thought-out plan that has been memorized will assist in ensuring a successful experience by the client; this is similar to using a checklist. The awareness of timing is important yet very difficult for individuals with executive dysfunction. Depending on the level of cognitive impairment, the conversations and training would need to include the client's partner. The more impairment that a person has, the more it might lead to limited carryover and memory. Thus, the client might need an additional person to receive the training to assist in implementing strategies in the bedroom.

Communication with the sexual partner is important so that all are comfortable indicating if they are in a sexual mood or not, and in a direct way. Interpreting nonverbal communication is often challenging for this type of client, and he or she might frequently feel rejected when he or she receives mixed messages. Four main communication dysfunctions occur after a stroke: (1) receptive aphasia, (2) expressive aphasia, (3) dysarthria, and (4) dyspraxia (NSA, 2012). These deficits can impede a sexual relationship and interaction, as communication is key for positive experiences for all parties. Alternative communication cues (e.g., hand signs, particular sounds) need to be established between the partners to communicate enjoyable feelings, painful feelings, and directions.

However, the most human of indicators that sex is desired (e.g., touching, stroking, kissing, eye-to-eye contact, nonverbal cues) apply to clients with CVA. Some clients may need to relearn these signs, and some may need to be reminded because they will not remember them.

Depression and Anxiety

When depression occurs after a stroke, it is very common for medications to be used in treatment. Often these medications can cause sexual arousal side effects (Korpelainen et al., 1999). This creates a dual impact on sexual desire. The client is not as intrinsically motivated for a sexual experience due to the depression as well as from the side effects from the medication for depression or other medical reasons.

Anxiety can also be a factor in preventing sexual activity. Often a fear of those who had a stroke is that sex will cause another stroke (Shah, 2009). It is significantly unlikely that sex will cause another stroke. NSA (2007) reported that a person is no more likely to have a stroke during sex than during other activities completed in life. It is even recommended that an active life is healthy, including having a healthy sex life.

Visual–Perceptual Issues

The most significant visual or perceptual deficits that will affect a person in his or her sexual role after a stroke are homonymous hemianopsia or visual–spatial inattention. The more impairing deficit is the visual–spatial inattention, as it can include a body-related unawareness in which the client has very poor awareness of one side of his or her body, leading to awkward or possibly uncomfortable positions. The challenge with these deficits is to increase awareness to the loss side. The partner must be acutely aware of this deficit and can help in compensating during sexual activity. Such compensation might be as simple as having awareness of the location of the neglected arm and leg to ensure safe and accurate positioning, or actually physically moving the neglected side to incorporate a whole-body experience.

Lubrication

After a stroke, women have reported having decreased lubrication during intercourse (NSA, 2007). This could be from the damage from the stroke or be a side effect of other medical management medications. The simplest accommodation for lack of lubrication is a water- or silicone-based lubricant. If this is not effective enough, it is recommended that the client consult her gynecologist.

Erectile Dysfunction

After a stroke, many men experience erectile dysfunction and ejaculation difficulty (Korpelainen et al., 1999; NSA, 2007). Like the lack of lubrication for a woman, the erectile dysfunction for a man can be caused from a change in the brain or from medication side effects. The primary accommodation for this difficulty is pharmacologically based, which requires a prescription from a physician.

If pharmacological options are not effective, the client might need assistance in exploring nonpenetrative sex, such as oral sex, or tool or device use.

Bowel and Bladder

Incontinence can be a significant barrier during oral sex (Kaufman et al., 2007) because of the proximity between one's face and another's peritoneal region. When sexually excited, it is common for one's body to release urine or feces. The most effective compensations for this difficulty are to ensure complete emptying of the bladder or rectum before sex. If catheterization is an option, this can also be done prior to sexual activity. Avoiding alcohol and caffeine before oral sex is also helpful, as both are diuretics and increase the sense of bowel and bladder voiding urgency.

If bladder incontinence is a concern for a male, a catheter can be used during penetration with a condom to hold it in place. Intercourse can also be performed in a bathtub, shower, or other wet environment to deal with other bodily fluids (Kaufman et al., 2007).

Sexual positions can affect the pressure on the bowel and bladder as well. Being on one's side with the person with incontinence on top might be helpful. Finally, numerous medications affect the function of bowel and bladder (Kaufman et al., 2007). Clients should discuss these concerns with both their doctors and pharmacists. Medications that are taken regularly could be the cause of the problem, and in some circumstances, might be easily exchanged for another. A combination of medications might also cause side effects, and a pharmacist might be able to identify the combination. This might require prompting and a note from the therapist to assist in facilitating the conversation and problem-solving process.

Educating Others

Another area in which the occupational therapist can assist in providing education is by discussing sexuality with a client's attendant, caregiver, spouse, or anyone other than the client. This communication would clearly require the appropriate clearances and releases. Although it is not the role of an attendant to have sexual contact with a client, it might be part of his or her role to assist in facilitating sexual play for the person on his or her own or with somebody else (Kaufman et al., 2007). This might include assisting with equipment or prophylactic setup. Addressing this topic requires significant tact and planning on the client's behalf. The key concepts to remember are that each person has his or her own views about sexuality, and these views need to be respected (Kaufman et al., 2007). An open and direct conversation needs to occur about what is needed and not needed, as well as setting up defined boundaries.

Occupational therapy practitioners are in the position of promoting and facilitating open, objective, and direct conversations with clients and between clients and their partners. Occupational therapy communication and education is a valuable service to staff of home health agencies, hospitals, and nursing facilities. As a member of the client's team, occupational therapy practitioners can play a vital role assisting a client in achieving his or her sexual objectives.

In facilitating conversation, therapists can discuss defined boundaries between staff and the client or between the client and his or her partner. Barriers include location and time factors that influence the client's comfort and personal needs. Other barriers could be general communication and comfort levels of the conversation participants. Guidance for open and direct conversations should be encouraged and protected.

Sex Education and Reimbursement

Much like all areas of medical practice, reimbursement is important. The following is offered only as a suggestion not as an insurance rule. Please refer to your facility policies and the insurance regulations for specific situations. As sex is categorized as an ADL, it is reasonable to bill under the *Current Procedural Terminology*™ (*CPT;* American Medical Association, 2011) for *self-care* (97535) or *therapeutic activities* (97530). If you are educating on tone management, it is reasonable to bill under *neuromuscular re-education* (97112). Note that this is a guide, and the occupational therapy practitioner's professional judgment is required to assign the appropriate *CPT* code.

Summary

Occupational therapy practitioners clearly have a role in assisting and guiding stroke survivors through the sexuality process if desired by the client, or at least open the door for communication about sexuality. Not only is doing so part of the *Framework* (AOTA, 2008), it is also part of treating the client in a holistic manner. As an occupational therapist who has had this conversation with numerous clients, my advice is this: Clients do have questions about sexuality, and they will open up if given the opportunity. Finding the right environment and the correct time will ensure a positive experience for therapist and client. Sex can be an uncomfortable topic, but with practice, therapists will be able to broach the subject with ease, and clients will sense your comfort level (see Case Example 8.1).

Case Example 8.1. Jane: Stroke

Jane, 55 years of age, survived a right CVA and presented with neglect of the left side of her body, muscle weakness, and fatigue, and she started to develop spasticity in her left upper and lower extremities. In an outpatient setting, the occupational therapist brought up the topic of sexuality. Jane confirmed that sexual activity was a meaningful activity for her prior to her stroke but that she hadn't felt up to engaging in it since the CVA. She also indicated that she feared her husband of 30 years felt overburdened with her care and was no

---

(Continued)

Case Example 8.1. Jane: Stroke *(cont.)*

longer sexually interested in her. He also indicated that he is afraid that she may have another stroke if she becomes "overexcited or overworked."

The occupational therapist told Jane that she could provide some education on sexuality after stroke, if she was interested. Jane affirmed that she wanted to know more. In talking together, the occupational therapist learned that Jane felt that she had the most energy in the morning. The occupational therapist suggested that Jane and her husband plan sexual activity for that time frame and to go very slowly. The occupational therapist offered to educate Jane's husband as well, but Jane felt that discussion of sexuality would be better coming from her. Jane and her occupational therapist discussed communication strategies that could facilitate comfort between Jane and her husband, so he would not fear hurting her and to maximize enjoyment for both of them. Communication strategies included using verbal and physical cues. The occupational therapist explained the concept of body mapping and suggested that Jane and her husband use that strategy to better communicate, intimately engage with each other, and determine what areas of Jane's body could feel pleasurable sensation. For fun and to assist in learning the process, Jane could also "map" the body of her husband. Body mapping was also promoted to encourage awareness of Jane's left-sided inattention and what her sensation and tolerance were for touch.

During her next visit, Jane said that the body mapping had been enjoyable for both her and her husband and that she was anxious to try intercourse. The occupational therapist explained that left side-lying positions would be least likely to fatigue her and would allow her to increase the weight bearing on her left side to manage spasticity. She also suggested a silicone-based lubricant to decrease any potential vaginal pain or dryness. Finally, the occupational therapist reminded Jane to communicate openly with her husband, so he could better get to know what she enjoyed—and vice versa.

Questions to Consider

1. How did the occupational therapist use the PLISSIT model?
2. How would the intervention have changed if Jane also presented with oral–motor difficulties?
3. How would the occupational therapist seek reimbursement with *CPT* coding?

References

American Medical Association. (2011). *CPT 2012.* Chicago: Author.

American Occupational Therapy Association. (2008). Occupational therapy practice framework: Domain and process (2nd ed.). *American Journal of Occupational Therapy, 62,* 625–683. doi:10.5014/ajot.62.6.625

American Speech and Hearing Association. (2004). *Communication facts: Special populations—Stroke.* Retrieved February 3, 2012, from http://www.asha.org/Research/reports/stroke/

American Stroke Association. (2012). *Warning signs.* Retrieved February 3, 2012, from http://www.strokeassociation.org/STROKEORG/WarningSigns/Warning-Signs_UMC_308528_SubHomePage.jsp

Annon, J. (1976). The PLISSIT model: A proposed conceptual scheme for the behavioral treatment of sexual problems. *Journal of Sex Education and Therapy, 2*(2), 1–15.

Bosworth, K. (2012). *Chronic obstructive pulmonary disease (COPD) energy conservation techniques.* Retrieved February 25, 2012, from http://www.ehow.com/way_5179759_chronic-_copd_-energy-conservation-techniques.html

Crepeau, E. B., Cohn, E. S., & Schell, B. A. B. (Eds.). (2003). *Willard and Spackman's occupational therapy* (10th ed.). Philadelphia: Lippincott Williams & Wilkins.

Fulbright, Y. K. (2009). *Lovers with disabilities become liberated with tantric sex.* Retrieved February 24, 2012, from http://devoteedisabled.multiply.com/journal/item/163

Gillen, G. (2006). Coping during inpatient stroke rehabilitation: An exploratory study. *American Journal of Occupational Therapy, 60,* 136–145. doi:10.5014/ajot.60.2.136

Gutman, S. A., & Schonfeld, A. B. (2009). *Screening adult neurologic populations: A step-by-step instruction manual* (2nd ed.). Bethesda, MD: AOTA Press.

Hattjar, B. (2007). *Occupational therapy practitioners' perspectives related to addressing sexual activity with chronic, physically disabled clients.* Unpublished Capstone Project, Fort Lauderdale–Davie, FL: Nova Southeastern University.

Hattjar, B. (2011). Sexuality and people with chronic disability. In C. H. Christiansen & K. M. Matuska (Eds.), *Ways of living: Intervention strategies to enable participation* (4th ed., pp. 457–470). Bethesda, MD: AOTA Press.

Hinojosa, J., & Kramer, P. (1997). Fundamental concepts of occupational therapy: Occupation, purposeful activity, and function [Statement]. *American Journal of Occupational Therapy, 51*(10), 864–866.

Kaufman, M., Silverberg, C., & Odette, F. (2007). *The ultimate guide to sex and disability* (2nd ed.). San Francisco: Cleis Press.

Klein, M. J., & Merritt, L. (2011). *Sexuality and disability.* Retrieved March 16, 2012, from http://www.emedicine.com/pmr/topic178.htm

Korpelainen, J. T., Nieminen, P., & Myllylä, V. V. (1999). Sexual functioning among stroke patients and their spouses. *Stroke, 30,* 715–719.

Linder, S. (2007). *The missing activity of daily living.* Retrieved June 3, 2007, from http://www.occupational-therapy.advanceweb.com

McVeigh, A. (2009). *Redefining sexuality after stroke.* Retrieved February 13, 2010, from http://www.stroke.org/site/PageServer?pagename=SS_MAG_jf2009_feature_sexuality

Mosby's Medical Dictionary (8th ed.). (2008). Philadelphia: Mosby/Elsevier.

National Stroke Association. (2007). *HOPE: The stroke recovery guide.* Centennial, CO: Author.

Nelson, D. L., & Jepson-Thomas, J. (2003). Occupational form, occupational performance, and a conceptual framework for therapeutic occupation. In P. Kramer, J. Hinojosa, & C. B. Royeen (Eds.), *Perspectives in human occupation: Participation in life* (pp. 87–157). Philadelphia: Lippincott Williams & Wilkins.

Rees, P. M., Fowler, C. J., & Maas, C. P. (2007). Sexual function in men and women with neurological disorders, *The Lancet, 369,* 512–525.

Shah, M. V. (2009). Sexuality after stroke. In J. Stein, R. L. Harvey, R. F. Macko, C. J. Winstein, & R. D. Zorowitz (Eds.), *Stroke recovery and rehabilitation* (pp. 721–734). New York: Demos Medical Publishing.

Stone, J., Townend, E., Kwan, J., Haga, K., Dennis, M. S., & Sharpe, M. (2004). Personality change after stroke: Some preliminary observations. *Journal of Neurological and Neurosurgical Psychiatry, 75*(12), 1708–1713. doi: 10.1136/jnnp.2004.037887

Ueda, S., & Okawa, Y. (2003). The subjective dimension of functioning and disability: What is it and what is it for? *Disability and Rehabilitation, 25*(11–12), 596–601.

Vega, J. (2008). *Interesting facts and statistics about stroke.* Retrieved February 11, 2012, from http://stroke.about.com/od/strokestatistics/a/StrokeStats.htm

Vaughan, D. (2009, August 31). The unspoken ADL: Helping patients regain their sex lives. *Today in OT,* p. 24–25.

Warren, M. (2011). Intervention for adults with vision impairment from acquired brain injury. In M. Warren & E. A. Barstow (Eds.), *Occupational therapy interventions for adults with low vision* (pp. 403–448). Bethesda, MD: AOTA Press.

Woodson, A. M. (2008). Treatment to promote occupational function for selected diagnostic categories: Stroke. In M. V. Radomski & C. A. Trombly (Eds.), *Occupational therapy for physical dysfunction* (6th ed., 1001–1041). Philadelphia: Lippincott Williams & Wilkins.

9

Mental Disorders and Sexuality

Christine Linkie, MS, OTR/L

Key Terms and Concepts

- Bipolar disorder
- Client-centered practice
- Comorbidity
- Depression
- HIV/AIDS
- Major depression
- Posttraumatic stress disorder
- Recovery model
- Serious mental illness
- Schizophrenia
- Substance abuse
- Therapeutic use of self.

Upon completion of this chapter, readers will be able to

- Identify mental disorders and their characteristics;
- Identify issues related to sexuality, intimacy, and quality of life associated with mental disorders;
- Discuss compatibility of the *International Classification of Functioning, Disability and Health* (World Health Organization, 2001) and

the Recovery Model with client-centered practice in occupational therapy;

- Understand the role of occupational therapy in helping clients develop healthy sexuality;

- Understand the risk of HIV/AIDS among clients with mental disorders;

- Select appropriate assessment tools related to sexuality for clients with mental disorders; and

- Synthesize evaluation results into meaningful and appropriate treatment goals.

Introduction

Mental disorders are "conditions that affect cognition, emotion, and behavior" (Manderscheid et al., 2010, p. 2) and include diagnoses such as bipolar disorder, depression, posttraumatic stress disorder (PTSD), schizophrenia, and substance abuse. Mental disorders are the leading cause of disability among adolescents and adults ages 15–44 years in the United States and Canada (National Institute of Mental Health [NIMH], 2009a).

Having a mental disorder can negatively affect a person in all areas of his or her occupational functioning (e.g., work, leisure, interpersonal relationships) and, thus, can affect his or her quality of life (QoL). The concept of QoL has become an important concept in mental health care not only for humanitarian reasons but also as an approach to treatment planning and outcome measurement (Schmidt, Staupendahl, & Vollmoeller, 2004). This chapter examines one component of QoL—sexuality—as it relates to people who have mental disorders.

Although a comprehensive discussion of all mental disorders and issues of sexuality is beyond the scope of this chapter, a general overview of some of the common diagnoses that occupational therapists might encounter are included, along with a discussion of occupational therapy principles, the Recovery Model, risky sexual behaviors and HIV/AIDS, assessments, and interventions.

Occupational Therapy Principles and the Recovery Model

Two important principles of occupational therapy underlie this discussion: (1) client-centered practice and (2) therapeutic use of self. *Client-centered practice* is "a process in which the client is the focal point around which occupational therapy treatment evolves" (Maitra & Erway, 2006, p. 298).

Therapeutic use of self is defined as intentionally interacting with a client in a manner that is caring, respectful, and therapeutic (Taylor, 2008).

Maintaining professional boundaries is also very important. Clinicians who address issues of sexuality must acknowledge their own personal feelings, along with any biases they might have (Gordon, Tschopp, & Feldman, 2004). Like other rehabilitation practitioners, some occupational therapists might have had limited exposure to the area of sexuality; after assessing their attitudes and skills, they might need further information and education. Collaboration with other professionals (e.g., social workers, psychologists, physicians) is often essential. Although occupational therapy might be helpful in addressing the development of healthy sexuality for many people who have mental disorders, therapists should not hesitate to refer clients to other health professionals when their services would be more appropriate.

Two clients with the same diagnosis can have different levels of functioning (Bonder, 2010). For example, one person who has depression might have great difficulty with his or her role as a partner, but another person with depression might not. An occupational therapy approach to clients with mental disorders focuses on the person—his or her functional abilities and occupational roles.

In occupational therapy, health is viewed not as an absence of disorder or disability but rather as a state of adaptation in which individuals have the supports needed to fulfill life roles in their environments, including the role of intimate partner. Practitioners need to take a wellness approach to mental disorders (Manderscheid et al., 2010). Rather than focusing only on the disease (i.e., the disabling aspects), treatment needs also to focus on recovery—"a life-long process in which a person with a mental disorder and disability strives to participate fully in community life, even in the presence of continuing symptoms and disabilities" (Manderscheid et al., 2010, p. 2).

A shift in mental health practice is being made from a medical model, in which treatment is directed by a clinician to ameliorate symptoms, to a wellness and recovery model in which goals are set with the client, with the ultimate goal of maximum participation in community and daily life occupations. In 2006, the Substance Abuse and Mental Health Service Administration (SAMHSA) published its Consensus Statement on Mental Health Recovery, which outlined 10 components for recovery-based treatment of mental disorders and disabilities. The following components were included:

- Self-direction
- Individualized and person-centered care

- Empowerment
- Holistic approach
- Understanding of nonlinear process
- Strengths-based approach
- Peer support
- Respect
- Responsibility
- Hope.

All of these components resonate with occupational therapy practice and might be applied to occupational therapy interventions that address sexual health. SAMHSA (2006) elaborated on the strengths-based approach component by stating,

> Recovery focuses on valuing and building on the multiple capacities, resiliencies, talents, coping abilities, and inherent worth of individuals. By building on these strengths, consumers leave stymied life roles behind and engage in new life roles (e.g., partner, caregiver, friend, student, employee). The process of recovery moves forward through interaction with others in supportive, trust-based relationships. (p. 2)

Occupational therapy fits well with a recovery and wellness service delivery model for mental disorders, as it "guides [clinicians] to see the person from a holistic point of view, and to provide interventions in kind" (Wollenberg, 2001, p. 101).

Several well-known publications help guide occupational therapy approaches to recovery and wellness. The *Diagnostic and Statistical Manual of Mental Disorders (DSM–IV–TR;* American Psychiatric Association [APA], 2000) is commonly used in the United States to diagnose and describe mental disorders, and occupational therapy practitioners can use it as a valuable reference tool. The current *DSM–IV–TR* is under revision; a new edition is expected in 2013. The World Health Organization's (WHO's; 2010) *International Classification of Diseases (ICD–10)* is the most widely used tool worldwide to describe diagnoses (Cara & MacRae, 2005), although the American Occupational Therapy Association (AOTA; 2009) has pointed out its lack of functional diagnoses. Medicare has delayed implementation of the *ICD–10* until October 2013 due to its heavy compliance burden on service providers (AOTA, 2009).

WHO's (2001) *International Classification of Functioning, Disability and Health (ICF)* also includes activity engagement and acknowledges that both personal and environmental factors can influence a person's functional abilities. *ICF* includes four sections: (1) body functions, (2) body structures, (3) activities and participation, and (4) environmental factors. This structure and approach to classification is congruent with the *Occupational Therapy Practice Framework: Domain and Process (Framework;* AOTA, 2008). Occupational therapy's domain includes areas of occupation, client factors, performance skills and patterns, context and environment, and activity demands, and the *Framework* classifies sexual activity as an activity of daily living.

Sexuality and Quality of Life

Sexuality encompasses much more than physical contact. WHO (2012) defined *sexual health* as a sense of well-being that encompasses a person's social–emotional and physical functioning with regard to his or her sexuality. Sexual health entails safety, pleasure, and respect, nonviolence, and freedom from oppression and discrimination. Items about sexuality are included in the World Health Organization Quality of Life Questionnaire (WHO, 2004), including satisfaction with both sex and personal relationships.

Sexuality includes a person's perception of himself or herself as an attractive and sexual being, as well as his or her ability to connect with another person in a relationship that is marked by both physical and emotional intimacy. *Sexuality* here refers not only to sexual behaviors but also to "achievement of an emotional closeness" (Esmail, Darry, Walter, & Knupp, 2010, p. 7) the visual connections, caring words, and physical touches that constitute the language of intimacy. Writing of friendship and sexuality among people with mental disorders and disabilities, Whetstone and Rich (1999) stated, "Without the joy and pleasures of warm friendships, caring intimacy, and sexual expression, the quality of life for anyone is less than what should be acceptable" (p. 4).

Mental disorders can have a profound impact on sexuality and relationships in many ways. For example, both women and men with severe mental illness (SMI) are less likely to marry, although women with SMI have a greater number of sexual partners over their lifetimes (Dickerson et al., 2004). People with mental disorders face many obstacles to establishing satisfying personal relationships, expressing their sexuality, and achieving sexual fulfillment. These obstacles reflect both person and environment factors and might include social stigma, marginalization, poverty, unemployment, agency policies and practices, cognitive impairment, and poor social skills (Ace, 2007).

Mental Disorders

This section discusses the demographics and diagnoses for mood disorders (i.e., major depressive and bipolar), substance use disorders (i.e., dependence and abuse), and schizophrenia, as well as occupational therapy strategies for managing them in the context of sexuality and intimate personal relationships.

According to NIMH (2009a), 1 in 4 adults in the United States experiences symptoms of a diagnosable mental disorder in a given year. About 6% of the population, or 1 in 17 people, have an SMI that significantly impairs functioning. Table 9.1 shows recent demographics of mental disorders in the United States.

Mood Disorders

Mood disorders are characterized by periods of depression, elation, or both. The two main types of mood disorders are major depressive and bipolar disorders (APA, 2000). To be diagnosed with a mood disorder, a person would have to experience at least one episode that would meet the criteria for that disorder. Exhibits 9.1 and 9.2 provide an overview of two types of episodes in mood disorders—depression and mania.

Major depression is characterized by a combination of symptoms (e.g., persistent sadness, hopelessness, irritability, feelings of guilt) that interfere with a person's ability to work, sleep, study, eat, and enjoy once-pleasurable activities, including sex (NIMH, 2011). *Bipolar disorder* is characterized by cycling mood changes, which shift from extreme highs (e.g., mania) to extreme lows (e.g., depression; NIMH, 2009b). Bipolar disorder includes *both* mania and depression.

Table 9.1. Demographics of Mental Disorders in the United States

Diagnosable mental disorder	57.7 million adults[a]
Schizophrenia	2.4 million adults[b]
Major depressive disorder	14.8 million adults[b]
Bipolar disorder	5.7 million adults[b]
Posttraumatic stress disorder	7.7 million adults[b]
Substance abuse and dependency	22.2 million children and adults ages 12 and older[c]

Note. [a]National Institute of Mental Health (2009a), [b]National Institute of Mental Health (2008), [c]Substance Abuse and Mental Health Service Administration (2008).

Exhibit 9.1. Depression Signs and Symptoms

The signs and symptoms of depression include

- Persistent sad, anxious, or "empty" feelings
- Feelings of hopelessness or pessimism
- Feelings of guilt, worthlessness, or helplessness
- Irritability, restlessness
- Loss of interest in activities or hobbies once pleasurable, including sex
- Fatigue and decreased energy
- Difficulty concentrating, remembering details, and making decisions
- Insomnia, early-morning wakefulness, or excessive sleeping
- Overeating or appetite loss
- Thoughts of suicide, suicide attempts
- Aches or pains, headaches, cramps, or digestive problems that do not ease even with treatment.

Note. National Institute of Mental Health (2011).

For major depression to be diagnosed, two depressive episodes must have occurred, and a significant change must have occurred in the affected person's level of social or occupational functioning. For diagnoses of depressive or bipolar disorders, symptoms must not be able to be accounted for by another reason (e.g., medication side effects, medical condition).

To be diagnosed with mania, mood change must cause a significant impairment to functioning (occupational or relational social). Alternatively, hospitalization might be indicated because of psychotic features or a threat to self or others.

Sexuality and intimacy

Although study results vary, up to 70% of people who have depression experience some type of associated sexual dysfunction (Balon, 2007). Dysfunction might occur in sexual interest, arousal, or orgasm. Sexual dysfunction often takes the form of reduced sexual desire and response, separate from any side effects of medication (Kennedy, Dickens, Eisfeld, & Bagby, 1999). It is

Exhibit 9.2. Manic Episode Signs and Symptoms

Mood Changes

- A long period of feeling "high" or an overly happy or outgoing mood
- Extremely irritable mood, agitation, feeling "jumpy" or "wired."

Behavioral Changes

- Talking very fast, jumping from one idea to another, having racing thoughts
- Being easily distracted
- Increasing goal-directed activities, such as taking on new projects
- Being restless
- Sleeping little
- Having an unrealistic belief in one's abilities
- Behaving impulsively and taking part in many pleasurable, high-risk behaviors, such as spending sprees, impulsive sex, and impulsive business investments.

Note. National Insittute of Mental Health (2009b).

estimated that 40%–50% of people experience decreased sexual interest and arousal when depressed (Lykins, Janssen, & Graham, 2006).

During a depressive episode, women might be more likely to experience less desire than men might experience (Lykins et al., 2006); however, men might have more difficulty with sexual response. Kennedy et al. (1999) found that 22% of men reported delayed ejaculation, and 15% of women reported difficulty in achieving orgasm. These findings were independent of the severity of depression.

It is important to note that there are individual differences. For example, Kennedy et al. (1999) reported that depressed women who are introverted are more likely to have difficulty with arousal and orgasm. Their study found that about 40% of people do not experience changes in sexual interest and arousal when depressed. It is very important to consider sexuality as it relates to people who have mood disorders, as sexual dysfunction might be associated with an increased risk of suicidal ideation (Dell'Osso et al., 2009).

Some people experience an increased interest in sex during episodes of depression. Lykins et al. (2006) found that 9.5% of women with nonclinical depression experience increased sexual desire and response. Similar results have been found with men. Increased interest in sex might be a reflection of the depressed person's decrease in self-esteem; he or she might be seeking validation and reassurance (Bancroft et al., 2003). Depression might put individuals at risk for increased sexual risk-taking behaviors because an individual in a depressed state might be more prone to apathy about consequences (Bancroft et al., 2003).

Increased sexual activity is associated with manic episodes in bipolar disorder. Research suggests that 57% of people who have bipolar disorder experience *hypersexuality* (Solovitch, 2009)—impulsive new relationships or sexual acts—which can lead to risky behaviors (e.g., unprotected sex, sex with strangers; see below for information on HIV/AIDS) and can severely disrupt partner and family relationships. Internet dating sites and online chat rooms might also pose potential risks for individuals who present with impulsive behaviors or social skill deficits, regardless of their mental health diagnoses.

Occupational therapy is concerned with helping people fulfill their life roles, and both depression and mania can significantly affect an individual's ability to fulfill his or her role as a partner. Green, Knysz, and Tsuang (2000) stated, "Bipolar disorder is arguably one of the most difficult of mental disorders and disabilities for intimate relationships. Families must endure episodic and recurrent mood swings and might experience the patient as unreliable and/or unavailable" (p. 1396).

For the person with depression, even having a general conversation might sometimes be difficult, let alone expressing himself or herself sexually. However, in a qualitative study of people with severe depression and their partners, affected individuals "focused on their deeply felt desire for intimacy and sexual contact with their partner, in spite of their mental illness" (Ostman, 2008, p. 358). People with depression reported feelings of anger, abandonment, helplessness, or aversion resulting from unresolved difficulties with sexuality. Partners reported suppressing their sexuality or trying to engage their partner sexually that resulted in sex feeling "forced and artificial" (Ostman, 2008, p. 359) to both parties. Symptoms of depression—lack of motivation, changed sexual interest, anhedonia (the inability to feel pleasure or sustain interest)—can be confusing and frustrating for both people with depression and their partners (see Case Example 9.1).

Case Example 9.1. Jaclyn: Depression

Jaclyn, age 30, has been working with her occupational therapist to help establish routines and set small goals during this episode of depression. She is working with a psychiatrist to help her manage her medications. Jaclyn stated that her self-esteem is at a low point and that she feels guilty about the strain that her sadness and lack of motivation puts on her relationship with her husband Ben. She shared that, although she did not want to have sex, she missed being intimate with him. During therapy, Jaclyn's occupational therapist might consider the following interventions:

- Role-play conversations to increase Jaclyn's comfort in discussing issues with her husband.
- Discuss side effects of medication, and help Jaclyn identify questions to ask doctor.
- Use a journal to address coping and self-esteem.
- Use sexual function assessment to track changes in sexual behavior.
- Suggest other ways to be intimate (e.g., sensual massage).
- Suggest ideas for activities couple can make part of their routine (e.g., taking nightly walks).
- Encourage the couple to laugh together at times when depression momentarily eases.
- Explore leisure activities, including exercise, to develop more positive sense of self.
- Refer to counseling for Jaclyn and her husband, if indicated.

Questions to Consider

1. How does Jaclyn's depression affect her sexuality?
2. At what stage of recovery is Jaclyn in?
3. What are Jaclyn's strengths and challenges, and how might treatment address them?
4. What are Jaclyn's goals?

Medication side effects

Many medications used to treat depression have sexual side effects (e.g., decreased desire, difficulty with erection or lubrication, delayed orgasm; Kennedy & Rizvi, 2009). Side effects that affect sexuality can have serious consequences in the long term for people with depression for two reasons. First, as sexuality is related to well-being, not being able to enjoy sexual contact can harm self-esteem and intimate relationships, which in turn can exacerbate depression (Kennedy & Rizvi, 2009). Second, sexual side effects are often a cause of medication noncompliance (Hirschfield, 1999).

Occupational therapists working with people who are being treated pharmacologically for mental disorders and disabilities can help clients to understand the sexual side effects of their medications. Clients can then discuss strategies with their prescribing physicians. Strategies considered might include changing medications, reducing dosages, adding medications to ameliorate side effects, and drug holidays (Balon, 2007). These strategies have associated risks, and they should never be attempted except under the guidance of the prescribing physician.

Occupational therapists might help manage sexual side effects by suggesting nonpharmaceutical strategies, such as planning for sexual activities as dosages are wearing off and using sexual aids (e.g., rings, vibrators, lubricants). When pharmaceutical strategies are used, occupational therapists can help clients track their sexual functioning using an assessment tool such as the Arizona Sexual Experience Scale (ASEX; McGahuey et al., 2000), a short rating scale that includes interest, arousal, responsivity, orgasm, and satisfaction.

Substance Use Disorders

There is a high rate of comorbidity in mental disorders and disabilities. NIMH (2009a) estimated that almost half (45%) of people with a mental disorder also have at least one other mental disorder; dual diagnosis is related to increased severity of the mental disorder. Often, the co-occurring condition is substance abuse—drug or alcohol. In its National Survey of Drug Use and Health, SAMSHA (2008) found that 25.2% of adults with an SMI also had a substance use disorder (see Case Example 9.3).

Case Example 9.2. Lea: Bipolar Disorder

Lea, age 30, has bipolar disorder and has recently stabilized after experiencing a manic episode with psychotic features. She currently lives with her parents and attends a program for outpatient day treatment that includes occupational therapy. Lea is anxious and occasionally highly reactive; she sometimes does not understand how her behaviors affect others. Lea has been in an "on-again-off-again" sexual relationship with a much older man since she was a teenager. She senses that the relationship is not healthy and has said that she would like to have a "real" relationship. Lea's interests include art and technology.

Questions to Consider

1. What are the characteristics of bipolar disorder?

2. What are Lea's goals?

3. How might an occupational therapy practitioner integrate Lea's interests in art and technology into an intervention?

4. How might the occupational therapy practitioner collaborate with other health care professionals to meet Lea's needs?

5. What interventions might occupational therapy provide?

Case Example 9.3. Samuel: Substance Use and Depression

Samuel, age 34, has a dual diagnosis of substance dependency and depression. He presently lives in a homeless shelter and has been sober for 4 months. Samuel participates in a 12-step program, meets individually with his occupational therapist, and attends daily therapeutic groups. Occupational therapy groups focus on self-care, goal setting, coping skills, productive leisure activity, prevocational skills, social interaction, and household management. During his individual sessions with his occupational therapist, he increasingly talks about how much he wants to find a girlfriend. Samuel will be starting a vocational program soon and wonders what to do if he meets a woman there.

After meeting with the treatment team, Samuel's occupational therapist and a social worker at the shelter plan to co-lead a group to help shelter residents develop healthy sexuality and related behaviors. Small groups are divided by gender, as a leader of the same gender will address some topics. The occupational therapist and social worker have discussed inclusion criteria for the group and the need to tailor it to the readiness level of members. The following topics are some of the many that they are considering to address:

- Hygiene and grooming
- Maintaining and respecting personal boundaries
- Dating etiquette
- Assertive vs. aggressive behaviors
- HIV/AIDS transmission
- Safer sex practices
- Gender roles
- Verbal and nonverbal communication
- Healthy relationship attributes.

Questions to Consider

1. What are some of the risks associated with substance abuse and sexual activity?

2. How might substance abuse have affected Samuel's sexuality?

3. At what stage of recovery is Samuel?

4. How can the occupational therapy practitioner balance Samuel's desire to be in a relationship with the need to ensure that he does not put himself or others at risk?

Exhibit 9.3. Substance Abuse and Dependency Signs and Symptoms

Some of the symptoms and behaviors of substance abuse and dependence can include

- Confusion
- Continuing to use drugs even when health, work, or family are being harmed
- Episodes of violence
- Hostility when confronted about drug dependence
- Lack of control over drug abuse—being unable to stop or reduce intake
- Making excuses to use drugs
- Missing work or school, or a decrease in performance
- Needing daily or regular drug use to function
- Neglecting to eat
- Not caring for physical appearance
- No longer taking part in activities because of drug abuse
- Secretive behavior to hide drug use
- Using drugs even when alone.

Source. National Institutes of Health (2012).

The *DSM–IV–TR* (APA, 2000) categorized substance use disorders into two types: (1) substance abuse and (2) substance dependence. *Dependence* referred to addiction (e.g., increased tolerance, compulsive use, withdrawal symptoms), while *abuse* refers to the destructive effects of the recurring use of alcohol or drugs (National Institute on Drug Abuse, 2011). Exhibit 9.3 lists the signs and symptoms of substance abuse.

If an individual is experiencing *tolerance* (needing more of the substance to get the same effect) and *withdrawal* (symptoms of discontinued use associated with specific substances), only one of the above criteria is needed for diagnosis. Both tolerance and withdrawal can become medical emergencies, as withdrawal can lead to hospitalization, and tolerance can lead to overdose and death (Cara & MacCrae, 2005).

Sexuality and intimacy

Substance abuse disorders can physically and emotionally affect sexuality and intimacy, but it is difficult to determine the extent to which substance abuse alone influences sexuality, or whether issues are caused by medications or comorbidities. The type of abused substance also is a factor. Dissatisfaction with sexual intimacy has a high incidence rate among those with substance abuse disorders and their partners (Hussaarts, Roozen, Meyers, van de Wetering, & McCrady, 2012). However, research findings give a varied picture of how substance use affects sexuality. For example, one study found the majority of participants who previously abused heroin thought it improved premature ejaculation, but the same study found opiate misuse related to worsened premature ejaculation (Chekuri, Gerber, Brodie, & Krishnadas, 2012). Alcohol dependency consistently correlates with erectile dysfunction in men, interrupted menstruation in women, and decreased orgasm in both men and women (Mayo Clinic, 2010).

However, in general, alcohol and drugs negatively affect sexual performance and pleasure, most commonly by

- Altering levels of certain neurotransmitters in the brain (especially serotonin, norepinephrine, and dopamine) that are related to pleasure, relaxation, pain relief, mood elevation, and increased physical activity;
- Changing how hormones linked to sexual arousal are released; and
- Changing blood flow or neural signals to or from the sex organs (National Center on Addiction and Substance Abuse at Columbia University [CASA], 1999).

Ironically, many people use alcohol and drugs to facilitate sex in spite of the physiological effects that show clear decreases in functioning (CASA, 1999).

Most research focusing on sexuality and substance abuse disorders highlights the risk that the combination of drugs and sex poses (e.g., practicing unsafe sex, significantly increased numbers of partners; CASA, 1999). Therefore, safety of the client and his or her partners is of the utmost importance. Healthy expression of sexuality cannot occur without simultaneous treatment of the substance abuse disorder. Although substance abuse disorders are intrinsically resistant to treatment and clients are vulnerable to relapse, the evidence clearly shows that treatment for substance abuse significantly decreases rates of relapse (O'Day, 2009).

In an evidence-based review of literature focused on interventions with persons with substance use disorders, Stoffel and Moyers (2004) found four main intervention methods that could be modified with an occupational perspective:

1. *Brief interventions:* 5-minute to 1-hour sessions that may lead the client to self-directed change or seek further treatment.

2. *Cognitive–behavioral therapy:* Treatment approach that uses principles of behavioral and cognitive therapy, focusing on developing successful coping behaviors.

3. *Motivational strategies:* Strategies that identify the client's readiness to change, improve motivation to change, and promote moving to the next stage of change.

4. *12-step treatment programs:* Programs consistent with the principles of self-help programs, such as Alcoholics Anonymous.

Brief interventions. Brief interventions can be very effective in detecting and addressing alcohol abuse (studies have not focused on their effectiveness for other substances; Stoffel & Moyers, 2004). Occupational therapists working with clients in various practice settings might realize substance abuse is affecting rehabilitation and occupations, including sexual performance and satisfaction. Because substance abuse can affect sexuality and intimacy, among other valued roles and occupations, therapists can gently bring up the topic and provide factual information or, if necessary, refer or persuade the client to full treatment.

Cognitive–behavioral interventions. Cognitive–behavioral interventions that focus on relapse prevention are highly effective (Stoffel & Moyers, 2004). Using such an approach, an occupational therapist would include coping strategies and help the client to develop free-time activities. The substance *will* leave a void for the client; although occupational therapy is effective in helping clients stop drug use, it also assists them in filling the void the substance leaves behind with productive occupation (Opp, 2009).

Evidence shows that learning skills such as anger management, coping, relapse prevention (e.g., avoiding high-risk environments), and other skills needed for daily living in the community results in decreased depression, aggressiveness, and passiveness and increases self-esteem, life satisfaction, and assertiveness (Stoffel & Moyers, 2004). These characteristics better prepare clients to be engaged, fully participatory partners in sexual relationships.

Motivational strategies. Stoffel and Moyers (2004) describe motivational strategies as having two parts. In early intervention, such strategies are used as part of a brief intervention to propel the client to treatment or change. Later, motivational interventions are used as part of larger therapeutic interventions, including achieving and maintaining sobriety.

Motivational strategies can include motivational interviewing, such as asking the client about his or her interests and valued roles. A client who enjoyed sexuality activity and values his or her role as a partner could be particularly motivated to maintain sobriety. For example, a woman's ability to achieve orgasm is significantly improved when she is not abusing drugs or alcohol (CASA, 1999). Educating clients on how drug abuse negatively affects sexual pleasure and intimacy, and providing clear instruction on safe sex practices, can assist in motivating clients to remain sober and enjoy greater occupational performance.

12-step treatment programs. Evidence shows 12-step programs to be effective in creating and maintaining health in cases of substance abuse disorders, and self-help groups in particular contribute to better outcomes in terms of drug abstinence (Stoffel & Moyers, 2004). Occupational therapy practitioners facilitating such programs or working with clients in them can help clients and family members integrate a 12-step philosophy into occupations, including those related to sexuality. For clients who identify sexuality as an important occupation, occupational therapy practitioners can use this to develop meaning that reinforces clients' progress toward sobriety.

Medication side effects

Some medications used to treat substance abuse (e.g., Antabuse, methadone) are reported to cause sexual problems, such as premature ejaculation or inability to achieve orgasm (Cohen, Kühn, Sträter, Scherbaum, & Weig, 2010). However, because of the high incidence of sexual problems due to substance abuse itself, it is difficult to determine the extent to which medication contributes to sexual dysfunction (Chekuri et al., 2012). When pharmaceutical strategies are included as part of treatment, clients can track their sexual functioning with the ASEX scale (McGahuey et al., 2000).

Posttraumatic Stress Disorder

Many types of anxiety disorders are described in the *DSM–IV–TR* (APA, 2000), including obsessive–compulsive disorder, generalized anxiety disorder, and PTSD. Although the different anxiety disorders have their own etymologies, signs, and symptoms, they share a common factor: an experience of stress that is debilitating. Stress from anxiety can manifest itself emotion-

Exhibit 9.4. PTSD Signs and Symptoms

PTSD can cause many symptoms. These symptoms can be grouped into three categories:

1. Re-experiencing symptoms

- Flashbacks—reliving the trauma over and over, including physical symptoms like a racing heart or sweating
- Bad dreams
- Frightening thoughts.

Re-experiencing symptoms might cause problems in a person's everyday routine. They can start from the person's own thoughts and feelings. Words, objects, or situations that are reminders of the event can also trigger re-experiencing.

2. Avoidance symptoms

- Staying away from places, events, or objects that are reminders of the experience
- Feeling emotionally numb
- Feeling strong guilt, depression, or worry
- Losing interest in activities that were enjoyable in the past
- Having trouble remembering the dangerous event.

Things that remind a person of the traumatic event can trigger avoidance symptoms. These symptoms might cause a person to change his or her personal routine. For example, after a bad car accident, a person who usually drives might avoid driving or riding in a car.

3. Hyperarousal symptoms

- Being easily startled
- Feeling tense or "on edge"
- Having difficulty sleeping or having angry outbursts.

Hyperarousal symptoms are usually constant instead of being triggered by things that remind one of the traumatic event. They can make the person feel stressed and angry. These symptoms might make it hard to do daily tasks, such as sleeping, eating, or concentrating.

Source. National Institute of Mental Health (2009c).

ally (e.g., feeling extremely frightened, helpless, overwhelmed), behaviorally (e.g., disconnection, irritability, flight–fright–freeze response), cognitively (e.g., distractibility, memory lapse, difficulty thinking clearly), or physiologically (e.g., increased blood pressure or heart rate, gastrointestinal distress, decreased sexual interest).

Anxiety disorders might interfere with functioning and life roles, including sexuality and ability to participate as a partner. Withdrawal from relationships is one of the symptoms of PTSD and has been the subject of recent attention because of its impact on people who have served in military combat.

As described by *DSM–IV–TR* (APA, 2000), a person who has been diagnosed with PTSD has a history of being exposed to a traumatic event (or events). Traumatic events include but are not limited to violent assault, sexual abuse, torture, military combat, being diagnosed with a life-threatening illness, learning about the death or serious disease of a loved one, and witnessing a violent event. Exhibit 9.4 describes the signs and symptoms of PTSD.

Symptoms of PTSD usually begin within 3 months after a traumatic event, but the onset might take place after 6 months or more. The traumatic events and related onset of PTSD can occur at any age. PTSD is considered *acute* if symptoms last for fewer than 3 months and *chronic* if they persist longer. Depression is often comorbid with PTSD; each condition might exacerbate symptoms of the other (O'Donnell, Creamer, & Pattison, 2004).

Sexuality and intimacy

PTSD has been associated with decreased relationship satisfaction (Schnurr, Lunney, Bovin, & Marx, 2009) and has been found to significantly affect family and intimate relationships. Lyons (2009) stated, "PTSD is one of the best predictors of relationship problems" (p. 377).

War veterans

Symptoms of concurrent PTSD and depression have been found among veterans of Operation Enduring Freedom (Afghanistan) and Operation Iraqi Freedom (OEF/OIF; Greiger et al., 2006; Lapierrre, Schwegler, & LaBauve, 2007), as well as among veterans of military operations in other areas (e.g., Somalia, Rwanda, the former Yugoslavia; Ray & Vanstone, 2009). Trauma associated with combat experiences puts soldiers at a higher risk of developing PTSD; prevalence for returning OEF/OIF Veterans has been reported at 14% (Schnurr et al., 2009).

PTSD might be triggered by circumstances that remind the individual of the event that he or she experienced. For example, in the case of a war veteran who has returned home, a car backfiring or other loud noise might remind him or her of a bomb explosion and trigger symptoms of PTSD.

Carolyn Baum, Past President of AOTA, testified before the House Veterans' Affairs Subcommittee on Health in 2008 about the unique role of occupational therapy in treating veterans with PTSD. In her presentation, Baum (2008) emphasized performance of daily life activities, community reintegration, and inclusion of family relationships in treatment: "Occupational therapists might address issues of cognitive executive function, such as memory, planning or organizational skills. . . . Therapists also work with veterans with PTSD to engage in activities that will help them manage or ameliorate depressive symptoms and/or excessive anxiety, and address issues of substance abuse." Although treating anxiety and other symptoms of PTSD is vital, "improved quality of life should be prioritized as a goal of treatment" (Schnurr et al., 2009, p. 734).

Baum (2008) noted, "Occupational therapy . . . can help veterans regain control of their anxiety and their future so that they can return to relationships and activities of meaning and purpose in their lives." Occupational therapists, in individual and group sessions, can provide information about combat-related PTSD and the stress it places on relationships, teach anger management techniques and coping strategies, facilitate discussions on intimacy, provide outlets for stress relief, and support development of leisure occupations to facilitate relationship-building in couples and families.

People with PTSD who have served in the military are at a higher risk of having problems with intimate relationships when compared to civilians with PTSD (Taft, Watkins, Stafford, Street, & Monson, 2011). Soldiers who return to their home communities face many challenges: finding a job, reintegrating into family and social life, learning to live with injuries, and dealing with the loss of friends and colleagues.

The support of loving partners and fulfillment found in dating and relationships can be invaluable. However, for many war veterans, combat-related PTSD sets up impediments to establishing or maintaining fulfilling and healthy relationships. Emotional withdrawal and anger can make it difficult for the veteran with PTSD to get the support from his or her partner that might aid the healing process (Ray & Vanstone, 2009). Although the emotional numbness and withdrawal that are symptomatic of PTSD might have the greatest negative impact (Gavloski & Lyons, 2004; Schnurr et al., 2009), anger and verbal or physical aggression might also get in the way of close relationships (Lyons, 2009; Solomon, Deckel, & Zerach, 2008; Taft et al., 2011). Ray and Vanstone (2009) quote a veteran diagnosed with PTSD who had returned from deployment as a peacekeeper:

> I was more anxious . . . stressed; I had a lot more anger. I was making my family and wife suffer with some physical and psychological abuse. I was still closed up in what I was saying or doing. I was trying to find the answers in my head as to why I'm like that and what's happening with me. My wife said . . . you've changed, you're different. I said no. Three times my marriage almost broke up. Part of it is a couple, but a big part was me. I never realized they were symptoms of PTSD, but now I know that was the reason. (p. 842)

Veterans with PTSD might also have difficulty with sexual functioning. Compared to Vietnam War veterans who did not have PTSD, Vietnam veterans with PTSD have been found to have more difficulty with erections, with trusting and communicating with women, and even with feeling that they were worthy of love (Garte, 1989). Gavloski and Lyons (2004) described the difficulty that couples might have in re-establishing their roles after a veteran returns home. While the soldier is away, the partner who is home independently manages the house, children, money, and social network. When the veteran returns, roles often shift again. At the same time that the veteran is dealing with the symptoms of PTSD and trying to adjust to civilian life, he or she might feel pressured to take on family responsibilities, or might find that the partner has taken over responsibilities that the veteran used to enjoy. If coping skills are not adaptive (on the part of both partners), the veteran might emotionally withdraw, which might lead to weakened relational bonds (Gavloski & Lyons, 2004).

Many couples show great resiliency and can maintain strong partnerships. Self-disclosure has been found to mediate the relationship between PTSD and marital intimacy in that opening up to a spouse was associated with increased intimacy (Solomon et al., 2008; see Case Example 9.4). Treatment approaches to improve PTSD symptoms and partner relationships include cognitive–behavioral therapy, cognitive–behavioral conjoint therapy, psychoeducational groups, individual therapy, and social activities (Lyons, 2009; Monson, Taft, & Fredman, 2009). The National Center for PTSD at the Veterans Administration provides free resources for clinicians and families at www.ptsd.va.gov.

Case Example 9.4. John: PTSD

John, age 27, returned from combat in Iraq with multiple injuries, including an amputated arm. He has been participating in occupational therapy to learn to use and care for his prosthesis. In talking with John, his occupational therapist learned that "things weren't good" at home and that he often became angry over seemingly minor incidents.

The occupational therapist thanked John for sharing his thoughts, acknowledged the difficulty of what he was experiencing, and said that she would like to pursue getting him more help. She mentioned her concerns to his case manager. John was evaluated by a clinical psychologist, diagnosed with PTSD, and began treatment.

In occupational therapy, John's therapist worked with him to both use his prosthesis and manage PTSD symptoms to participate in his daily life occupations. John also joined a coping skills group co-led by an occupational therapist and a psychologist, who were concurrently leading a group for spouses of veterans. Soon afterward, John and his wife began psychological counseling as a couple.

Questions to Consider

1. In what ways might PTSD affect sexuality?

2. How might the occupational therapy practitioner bring up the topic of sexuality?

3. How could the occupational therapy practitioner collaborate with the psychologist to address sexuality in the group setting?

Civilians

Civilians who are affected by wartime violence might also be at risk for developing PTSD. Tuchner, Meiner, Parush, and Hartman-Maeir (2010) described a woman who developed PTSD subsequent to sustaining multiple serious injuries during a terrorist attack. The researchers suggest that an occupational therapy group that addresses social isolation and occupational role withdrawal might be beneficial, as the woman had withdrawn from her husband, children, and friends.

Exhibit 9.5. Schizophrenia Signs and Symptoms

Positive symptoms—psychotic behaviors not seen in healthy people:

- Hallucinations
- Delusions
- Though disorders
- Movement disorders.

Negative symptoms—associated with disruptions to normal emotions and behaviors. These can be mistaken for depression or other conditions:

- "Flat affect" (a person's face does not move, or he or she talks in a dull or monotonous voice)
- Lack of pleasure in everyday life
- Lack of ability to begin and sustain planned activities
- Speaking little, even when forced to interact.

Cognitive symptoms—difficult to recognize, often detected after other tests are performed:

- Poor executive functioning (the ability to understand information and use it to make decisions)
- Trouble focusing or paying attention
- Problems with working memory (the ability to use information immediately after learning it).

Note. National Institute of Mental Health (2009d).

Schizophrenia

Schizophrenia is a relatively common SMI characterized by significant alterations in cognition, affect, and behaviors. Perception, thought, and emotion can become changed so that a person's sense of self is changed.

Schizophrenia is also classified according to positive and negative symptomology, known as Type 1 and Type 2 schizophrenia, respectively. People with

Type 1 schizophrenia, characterized by positive symptoms and little or no cognitive defect, generally have better outcomes than those with *Type 2 schizophrenia,* which is characterized by negative symptoms, cognitive deficits, and ongoing difficulty with functioning (Cara & MacRae, 2005). As defined by the *DSM–IV–TR* (APA, 2000), positive symptoms are excesses or distortions of normal mental functions, while negative symptoms represent a loss or reduction of normal functioning (see Exhibit 9.5 for positive and negative symptoms).

The onset of schizophrenia is usually in late adolescence or early adulthood, although it can present in childhood, middle age, or late adulthood. Diagnosis can be challenging because no one symptom defines the disorder, and other mental disorders and disabilities share similar symptoms (National Alliance on Mental Illness [NAMI], 2007).

Although schizophrenia can disrupt a person's ability to engage in occupations ranging from activities of daily living (ADLs; e.g., grooming, dressing) to life roles (e.g., spouse, worker), it is treatable and can be managed as a chronic disorder. Treatment approaches include medication (e.g., antipsychotics), recovery supports or relapse prevention (e.g., peer support), caregiver support, hospitalization (when acute symptomology is present), psychosocial rehabilitation, counseling, housing, work, education, and skill development (NAMI, 2007). With the exception of prescribing medications, occupational therapy can play a role in all of these treatment approaches, including helping people with schizophrenia to be active community members and to develop meaningful social relationships.

Fully participating in community and social life can be challenging for people with schizophrenia because of the many myths that persist about the condition. NAMI (2007) noted that the discrimination against people with schizophrenia is fueled by these misconceptions. Cara and MacRae (2005) debunked these myths, explaining, for example, that people with schizophrenia tend not to be dangerous or violent and do not necessarily need to live in institutions or other highly structured facilities. For some people with schizophrenia, the prognosis is promising. They might have active and successful family, work, and community lives; there is evidence of recovery rates of more than 50% (Kruger, 2000). Citing data from a longitudinal study of people with schizophrenia, Kruger noted,

> Over the very long term of 2 to 4 decades the majority of persons diagnosed with schizophrenia not only did not deteriorate in functioning (as the accepted received body of psychiatric research would have it), but that their symptoms were seen to ameliorate and improve; and their functional levels were observed to return to premorbid or even higher levels. (p. 32)

Although this might seem overly optimistic for some, many people who have schizophrenia lead fulfilling and productive lives (Cara & MacRae, 2005). Clinicians need to include clients in the treatment process and ask clients themselves what makes them feel better; subjective measures of wellness (e.g., QoL assessments) might be helpful (Strauss, 2008). Collaborating with individuals to name what is important to them and what helps, identify meaningful goals, and obtain the skills and supports that they want and need are at the core of the Recovery Model.

Sexuality and intimacy

People with schizophrenia have identified relationships and sexuality as unmet needs in terms of QoL (Assalian, Fraser, Tempier, & Cohen, 2000; Fan et al., 2007; Schmidt et al., 2004). Managing time and connecting with others, including having an intimate relationship, have been identified as essential to QoL in people with schizophrenia: "'Having a good sexual relationship with someone,' realizing such life goals as having children and the fact that 'you grow old together, you learn together, you go through things together, phases'" is important (Laliberte-Rudman, Yu, Scott, & Pajouhandeh, 2000, p. 141). Occupational therapists who work with people with schizophrenia, therefore, need to address time management and daily structure, as well as social interaction and relational skills that lead to quality personal connections.

Perry and Wright (2006) found that people with SMIs were more likely to have longer-term relationships (i.e., more than 1 month) that do not lead to marriage or living together than are people without SMIs. They are also more likely to have more than one sexual partner at a time, less likely to wait 1 month before having intercourse with a new partner, and more likely to always use condoms during vaginal sex (Perry & Wright, 2006). Overall, their research revealed that people with SMI are less happy with their intimate relationships, and

> seem to take what they can get in terms of where, when, and with whom they have sex. This not only results in relationships that are less satisfying, less intimate, and much shorter-lived, but [it] also increases HIV risk by concentrating sexual activity within high-risk populations like IV drug users, sex workers, and others with serious mental illness. (p. 180)

One obstacle that gets in the way of people with SMI achieving the life goal of finding a partner is social stigma: "If you want a relationship with the opposite sex and they find out you're mentally ill . . . that will ruin everything'" (Laliberte-Rudman et al., 2000, p. 141). Aside from the difficulties that social stigma creates, schizophrenia has been associated with sexual dysfunction and relationship difficulties (Assalian et al., 2000; Fan et al., 2007; Kelly & Conley, 2004; Perry & Wright, 2006). Another difficulty for some people with schizophrenia in developing intimate relationships might be related to onset of the condition. When onset is during adolescence, a young person with SMI might have limited opportunities to date; therefore, he or she might also have limited opportunities to develop social skills, relational skills, and self-confidence. This limitation might leave him or her vulnerable to making risky sexual choices and to being sexually taken advantage of.

Medication side effects

Similar to depression, schizophrenia is associated with sexual symptoms that might be attributable to the condition itself or to the side effects of medication. Although some studies show increased sexual activity at the prodomal and early onset stages, schizophrenia has been associated with decreased desire (Assalian et al., 2000). However, Perry and Wright (2006) reported that people with schizophrenia might not have decreased desire overall and have the same needs to be sexually active as do all people.

Policies as barriers to healthy sexuality

Another challenging barrier for people with SMI to developing healthy intimate relationships might be "the generally negative sexual culture of treatment facilities . . . [that] can constrain behavior and opportunity for sexual interaction and can shape sexual activity when it does occur" (Perry & Wright, 2006, p. 179). Administrators and clinicians in residential, inpatient, and outpatient settings must balance consumers' rights to privacy and to association with people of their own choosing with their "right to be protected from sexual assault, sexual exploitation, or sexually transmitted disease" (Torkelson & Dobal, 1999, p. 157). Residential facilities can support QoL by including sexuality in both treatment and policy: "The long-term, residential environment can help or hinder the seriously mentally ill persons in their pursuit of their right to express and enjoy healthy sexual interactions" (Torkelson & Dobal, 1999, p. 156). Occupational therapists are in a position to help people with SMI not only through individual treatment and group work by helping to shape policies and programs in residential facilities and treatment centers:

> Occupational therapists [need] to attend to not only the barriers
> to occupation identified within a person, but also to the impact
> of external environments on occupation and quality of life. . . .
> Social and institutional environments can create handicaps for per-
> sons with mental illness. There is a potential advocacy role for
> occupational therapists to work with consumers to provide educa-
> tion aimed at changing attitudes regarding mental illness and to
> inform policy development relevant to those with mental illnesses.
> (Laliberte-Rudman et al., 2000, p. 145)

At the same time, sexual behaviors can pose risks for clients, which
must be taken into account. Supporting the sexuality of clients with mental
disorders while simultaneously protecting individuals from inappropriate or
abusive behaviors and sexually transmitted diseases makes sexuality a complex issue.

Mental Disorders and HIV/AIDS

Most mental disorders have been associated with risky sexual behaviors in
many populations, including those with substance abuse, major depression,
bipolar disorder, and schizophrenia, as well as with comorbid conditions.
These behaviors can lead to HIV/AIDS.

Risky Behaviors and Sexual Victimization

Risky sexual behaviors include having multiple partners, having intercourse
without using condoms, or exchanging sex for money. Substance use has
been associated with risky sexual behaviors, including users of stimulants,
intravenous drugs, and alcohol (Bousman et al., 2009; Calsyn et al., 2009;
Rotheram-Borus, Desmond, Comulada, Arnold, & Johnson, 2009). Drugs and
alcohol might lower inhibition, making it more likely that users participate in
sexual behaviors that they would avoid were they not intoxicated. Recently,
the use of methamphetamine has been a concern, as it is relatively readily available, highly addictive, and might both lower inhibitions and increase sexual
arousal (Centers for Disease Control and Prevention [CDC], 2007).

Adolescents and adults who are substance users and also have depressive symptoms are at an even higher risk of engaging in risky sexual behaviors (Bousman et al., 2009; Lee, Salman, & Fitzpatrick, 2009; Shrier, Harris,
Sternberg, & Beardslee, 2001).

Program components that have had positive outcomes for helping to decrease risky sexual behaviors in people who use substances include discussion

of social norms, use of role play, and development of coping strategies (Calsyn et al., 2009). Depression has been associated with risky sexual behaviors in people who use substances; therefore, therapeutic activities that develop self-efficacy, increase self-esteem, and instill a sense of hope are important to consider (Lejuez, Simmons, Aklin, Daughters, & Dvir, 2004).

In general, people with SMIs as a group are more likely to engage in risky sexual behaviors than people who do not have mental disorders (Senn & Carey, 2009). Senn and Carey (2009) identified difficulty with communication skills, lack of knowledge about safer sex practices, and decreased opportunity for long-term relationships as possible risk factors for unsafe sexual behaviors. People with SMI are also at risk of experiencing social factors that are associated with risky sexual behaviors (e.g., poverty, homelessness, living in neighborhoods with high rates of drug use, and estrangement from family and other social supports; Kloos et al., 2005). Mood disorders and substance use have also been associated with increased risk of sexual victimization in women (Meade et al., 2009; Messman-Moore, Coates, Gaffey, & Johnson, 2008).

Risky Behaviors and HIV/AIDS

The CDC (2007) and the WHO (2006) have identified both risky sexual behaviors and substance use as risk factors in the transmission of HIV/AIDS. When individuals use drugs or alcohol, they might be more likely to engage in risky sexual behaviors and thus are at a greater risk of contracting or transmitting HIV. Research has demonstrated this in many populations, including adolescents (Howard & Wang, 2004; Levy, Sherritt, Gabrielli, Shrier, & Knight, 2009), homeless and marginally housed adults (Rotheram-Borus et al., 2009), and adults in residential treatment (Lejuez et al., 2004).

Clinicians are encouraged by the WHO (2006) to involve clients with comorbid substance dependency and HIV/AIDS in treatment planning, intervention and service evaluation, along with providing peer support, advocacy, and community activities. This is compatible with occupational therapy's emphasis on client-centered practice. Programs that include motivational interviewing (e.g., open-ended questioning, empathy, reflection) have been found to be more effective than those that take a didactic-education-only approach (Mausbach, Semple, Strathdee, Zians, & Patterson, 2007; Morgenstern et al., 2009). Additional best practice components include repeated sessions, direct questions about sexuality (scripted if necessary), and appropriate medical interventions (e.g., antiretroviral therapy; Schreibman & Friedland, 2003).

Persons with SMIs are also at an increased risk of having HIV infection (Carey et al., 2004). SMIs are associated with persistent occupational and social dysfunction (Kloos et al., 2005). Individuals with SMIs have a wide range of abilities and challenges and may live in or receive services through inpatient hospitalization, outpatient clinics, day treatment programs, supportive housing, and community-based treatment. Occupational therapists who work with this population need to have a basic awareness of three areas related to SMI and HIV: (1) factors that affect risky sexual behaviors; (2) laws and policies regarding HIV testing, transmission, and reporting; and (3) best practices that are currently being studied.

SMIs reflect a heterogeneous population with varying symptoms and risk factors. Substance use, childhood sexual abuse, and sex trading have been identified as among the correlates of HIV infection in people with SMI (Meade & Sikkema, 2007). In their study of people with SMI, McKinnon, Cournos, and Herman (2001) found that a lifetime history of alcohol or drug dependency or abuse significantly increased the probability of having HIV. The authors examined the associations between specific psychiatric symptoms and risky sexual behaviors. For example, more severe cognitive symptomology (e.g., difficulty with abstract thinking, conceptual disorganizations, poor attention) was associated with increased probability of trading sex but was not associated with lifetime alcohol or drug use. The authors suggested that the association between cognitive difficulties and risky sex in people with SMIs might be explained by a perceived need to trade sex for housing or other survival needs or by vulnerability to coercion. Meade and Sikkema (2005) provide a review of risk factors associated with HIV transmission in people with SMIs, finding a correlation between risk behaviors (e.g., unprotected intercourse, multiple partners, injection drug use) and psychiatric illness, childhood abuse, substance use, and cognitive–behavioral issues.

HIV/AIDS Laws and Policies

All health care providers are required to follow policies and laws regarding patient confidentiality with regard to HIV status. However, laws and policies related to HIV testing, partner notification, and HIV transmission vary from state to state. Therefore, legal issues and ethical discussions are also part of the current landscape of SMI and HIV.

HIV transmission and partner notification

Therapists need to be aware of the laws and regulations regarding HIV transmission, partner notification, provider reporting, and patient confidentiality in their states, as well as the policies and mechanisms that operationalize these laws and policies in the workplace. In general, most states have laws that dictate criminal consequences for the knowing transmission of HIV (Lambda Legal, 2010). However, laws do vary widely from state to state.

New York, for example, has a partner notification law. According to the New York City Department of Health and Mental Hygiene (2012), doctors and those individuals who make medical diagnoses or laboratories that perform diagnostic tests, but not other service providers, report the names of people who have HIV. People with HIV are not required by law to reveal the names of people with whom they have had sexual contact. If a mental health provider is aware that client with HIV is having sexual contact with others and not informing them of his or her HIV status, confidentiality laws prohibit the clinician from warning those individuals. However, the clinician may inform the physician on the team, who then has the option but not the legal duty to warn (J. Satriano, Director of HIV/AIDS Programs, New York State Office of Mental Health, personal communication, February 27, 2012).

There is a specific protocol for partner notification that the physician needs to follow. Mental health professionals can counsel the client, encourage him or her to protect the health of partners by telling them of his or her HIV status and using safer sex practices, and provide access to condoms with instructions for their use. In an inpatient environment in which sexual contact has occurred, clinicians may warn patients to be aware of the risk of HIV transmission but may not identify people who are infected with HIV (J. Satriano, personal communication, February 27, 2012). The New York State Department of Health AIDS Institute (2007) provides guidelines for health care professionals who treat people with SMIs and HIV infection.

New York's laws and protocols are different from (and, in many cases, more liberal than) those of other states. In Michigan, for example, doctors are required by law to notify known sexual partners of people with HIV. People who know they are infected with HIV and have sexual contact without first informing partners of their HIV status (and having consent) are subject to criminal prosecution as felons (Michigan Department of Community Health Division of Health, Wellness, and Disease Control, 2006). Therefore, the obligations of mental health providers in Michigan may be different from those in New York. In both states, assistance is available for people with HIV to inform their partners. Lamba Legal (2010) provides an online summary of laws (which is not a substitute for legal advice).

HIV testing

Given the increased rate of HIV infection among people with SMIs, leaders in the mental health community have advocated for "more strenuous promotion of voluntary HIV testing programs" (Walkup, Satriano, Barry, Sadler, & Cournos, 2002, p. 1937) for people with SMIs. Testing would allow people with SMIs to get appropriate treatment and would have benefits for public health. In New York, although HIV screening is now required for every medical contact unless patients opt out in writing, mental capacity is an issue for psychiatric patients upon their admission to hospitals. The policy for these patients, therefore, is to first help them become stabilized and then to offer HIV testing prior to discharge (J. Satriano, personal communication, February 27, 2012).

The NAMI (2011) asserts in its public policy platform that "all persons with serious mental illnesses should be encouraged to be tested for HIV" (p. 9). Those who test positive should be provided with treatment, education, counseling, and peer support.

HIV interventions

Although individuals with SMIs are at an increased risk of HIV infection, "relatively few interventions" have been targeted for this population thus far (Kloos et al., 2005, p. 358). Intervention research is at its beginning stages, and results for interventions have been mixed. However, research-based interventions do hold promise for increasing risk awareness and changing risky behaviors.

Results from small-group intervention in psychiatric outpatient treatment for people with SMI and alcohol or drug use found that women who increased their HIV knowledge and interaction skills had fewer casual sexual partners, engaged in less unprotected sex, talked more to their partners, and had fewer STDs (Carey et al., 2004). However, a randomized controlled trial did not yield significant reduction of risky sexual behaviors in men with SMI in outpatient and day hospital settings (Berkman et al., 2007).

Kloos et al. (2005) suggested that because people who live in supportive housing are ready to make changes in their lives, targeted interventions in this environment has potential for efficacy. Such interventions must also consider prevention strategies for when individuals leave supportive structures. The authors found that people with SMIs who lived in supportive housing had knowledge of HIV prevention and no cognitive limitations that would impede their abilities to learn strategies to protect themselves and others. Impediments may be related to motivational and emotional factors, as well as structural factors related to program implementation.

Interventions that address the prevention of HIV transmission among people with SMIs must consider factors that are specific to this group and their living situations (e.g., stigma, motivation, transitional living; Kloos et al, 2005). Program components that have been suggested include HIV education, assertiveness and social interaction training, inclusion of drug-related behaviors, problem-solving, and personal risk management; gender differences also need to be taken into account (McKinnon, Cournos, & Herman, 2002).

McKinnon et al. (2002) stated that to be considered comprehensive, treatment programs for people with SMI need to include HIV prevention; the authors suggested implementation of evidence-based intervention "similar to psychosocial rehabilitation programs" (p. 27). McKinnon et al. exhorted mental health professionals to take an active role and use interventions that help clients to "personalize the risk, find the motivation to act more safely, and believe in their capacity to execute the skills needed to make the appropriate changes" (p. 27).

HIV transmission and SMI is a complex issue that has legal, ethical, health, and practice implications. Collaboration with a team is essential to understand institutional policy and the ways in which state laws are implemented and also to provide interventions that address the prevention of HIV transmission and promote healthy sexual behaviors.

Mental health professionals must balance client confidentiality with public health concerns (Senn & Carey, 2009). Knowledge of the law is necessary, and working with a team may be the best approach to address ethical and legal concerns as well as client health and well-being. HIV prevention interventions that are integrated into existing mental health programming for adults with SMI have been found to be cost-effective (Johnson-Masotti, Pinkerton, Kelly, & Stevenson, 2000) and can be delivered in health care facilities, day treatment, supportive housing, and community-based programs.

Assessments

When addressing sexuality with people who have mental disorders, many assessment tools might be helpful in clarifying client needs and priorities and framing sexuality within the broader context of psychosocial treatment. Occupational therapists might use findings from assessments to help clients set goals, identify appropriate treatment interventions, and collaborate with other clinicians who are part of the treatment team. The following are assessment tools that can be used in a client-centered assessment process when sexuality and intimacy are areas of concern.

Adolescent and Adult Sensory Profile

The Adolescent and Adult Sensory Profile (AASP; Brown & Dunn, 2002) is a 60-item self-report questionnaire that assesses sensory responses to visual, auditory, tactile, taste and smell, activity level, and movement stimuli. The AASP is evidence-based and provides a measure of sensory responsivity and modulation. *Sensory modulation* is defined by Miller, Reisman, McIntosh, and Simon (2001) as "the capacity to regulate and organize the degree, intensity, and nature of responses to sensory input in a graded and adaptive manner" (p. 57).

The AASP organizes patterns of behavior that describe the interaction between neurological thresholds (amount of stimuli needed for response) and behavioral responses (active or passive responses to stimuli). Sensory modulation dysfunction might include oversensitivity, overarousal, or underregistration, which might functionally present as difficulty with emotion regulation, interpersonal relationships, and engagement in daily occupations (Champagne, Koomar, & Olson, 2010).

Differences in sensory processing have been long been associated with such developmental disabilities as autism spectrum disorders, but they also are associated with some mental disorders (Champagne et al., 2010). For example, people with schizophrenia and bipolar disorder have been found to present with a pattern of sensory avoidance; those with schizophrenia also demonstrated low sensory registration (Brown, Cromwell, Filion, Dunn, & Tollefson, 2002). Sensory processing differences have also been found in people who have PTSD (Stewart & White, 2008) and obsessive–compulsive disorder (Rieke & Anderson, 2009).

The AASP can help people with mental disorders understand sensory-processing issues that might impede their abilities to reach goals related to emotional and physical intimacy. For example, an individual who has high sensitivity (e.g., hypersensitivity to touch) might react negatively to a potential partner's light touch without understanding why. Occupational therapists can help clients understand the neural basis of their response patterns, use sensory-based and other strategies to treat them, teach cognitive and coping strategies to manage negative responses, and suggest environmental modifications. Wollenberg (2001) described a man with schizophrenia whose goal was to be involved in an intimate relationship:

> He wanted to increase his socialization and specifically, he wanted
> to get a girlfriend. It hurt his feelings as well as his chance to achieve

his goals when he heard others commenting on his poor hygiene. For this reason, he decided to explore the issue with his occupational therapist, even though he did not think the problem was that bad. . . . The results of . . . [the AASP] revealed that the consumer had low sensory registration. In other words, he required more sensory input than normal to recognize sensory triggers such as odors. . . . This shared knowledge between the occupational therapist and the consumer provided a strong foundation for working together to find a solution to the barriers that were keeping him from his goals. (pp. 105–106)

Arizona Sexual Experience Scale

The ASEX (McGahuey et al., 2000) is one of several self-report instruments that assesses sexual responses. Typically, these instruments are used to measure changes in sexual responses that are secondary to medication side effects. Occupational therapists who are working on issues of sexuality with people who are taking medications to treat depression, bipolar disorder, or schizophrenia might consider using such a checklist in collaboration with the client's physician. Information can then be shared as the physician adjusts medications to treat sexual side effects as well as the presenting mental disorder or disability.

Assessment of Communication and Interaction Skills

The Assessment of Communication and Interaction Skills (ACIS; Forsyth, Salamy, Simon, & Kielhofner, 1998) is an observation tool that provides a structured format to gather information about communication during social activity. The assessment looks at interaction in three domains: (1) physicality (e.g., gazes, postures), (2) information exchange (e.g., asserts, shares), and (3) relations (e.g., focuses, respects). The ACIS can be used to assess skills in both group and dyadic activities, which makes it useful for people who are working on developing healthy relationships. Data are recorded using a Likert-type scale to help identify communication habits that might obstruct positive social interactions.

Beck Depression Inventory

The Beck Depression Inventory, 2nd Edition (BDI–II; Beck, Steer, & Brown, 1996) is a 21-item self-report questionnaire. The BDI–II is not considered to be a diagnostic tool; rather, it assesses the presence or severity of symptoms in a person who has been diagnosed with depression. Respondents rate themselves on individual items on a 0–3 scale, depending on how they have felt in the preceding 2 weeks. Item scores are then added, yielding a total score that corresponds to a category of depression: mild, borderline, moderate, severe, or extreme. Some items on the scale are related to issues of sexuality and intimacy (e.g., decreased libido, social withdrawal, body image).

Canadian Occupational Performance Measure

The Canadian Occupational Performance Measure (COPM; Law et al., 2005) is an outcome measure that follows a semistructured interview format and uses structured scoring. Using a client-based approach, clinicians obtain information about clients' perceptions of their performance and satisfaction in many occupational domains, including self-care, productivity, and socialization. The client might bring up issues related to sexuality, or the clinician might gently introduce them. Goals are then collaboratively determined based on the client's priorities. The COPM is designed to be used with people with a variety of developmental levels and disabling conditions and could also be used with their caregivers and family members.

Hamilton Rating Scale for Depression

The Hamilton Rating Scale for Depression (HRSD; Hamilton, 1960) is an inventory that assesses the severity of symptoms in people who have already been diagnosed with depression. The inventory is designed to be completed by a clinician. Items—insomnia, anxiety, work or activity, and so on—are rated on a scale of 0–4 or 0–2. One item refers to sexual functioning. Originally published in 1960, the HRSD is now in the public domain and exists in several versions that contain 17 or 21 items. Scoring depends upon the version that is used. The HRSD is available online at a variety of Web sites.

Quality of Life Instruments

Many instruments are available that measure self-perceived QoL. Health-related quality of life (HrQoL) instruments have also been developed to assess HrQoL for clients with specific conditions. Instruments generally use a Likert-type scale to collect quantitative data about many life domains, including sexuality. One example, the Quality of Life Inventory (Frisch, 1994), is composed of 16 areas of functioning that include self-esteem, health, and love.

It is important to note, however, that quantitative assessments might not always give an accurate picture of perceived QoL, including in the area of sexuality, for people who have mental disorders and disabilities (Fan et al.,

2007). Depending on the client, it might also be preferable to include more qualitative approaches (e.g., guided interviews).

Zung Depression Scale

The Zung Depression Scale (Zung, 1965) is a self-report symptom inventory for people who have been previously diagnosed with depression. Similar to the HRSD, the scale is designed to assess severity of depression rather than to diagnose the disorder. There are 20 items on the inventory, and each is rated on a scale of 1–4. One item relates to sexuality. The final score falls into a range that indicates one of four categories: normal, mild, moderate, or severe depression. Adaptations and scoring information are available online at many Web sites.

Summary

Sexuality is a QoL component that is part of humanity. This chapter provided an overview of several mental disorders and related issues of sexuality that might accompany them. Occupational therapy, with its emphasis on life roles and client-centered practice, is positioned to be one of the health care professions that address the development of healthy sexuality and fulfilling relationships in clients with mental disorders. More research, programming, and education is needed in the area of sexuality and mental health to better understand how occupational therapy can contribute to this practice area, and how best to help clients develop healthy sexual identities and fulfilling life roles as partners.

Acknowledgment

The author thanks Robin Kahan-Berman, OTR/L, for generously sharing her knowledge, expertise, and ideas in preparing to write this chapter.

References

Ace, K. J. (2007). Mental health, mental illness, and sexuality. In M. S. Tepper & A. F. Owens (Eds.), *Sexual health, Vol. 1: Psychological foundations* (Praeger Perspectives: Sex, Love, and Psychology, pp. 301–329). Westport, CT: Praeger/ Greenwood.

American Occupational Therapy Association. (2008). Occupational therapy practice framework: Domain and process (2nd ed.). *American Journal of Occupational Therapy, 62,* 625–683. doi:10.5014/ajot.62.6.625

American Occupational Therapy Association. (2009). *Medicare delays implementation of ICD–10 coding system to October 2013.* Retrieved July 12, 2012, from http://www.aota.org/Practitioners/Reimb/News/Archives/News-Archive/icd10. aspx

American Psychiatric Association. (2000). *Diagnostic and statistical manual of mental disorders* (rev. 4th ed.). Washington, DC: Author.

Assalian, P., Fraser, R., Tempier, R., & Cohen, D. (2000). Sexuality and quality of life of patients with schizophrenia. *International Journal of Psychiatry in Clinical Practice, 4,* 29–33.

Balon, R. (2007). Depression, antidepressants, and human sexuality. *Primary Psychiatry, 14*(2), 42–50. Retrieved April 9, 2010, from http://www.primarypsychiatry.com/aspx/article_pf.aspx?articleid=990

Bancroft, J., Janssen, E., Strong, D. Carnes, L., Vukadinovic, Z., & Long, J. S. (2003). The relation between mood and sexuality in heterosexual men. *Archives of Sexual Behavior, 32*(3), 217–230.

Baum, C. (2008). *Posttraumatic stress disorder (PTSD) treatment and research: Moving toward recovery.* Witness Testimony for House Committee on Veterans' Affairs, April 1, 2008. Retrieved April 24, 2010, from http://veterans.house.gov/hearings/Testimony.aspx?TID=560&Newsid=2071

Beck, A. T., Steer, R. A., & Brown, G. K. (1996). *Beck Depression Inventory* (2nd ed.). San Antonio, TX: Psychological Corporation.

Berkman, A., Pilowsky, D. J., Zybert, P.A., Herman, D. B., Conover, S., Lemelle, S., et al. (2007). HIV prevention with severely mentally ill men: A randomized controlled trial. *AIDS Care, 19*(5), 579–588.

Bonder, B. R. (2010). *Psychopathology and function* (4th ed.). Thorofare, NJ: Slack.

Bousman, C. A., Cherner, M., Ake, C., Letendre, S., Atkinson, J. H., Patterson, T. L., et al. (2009). Negative mood and sexual behavior among nonmonogamous men who have sex with men in the context of methamphetamine and HIV. *Journal of Affective Disorders, 119,* 84–91. doi:10.1016/j.jad2009.04.006

Brown, C., Cromwell, R. L., Filion, D., Dunn, W., & Tollefson, N. (2002). Sensory processing in schizophrenia: Missing and avoiding information. *Schizophrenia Research, 55*(1), 187–195.

Brown, C., & Dunn, W. (2002). *Adolescent/Adult Sensory Profile manual.* San Antonio, TX: Psychological Corporation.

Calsyn, D. A., Hatch-Mallette, M., Tross, S., Doyle, S. R., Crits-Christoph, P., Song, Y. S., et al. (2009). Motivational and skills training HIV/sexually transmitted infection sexual risk reduction groups for men. *Journal of Substance Abuse Treatment, 37,* 138–150.

Cara, E., & MacRae, A. (2005). *Psychosocial occupational therapy: A clinical practice* (2nd ed.). Clifton Park, NY: Delmar.

Carey, M. P., Carey, K. B., Maisto, S. A., Gordon, C. M., Schroder, K. E. E., & Vanable, P. A. (2004). Reducing HIV-risk behavior among adults receiving outpatient psychiatric treatment: Results from a randomized controlled trial. *Journal of Consulting and Clinical Psychology, 72*(2), 252–268.

Centers for Disease Control and Prevention. (2007). *Methamphetamine use and risk for HIV/AIDS* [CDC HIV/AIDS Fact Sheet]. Available at http://www.cdc.gov/hiv/resources/factsheets/meth.htm

Champagne, T., Koomar, J., & Olson, L. (2010). Sensory processing evaluation and intervention in mental health. *OT Practice, 15*(5), CE1–CE8.

Chekuri, V., Gerber, D., Brodie, A., & Krishnadas, R. (2012). Premature ejaculation and other sexual dysfunctions in opiate dependent men receiving methadone substitution treatment. *Addictive Behaviors, 37*(1), 124–126.

Cohen S, Kühn, K. U., Sträter, B., Scherbaum, N., & Weig, W. (2010). Adverse side-effects on sexual function caused by psychotropic drugs and psychotropic substances. *Nervenartz, 81*(9), 1129–1137.

Dell'Osso, L., Carmassi, C., Carlini, M., Rucci, P, Torri, P., Cesari, D., et al. (2009). Sexual dysfunctions and suicidality in patients with bipolar disorder and unipolar depression. *Journal of Sexual Medicine, 6,* 3063–3070. doi:10.111 1/j.1743-6109.2009.01455.

Dickerson, F. B., Brown, C. H., Kreyenbuhl, J., Goldberg, R. W., Fang, L. J., & Dixon, L. B. (2004). Sexual and reproductive behaviors among persons with mental illness. *Psychiatric Services, 55*(11), 1299–1301.

Esmail, S., Darry, K., Walter, A., & Knupp, H. (2010). Attitudes and perceptions towards disability and sexuality. *Disability and Rehabilitation, 32*(14), 1148–1155. doi:10.3109/0963820903419277

Fan, X., Henderson, D. C., Chiang, E., Briggs, L. B., Freudenreich, O., Evins, A. E., et al. (2007). Sexual functioning, psychopathology and quality of life in patients with schizophrenia. *Schizophrenia Research, 94,* 119–127.

Forsyth, K., Salamy, M., Simon, S., & Kielhofner, G. (1998). *The Assessment of Communication and Interaction Skills (ACIS).* Chicago: University of Illinois at Chicago, Model of Human Occupation Clearinghouse. Available at http://www.uic.edu/depts/moho/assess/acis.html

Frisch, M. B. (1994). *Quality of Life Inventory: Manual and treatment guide.* Minneapolis: National Computer Systems.

Garte, S. H. (1989). Sexuality and intimacy in Vietnam veterans with posttraumatic stress disorder (PTSD). *Psychotherapy in Private Practice, 7*(2), 103–112.

Gavloski, T., & Lyons, J. A. (2004). Psychological sequelae of combat violence: A review of the impact of PTSD on the veteran's family and possible interventions. *Aggression and Violent Behavior, 9,* 477–501.

Gordon, P. A., Tschopp, M. K., & Feldman, D. (2004). Addressing issues of sexuality with adolescents with disabilities. *Child and Adolescent Social Work Journal, 21,* 513–527.

Green, C. A., Knysz, W., & Tsuang, M. T. (2000). A homeless person with bipolar disorder and a history of serious self-mutilation. *American Journal of Psychiatry, 157*(9), 1392–1397.

Grieger, T. A., Cozza, S. J., Ursano, R. J., Hoge, C., Martinez, P. E., Engel, C. C., et al. (2006). Posttraumatic stress disorder and depression in battle-injured soldiers. *American Journal of Psychiatry, 163,* 1777–1783. doi:10.5014/ajot.54.2.137

Hamilton, M. (1960). A rating scale for depression. *Journal of Neurology, Neurosurgery, and Psychiatry, 23,* 56–62.

Hirschfield, R. M. (1999). Management of sexual side effects of antidepressant therapy. *Journal of Clinical Psychiatry, 60*(14), 27–35.

Howard, D. E., & Wang, M. Q. (2004). The relationship between substance use and STD/HIV-related sexual risk behaviors among U.S. adolescents. *Journal of HIV/AIDS Prevention in Children and Youth, 6*(2), 65–82.

Hussaarts, P., Roozen, H. G., Meyers, R. J., van de Wetering, B. J., & McCrady, B. S. (2012). Problem areas reported by substance abusing individuals and their concerned significant others. *American Journal on Addictions, 21*(1), 38–46.

Johnson-Masotti, A. P., Pinkerton, S. D., Kelly, J. A., & Stevenson, L. Y. (2000). Cost-effectiveness of an HIV risk reduction intervention for adults with severe mental illness. *AIDS Care, 12*(3), 321–332.

Kelly, D. L., & Conley, R. R. (2004). Sexuality and schizophrenia: A review. *Schizophrenia Bulletin, 30*(4), 767–779.

Kennedy, S. H., Dickens, S. E., Eisfeld, B. S., & Bagby, R. M. (1999). Sexual dysfunction before antidepressant therapy in major depression. *Journal of Affective Disorders, 56*, 201–208.

Kennedy, S. H., & Rizvi, S. (2009). Sexual dysfunction, depression, and the impact of antidepressants. *Journal of Clinical Psychopharmacology, 29*(2), 157–164.

Kloos, B., Gross, S. M., Meese, K. J.., Meade, C. S., Doughty, J. D., Hawkins, D. D., et al. (2005). Negotiating risk: Knowledge and use of HIV prevention by persons with serious mental illness living in supportive housing. *American Journal of Community Psychology, 36*(3/4), 357–372.

Kruger, A. (2000). Schizophrenia: Recovery and hope. *Psychiatric Rehabilitation Journal, 24*(1), 29–37.

Laliberte-Rudman, B., Yu, B., Scott, E., & Pajouhandeh, P. (2000). Exploration of the perspectives of persons with schizophrenia regarding quality of life. *American Journal of Occupational Therapy, 54*(2), 137–147. doi:10.5014/ajot.54.2.137

Lambda Legal. (2010). *HIV criminalization: State laws criminalizing conduct based on HIV status.* Retrieved from February 26, 2012, from http://www.lambdalegal. org/publications/fs_hiv-criminalization

Lapierre, C. B., Schwegler, A. F., LaBauve, B. J. (2007). Posttraumatic stress and depression symptoms in soldiers returning from combat operations in Iraq and Afghanistan. *Journal of Traumatic Stress, 20*(6), 933–943.

Law, M., Baptiste, S., Carswell, A., McColl, M. A., Polatajko, H., & Pollock, N. (2005). *Canadian Occupational Performance Measure manual* (4th ed.). Toronto: CAOT Publications ACE.

Lee, Y. H., Salman, A., & Fitzpatrick, J. J. (2009). HIV/AIDS preventive self-efficacy, depressive symptoms, and risky sexual behavior in adolescents: A cross-sectional questionnaire survey. *International Journal of Nursing Studies, 46*, 653–660.

Lejuez, C. W., Simmons, B. L., Aklin, W. M., Daughters, S. B., & Dvir, S. (2004). Risk-taking propensity and risky sexual behavior of individuals in residential substance use treatment. *Addictive Behaviors, 29*, 1643–1647. doi:10.1016/j. addbeh.2004.02.035

Levy, S., Sherritt, L., Gabrielli, J., Shrier, L. A., & Knight, J. R. (2009). Screening adolescents for substance use: Related high-risk sexual behaviors. *Journal of Adolescent Health, 45*, 473–477.

Lykins, A. D., Janssen, E., & Graham, C. A. (2006). The relationship between negative mood and sexuality in heterosexual college women and men. *Journal of Sex Research, 43*(2), 136–143.

Lyons, J. A. (2009). Intimate relations and the military. In S. M. Freeman, B. A. Moore, & A. Freeman (Eds.), *Living and surviving in harm's way: A psychological treatment handbook for pre- and post-deployment of military personnel* (pp. 371–394). New York: Routledge.

Maitra, K. K., & Erway, F. (2006). Perception of client-centered practice in occupational therapists and their clients. *American Journal of Occupational Therapy, 60*, 298–310. doi:10.5014/ajot.60.3.298

Manderscheid, R. W., Ryff, C. D., Freeman, E. J., McKnight-Eily, L. R., Dhinga, S., & Strine, T. W. (2010). Evolving definitions of mental health and wellness. *Preventing Chronic Disease: Public Health Research, Practice, and Policy, 7*(1), A19.

Mausbach, B. T., Semple, S. J., Strathdee, S. A., Zians, J., & Patterson, T. L. (2007). Efficacy of a behavioral intervention for increasing safer sex behaviors in HIV-negative heterosexual methamphetamine users: Results from the Fast-Lane study. *Annals of Behavioral Medicine, 34*(3), 263–274.

Mayo Clinic. (2010). *Alcoholism: Complications.* Retrieved July 12, 2012, from http://www.mayoclinic.com/health/alcoholism/ds00340/dsection=complications

McGahuey, C. A., Gelenberg, A. J., Laukes, C. A., Moreno, F. A., Delgado, P. L., McKnight, K. M., et al. (2000). The Arizona Sexual Experience Scale (ASEX): Reliability and validity. *Journal of Sex and Marital Therapy, 26*(1), 25–40.

McKinnon, K., Cournos, F., & Herman, R. (2001). A lifetime alcohol or other drug use disorder and specific psychiatric symptoms predict sexual risk for HIV infection among people with severe mental illness. *AIDS and Behavior, 5*(3), 233–240.

McKinnon, K, Cournos, F., & Herman, R. (2002). HIV among people with chronic mental illness. *Psychiatric Quarterly, 73*(1), 17–31.

Meade, C. S., McDonald, L. J., Graff, F. S., Fitzmaurice, G. M., Griffin, M. L., & Weiss, R. D. (2009). A prospective study examining the effects of gender and sexual/physical abuse on mood outcomes in patients with co-occurring bipolar I and substance use disorders. *Bipolar Disorders, 11*(4), 425–433.

Meade, C. S., & Sikkema, K. J. (2005). HIV risk behavior among adults with severe mental illness: A systematic review. *Clinical Psychology Review, 25*, 433–457.

Meade, C. S., & Sikkema, K. J. (2007). Psychiatric and psychosocial correlates of sexual risk behavior among adults with severe mental illness. *Community Mental Health Journal, 43*(2), 153–169.

Messman-Moore, T. L., Coates, A. A., Gaffey, K. J., & Johnson, C. F. (2008). Sexuality, substance use, and susceptibility to victimization: Risk for rape and sexual coercion in a prospective study of college women. *Journal of Interpersonal Violence, 23*(12), 1730–1746.

Michigan Department of Community Health Division of Health, Wellness, and Disease Control. (2006). *Michigan HIV laws: How they affect physicians and other health care providers.* Retrieved February 26, 2012, from http://michigan.gov/documents/mihivlaws_49845_7.pdf

Miller, L. J., Reisman, J., McIntosh, D., & Simon, J. (2001). An ecological model of sensory modulation: Performance of children with Fragile X syndrome, autistic disorder, attention deficit hyperactivity disorder, and sensory modulation dysfunction. In S. Smith Roley, E. Blanche, & R. Schaaf (Eds.), *Understanding the nature of sensory integration with diverse populations* (pp. 57–82). San Antonio, TX: Therapy Skill Builders.

Monson, C. M., Taft, C. T., & Fredman, S. J. (2009). Military-related PTSD and intimate relationships: From description to theory-driven research and intervention development. *Clinical Psychology Review, 29*(8), 707–714.

Morgenstern, J., Bux, D. A., Parsons, J., Hagman, D. T., Wainberg, M., & Milton, T. (2009). Randomized trial to reduce club drug use and HIV risk behaviors with men who have sex with men. *Journal of Consulting and Clinical Psychology, 77*(4), 645–656.

National Alliance on Mental Illness. (2007). *Mental illnesses: Schizophrenia.* Retrieved May 14, 2010, from http://www.nami.org

National Association of Mental Illness. (2011). *Public policy platform.* Retrieved February 26, 2012, from http://www.nami.org/Template.cfm?Section=NAMI_Policy_Platform&Template=/ContentManagement/ContentDisplay.cfm&ContentID=105506

National Center on Addiction and Substance Abuse at Columbia University. (1999). *Dangerous liaisons: Substance abuse and sex.* New York: Author.

National Institute of Mental Health. (2008). *The numbers count: Mental disorders in America.* Retrieved April 6, 2010, from http://nimh.nih.gov/health/publications/the-numbers-count- mental-disorders-in-America/index.shtml

National Institute of Mental Health. (2009a). *Statistics.* Retrieved March 31, 2010, from http://nimh.nih.gov/statisitcs/index.shtml

National Institute of Mental Health. (2009b). *What are the symptoms of bipolar disorder?* Retrieved August 11, 2011, from http://www.nimh.nih.gov/health/publications/bipolar-disorder/what-are-the-symptoms-of-bipolar-disorder.shtml

National Institute of Mental Health. (2009c). *What are the symptoms of PTSD?* Retrieved August 11, 2011, from http://www.nimh.nih.gov/health/publications/post-traumatic-stress-disorder-ptsd/what-are-the-symptoms-of-ptsd.shtml

National Institute of Mental Health. (2009d). *What are the symptoms of schizophrenia?* Retrieved August 11, 2011, from http://www.nimh.nih.gov/health/publications/schizophrenia/what-are-the-symptoms-of-schizophrenia.shtml

National Institute of Mental Health. (2011). *What are the signs and symptoms of depression?* Retrieved August 11, 2011, from http://www.nimh.nih.gov/health/publications/depression/what-are-the-signs-and-symptoms-of-depression.shtml

National Institute on Drug Abuse. (2011). *InfoFacts: Understanding drug abuse and addiction.* Retrieved February 11, 2012, from http://www.drugabuse.gov/pub lications/infofacts/understanding-drug-abuse-addiction

National Institutes of Health. (2012). *Drug abuse.* Retrieved April 11, 2012, from http://www.nlm.nih.gov/medlineplus/ency/article/001945.htm

New York State Department of Health, AIDS Institute. (2007). *Severe and persistent mental illness in HIV-infected patients.* Retrieved February 26, 2012, from http://www.hivguidelines.org/clinical-guidelines/hiv-and-mental-health/severe-and-persistent-mental-illness-in-hiv-infected-patients/

New York City Department of Health and Mental Hygiene. (2012). *HIV/AIDS Information: HIV reporting/partner notification law.* Retrieved February 26, from http://www.nyc.gov/html/doh/html/ah/ahn1.shtml

O'Day, K. (2009). *Effectiveness of treatment techniques for substance abuse in occupational therapy.* Retrieved July 13, 2012, from http://commons.paci ficu.edu/cgi/viewcontent.cgi?article=1005&context=otmh&sei-redir=1& referer=http%3A%2F%2Fwww.bing.com%2Fsearch%3Fq%3DEffectiveness %2Bof%2Btreatment%2Btechniques%2Bfor%2Bsubstance%2Babuse%2Bin %2Boccupational%2Btherapy%26src%3DIE-SearchBox%26FORM%3DIE8 SRC#search=%22Effectiveness%20treatment%20techniques%20substance% 20abuse%20occupational%20therapy%22

O'Donnell, M. L., Creamer, M., & Pattison, P. (2004). Posttraumatic stress disorder and depression following trauma: Understanding comorbidity. *American Journal of Psychiatry, 161*(8), 1390–1396.

Opp, A. (2009). *Recovery with purpose: Occupational therapy and drug and alcohol abuse.* Retrieved July 12, 2012, from http://www.aota.org/Consumers/Profes sionals/WhatIsOT/MH/Articles/RecoveryWithPurpose.aspx

Ostman, M. (2008). Severe depression and relationships: The effect of mental illness on sexuality. *Sexual and Relationship Therapy, 23*(4), 355–363.

Perry, B. L., & Wright, E. R. (2006). The sexual partnerships of people with serious mental illness. *Journal of Sex Research, 43*(2), 174–181.

Ray, S. L., & Vanstone, M. (2009). The impact of PTSD on veterans' family relationships: An interpretative phenomenological inquiry. *International Journal of Nursing Studies, 46,* 838–847.

Rieke, E. F., & Anderson, D. (2009). Adolescent/adult sensory profile and obsessive–compulsive disorder. *American Journal of Occupational Therapy, 63,* 138–145.

Rotheram-Borus, M. J., Desmond, K., Comulada, W. S., Arnold, E. M., & Johnson, M. (2009). Reducing risky sexual behavior and substance use among currently and formerly homeless adults living with HIV. *American Journal of Public Health, 99*(6), 1100–1107.

Schmidt, K., Staupendahl, A., & Vollmoeller, W. (2004). Quality of life of schizophrenic psychiatric outpatients as a criterion for treatment planning in psychiatric institutions. *International Journal of Social Psychiatry, 50,* 262– 273. doi:10.1177/0020764004043140

Schnurr, P. P., Lunney, C. A., Bovin, M. J., & Marx, B. P. (2009). Posttraumatic stress disorder and quality of life: Extension of findings to veterans of the wars in Iraq and Afghanistan. *Clinical Psychology Review, 29,* 727–735.

Schreibman, T., & Friedland, G. (2003). Human immunodeficiency virus infection prevention: Strategies for clinicians. *Clinical Infectious Diseases, 36,* 1171–1176.

Senn, T. E., & Carey, M. P. (2009). HIV testing among individuals with a severe mental illness: Review, suggestions for research, and clinical implications. *Psychological Medicine, 39,* 355–363.

Shrier, L. A., Harris, S. K., Sternberg, M., & Beardslee, R. W. (2001). Associations of depression, self-esteem, and substance use with sexual risk among adolescents. *Preventive Medicine 33,* 179–189.

Solomon, Z., Deckel, R., & Zerach, G. (2008). The relationships between posttraumatic stress symptom clusters and marital intimacy among war veterans. *Journal of Family Psychology, 22*(5), 659–666.

Solovitch, S. (2009, Spring). Opening the door on hypersexuality. *Bipolar Magazine, 5,* 24–32. Available at http://www.bphope.com/Item.aspx/522/opening-the-door-on-Hypersexuality

Stewart, L. P., & White, P. M. (2008). Sensory filtering phenomenology in PTSD. *Depression and Anxiety, 25,* 38–45.

Strauss, J. S. (2008) Prognosis in schizophrenia and the role of subjectivity. *Schizophrenia Bulletin, 34*(2), 201–203. doi:10.1093/schbul/sbn001

Stoffel, V. C., & Moyers, P. A. (2004). An evidence-based and occupational perspective of interventions for persons with substance use disorders. *American Journal of Occupational Therapy, 58,* 570–586. doi:10.5014/ajot.58.5.570

Substance Abuse and Mental Health Service Administration. (2006). *National consensus statement on mental health recovery.* Retrieved April 25, 2010, from http://store.samhsa.gov/shin/content//SMA05-4129/SMA05-4129.pdf

Substance Abuse and Mental Health Service Administration. (2008). *Results from the 2008 national survey on drug use and health: National findings.* Retrieved April 6, 2010, from http://www.oas.samhsa.gov/nsduh/2k8nsduh/2k8Results.pdf

Taft, C. T., Watkins, L. E., Stafford, J., Street, A. E., & Monson, C. M. (2011). Posttraumatic stress disorder and intimate relationship problems: A meta-analysis. *Journal of Consulting and Clinical Psychology, 79*(1), 22–33.

Taylor, R. R. (2008). *The intentional relationship: Occupational therapy and use of self.* Philadelphia: F. A. Davis.

Torkelson, D. J., & Dobal, M. T. (1999). Sexual rights of people with serious and persistent mental illness: Gathering evidence for decision making. *Journal of the American Psychiatric Nurses Association, 5,* 150–161.

Tuchner, M., Meiner, Z., Parush, S., & Hartman-Maeir, A. (2010). Relationships between sequelae of injury, participation, and quality of life in survivors of terrorist attacks. *Occupational Therapy Journal of Research: Occupation, Participation, and Health, 30*(1), 29–38.

Walkup, J., Satriano, J., Barry, M., Sadler, P., & Cournos, F. (2002). HIV testing policy and serious mental illness. *American Journal of Public Health, 92*(12), 1931–1940.

Whetstone, W. R., & Rich, A. C. (1999). Friendship, intimacy, and sexuality among person with serious mental illness. *Visions: BC's Mental Health Journal, 8.* Retrieved February 7, 2010, from http://www.cmha.bc.ca/files/08.pdf

Wollenberg, J. L. (2001). Recovery and occupational therapy in the community mental health setting. In C. Brown (Ed.), *Recovery and wellness: Models of hope and empowerment for people with mental illness* (pp. 97–114). New York: Haworth.

World Health Organization. (2001). *International classification of functioning, disability and health (ICF).* Geneva: Author. Available at http://apps.who.int/classifications/icfen/

World Health Organization. (2004). *The World Health Organization Quality of Life Questionnaire (WHOQOF–BREF).* Geneva: Author.

World Health Organization. (2006). *Basic principles for treatment and psychosocial support of drug dependent people living with HIV/AIDS.* Geneva: Author.

World Health Organization. (2010). *International classification of diseases (1CD–10).* Geneva: Author. Available at http://apps.who.int/classifications/apps/icd/icd10online/

World Health Organization. (2012). *Health topics: Sexual health.* Retrieved March 1, 2012, from http://www.who.int/topics/sexual_health/en/

Zung, W. W. (1965). A self-rating depression scale. *Archives of General Psychiatry, 12*(1), 63–70.

10

~

Adolescents With Disabilities and Sexuality

Christine Linkie, MS, OTR/L, and Bernadette Hattjar,
DrOT, MEd, OTR/L, CWCE

Key Terms and Concepts

- Egocentrism
- Erikson's eight stages of psychosocial development
- Intimacy
- Secondary sex characteristics
- Therapeutic use of self
- Use of groups.

Upon completion of this chapter, readers will be able to

- Identify components and stages of sexual development and sexual identity development;
- Compare the experiences of adolescents with and without disabilities related to the development of healthy sexual identity;
- Discuss the effect of chronic disability on the development and persona of the sexual self;
- Describe characteristics of chronic disabilities and conditions associated with childhood and adolescence and some of their effects on physical and psychosocial development;
- Illustrate the application of the *Occupational Therapy Practice Framework* in addressing sexuality with adolescents who have disabilities;

229

- Give examples of important factors to consider when addressing adolescent sexuality; and

- Integrate information about group approaches to address sexual activity and sexuality in young people.

Introduction

Physical and psychosocial development occurs in all living beings. Sexual maturation is, quite simply, a part of the life cycle. The maturation process usually proceeds in a specific manner and moves the individual from infancy to adulthood.

Adolescence, the bridge between childhood and adulthood, is often a time of stress and difficulty for typically developing children. Young people with chronic disabilities might also experience adolescence in a typical, sequential manner; however, issues associated with chronic disabilities can magnify the intensity of the maturation process. The process of developing a healthy sexual identity is a complex one for any adolescent. For an adolescent who has a chronic disability, gaining a positive self-concept as a sexual being can be even more challenging.

Sexuality is defined as "the characteristics of the male or female reproductive elements and/or the constitution of an individual in relation to sexual attitudes and behaviors" (*Dorland's Medical Dictionary*, 2007) and "the sum of the physical, functional, and psychological attributes that are expressed by one's gender identity and sexual behavior, whether or not related to the sex organs or to procreation" (*Mosby's Medical Dictionary*, 2009). The second edition of the *Occupational Therapy Practice Framework: Domain and Process (Framework;* American Occupational Therapy Association [AOTA], 2008) includes sexuality as an activity of daily living (ADL) that may be addressed by occupational therapy practitioners and defines *sexual activity* as "any activity that provides sexual pleasure" (p. 631).

Sexuality does not refer solely to physical acts, such as kissing, hugging, or having intercourse. Sexuality encompasses much more: seeing oneself as attractive and feeling worthy of being liked for who one is, feeling confident and secure around others, and feeling that there is something special and unique about oneself (Murphy & Elias, 2006). Perhaps most important is that sexuality is a component of *intimacy*, which is the bonding that occurs when one gives and receives affection and shares feelings, thoughts, and dreams for the present and future. Just like his or her peers without disabilities, an adolescent who has a disability might dream of having a boyfriend or girlfriend, getting married, becoming sexually intimate, and raising a family (Murphy & Elias, 2006).

The American Academy of Pediatrics (AAP) Council on Children with Disabilities recently reaffirmed its policy statement on the sexuality of children and adolescents with disabilities. The statement reaffirmed that, to optimize development, young people with disabilities need access to support and education in all areas of sexuality, including puberty, pregnancy, pregnancy prevention, and social interaction (AAP, 2010; Murphy & Elias, 2006). Such access is especially important, as "adolescents with disabilities seem to be participating in sexual relationships without adequate knowledge and skills to keep them healthy, safe, and satisfied" (Murphy, 2005, p. 640).

Furthermore, young people with disabilities are at a higher risk of being sexually abused than their peers without disabilities (Donvan & Gerhardt, 2012). Research has shown this to be the case for adolescents with physical and intellectual disabilities and those with chronic illnesses (Haydon, McRee, & Halpern, 2011; Jones & Lollar, 2008). Health and rehabilitation professionals who work with adolescents need to support their clients in developing healthy sexual identities and increasing their independence in the physical, cognitive, and psychosocial aspects of sexuality (Jurgens, 2009; Murphy, 2005). Therefore, this chapter aims to provide readers with information and useful tools to help young people with a variety of chronic conditions and disabilities develop healthy sexuality.

Occupational therapists work with young people who have a variety of conditions and disabilities. Young people in the following diagnostic categories are frequently served by the profession, which will be addressed in this chapter: juvenile rheumatoid arthritis (JRA); juvenile diabetes; cerebral palsy (CP); muscular dystrophy (MD); spina bifida (SB); and mental health populations, including intellectual disability (ID), autism spectrum disorders (ASDs), and attention deficit hyperactivity disorder (ADHD). A review of the condition demographics and characteristics, as well as discussion of considerations for healthy sexual development, will be presented.

Adolescent Development

Psychosocial Development

Erikson's (1964) model for the stages of psychosocial development offers a framework with which to understand psychosocial development from infancy to adulthood. The "age and stage" format interfaces well with occupational therapy's appreciation for considering clients' developmental stages when exploring their occupations and providing interventions (Cole, 2008). Table 10.1 provides an overview of Erikson's Eight Stages of Psychosocial Development and identifies the preeminent feature of each stage.

Table 10.1. Erikson's Eight Stages of Psychosocial Development

Age	Stage
Birth to infancy	Trust vs. mistrust
Ages 1–3 years: Toddlerhood	Autonomy vs. shame and doubt
Ages 3–5 years: Early childhood	Initiative vs. guilt
Ages 6–12 years: Middle childhood	Industry vs. inferiority
Ages 13–22 years: Adolescence	Identity vs. role confusion
Ages 23–35 years: Young adult	Intimacy vs. isolation
Ages 35–50 years: Adulthood	Generativity vs. stagnation
Ages 50 to death	Integrity vs. despair

Source. Erickson (1964).

Erikson's (1964) model is helpful in understanding how major psychosocial challenges contribute to human development throughout the lifespan. This section will discuss two psychosocial stages—childhood and adolescence—as they relate to the development of sexuality in children and adolescents with disabilities.

Industry vs. inferiority (middle childhood, ages 6–12)

During this period, children cooperate and compete with peers as they learn academic, daily, purposeful tasks. Play and learning are the focus of this stage. A sense of inferiority might develop when a child feels he or she cannot meet the expectations of others or of an activity (Ballard, 2008). For children with chronic disabilities, many tasks are more difficult. Feeling inferior might result in reclusivity or depression. Children with disabilities might also refuse to participate in activities to avoid rejection, ridicule, or negative feedback on their performance. If a child with a disability does not gain a sense of mastery, productivity, or pleasure in his or her accomplishments, *ego development*—the definition of who "I" am—might be impeded (Cole, 2011). The peak of this developmental stage is achieved by securing competence in tasks or relationships that are attempted by the child. Clinicians can provide support by scaffolding activities, facilitating friendships, and identifying meaningful occupations, all of which contribute to the development of healthy self-esteem.

Identity vs. role confusion (adolescence, ages 13–22)

Erikson (1968) postulated that adolescents in their tweens through late teens are in a stage of *identity vs. role confusion*, during which they struggle to answer the fundamental question of "Who am I?" In their quest, early adolescents try new things. They become more engaged with peers and less dependent on their parents. Toward the end of this stage, older adolescents establish a sexual identity. Erikson's view was that if an adolescent did not successfully resolve his or her "identity crisis" and come through this stage with a healthy sense of self, he or she would suffer role confusion. This would create great difficulty in the next stage, during which young people grapple with the developmental challenge of *intimacy vs. isolation*. An adolescent who does not develop a healthy sense of self—including a sexual identity— would find it difficult to put his or her fragile identity at risk to open up enough to form true connections. Thus, adolescents who do not have healthy identities would have difficulty forming the close intimate relationships that lead to lasting friendships and successful marriages.

Adolescents who have chronic disabilities have the same developmental tasks, but their disabilities might make achieving the goal of identity development more challenging. They potentially need support in many ways: access to opportunities to try new things, experimentation with definitions of self, exploration of career options, individuation from parents, permission to develop a sexual identity, time and space to be with friends, and so on. Clinicians can help by including their adolescent clients' needs, goals, and preferences in their treatment plans; considering groups as part of intervention; and helping parents understand the developmental challenges of this stage.

Physical Development

The evolution into a sexual being hinges upon progressive maturation in both psychosocial and physical development. In children and adolescents challenged by chronic disability or illness, the progression of psychosocial development might be thwarted, slowed, or ignored until secondary sex characteristics and puberty occurs. *Secondary sex characteristics*, the visible physical changes that distinguish male from female, provide a visible sign of sexual maturation and emerging sexuality. Exhibit 10.1 describes secondary sex characteristic development.

Adolescents who have chronic disabilities usually undergo the same pubertal changes and develop similar secondary sex characteristics to their typically developing peers. However, some conditions might include different developmental trajectories. Girls with CP, for example, tend to begin puberty earlier than girls who do not have CP and, depending on their race, might complete puberty later than typically developing girls (Worley et al., 2002). Occupational therapists who address sexuality with adolescents who have disabilities and chronic conditions need to educate themselves on the potential differences in developmental trajectories for their clients.

Exhibit 10.1. Secondary Sex Characteristics

Females: Breast and breast tissue develop, hair begins to grow in the pubic area and then under the arms, acne begins, and the onset of the menses occurs. The physical body begins to accommodate for childbearing as the waist narrows and the hips widen (this is when young girls begin to develop a "figure"). Physiologically, the body begins to produce female hormones that support the ongoing maturation process. Psychologically, the hormones produce monthly mood swings, emotional ups and downs (lability), fatigue, abdominal cramping, and the typical symptoms encountered with the monthly menstrual cycle.

Males: Physical changes at this time include an increase in scrotal size and the enlargement of the penis and testicles, hair growth in the pubic area and under the arms, and commonly a slight increase in breast tissue. Acne begins to appear, and the body develops a masculine appearance with a larger chest and narrower hips. Hair begins to grow on the face, and the voice lowers. Muscles also increase in size and strength throughout the body, and the "little boy" appearance disappears into the beginning of a manly body.

Signs and Symptoms: Similarities Among Diagnostic Groups

Each disability diagnosis addressed by this chapter has its own unique signs and symptoms. In general, all diagnoses presented include these common elements:

- Onset of the condition occurs during gestation, birth, or early in life.
- The condition might engender developmental challenges in physical, psychological, and social realms.
- The condition persists throughout life.
- The condition might inhibit active engagement in life activities and pursuits.
- The presence of the condition might create higher-than-normal stress levels within family, school, religious, community, and recreational settings.

Juvenile Arthritis or Juvenile Rheumatoid Arthritis

JRA refers to a chronic arthritis condition that affects individuals before age 16. The first signs often are joint pain, swelling, or reddened or warm joints (Kidshealth.org, 2010; National Institutes of Health [NIH], 2011b). Rheumatologists state that the fewer the number of joints involved, the more likely a *remission,* a decrease of symptom severity, or complete disappearance of symptoms will be. Conversely, greater joint involvement suggests less likelihood of partial or total symptom remission (NIH, 2011b). NIH (2011b) reported that children who have many joints involved or who have a positive rheumatoid factor are more likely to have chronic pain, poor school attendance, and physical disability. Initial signs might be quite subtle or readily apparent.

Approximately 5–18 children of every 100,000 children develop JRA each year. More than 65,000 young people in the United States are diagnosed annually with JRA, as young as 2 years of age. JRA is a lifelong condition but is seldom life-threatening (NIH, 2011b).

Sexuality and JRA

Children and adolescents with JRA may experience delayed growth and pubertal onset at a later age. Along with the changes associated with puberty, adolescents with JRA must also deal with changes in appearance (due to joint involvement), fatigue and pain, and physical disability. They may also present with emotional immaturity due to dependence on others (e.g., parent or caregiver doing for them) and decreased opportunity for social contact (Ostlie, Dale, & Moller, 2007). These factors may directly affect sexual identity development during adolescence and into adulthood.

Juvenile Diabetes

Juvenile diabetes, also known as *Type 1 diabetes,* is caused by an inability or decreased ability of the pancreas to produce insulin. The onset is sudden, and the child remains insulin-dependent for life. Insulin does not cure juvenile diabetes and does not prevent the potential associated devastation that might include vision loss, limb amputation, kidney failure, nerve damage and neuropathy, heart attack and cardiovascular issues, neurological problems, and stroke.

The common signs of juvenile diabetes include extreme thirst, frequent urination, drowsiness or lethargy, increased appetite, sudden weight loss for no reason and without restrictive dieting, sudden vision changes, sugar in urine, fruity odor on breath, heavy or labored breathing, and stupor or unconsciousness (Juvenile Diabetes Research Foundation [JDRF], 2010). Juvenile diabetes is a chronic condition; at this time, no cure is known for this disease.

In the United States, as many as 3 million Americans have Type 1 diabetes. Annually, more than 15,000 children and 15,000 adults (approximately 80 cases per day) are diagnosed with Type 1 diabetes (JDRF, 2011). This might be attributed to better diagnostic techniques or an actual rise in the number of diabetic cases overall. Approximately 1 in 400 American children and adolescents younger than 20 years of age is diagnosed with diabetes (American Diabetes Association [ADA], 2011). Approximately 2 million children and adolescents 12–19 years of age have prediabetic conditions or tendencies, including elevated glucose levels, obesity, and limited exercise tendencies (ADA, 2007). These factors have been identified as contributors to the development of diabetes.

Sexuality and Diabetes

Type 1 diabetes is an "invisible" disability and might not be brought up for discussion with nonfamily members until a need is present. A peer or nonfamily member may not understand the disease and the necessity of consistently and diligently attending to it. During adolescence, a time when "fitting in" is essential, diabetes may place the individual under peer scrutiny (Gordon, Tschopp, & Feldman, 2004). The adolescent may be evaluated for his or her suitability as a friend or mate and may be devalued by peers and others who do not understand the disease (Gordon et al., 2004).

Because of his or her limited social interaction, the child or adolescent with diabetes may have unrealistic or romanticized expectations of interpersonal and sexual relationships. Images provided through the media may further distort the meaning and essence of healthy and positive relationships with others (Howland & Rintala, 2001). The child or adolescent with diabetes might be assessed and treated for areas related to physical and emotional maturity, as diabetes can affect these areas that then affect occupational performance.

Cerebral Palsy

A common developmental disorder, *CP*, has the potential to cause long-term physical impairment (Aisen et al., 2011). The disorder is characterized by nonprogressive abnormalities in the developing brain that create a cascade of neurologic, motor, and postural deficits in the developing child (Rogers, Gordon, Schanzenbacher, & Case-Smith, 2001). Seizures may accompany CP, and cognitive, ocular–motor, visual–perceptual, oral–motor, and speech deficits may be present, and differentiating between cognition and communication difficulties is very important (Aisen et al., 2011). The nature of the associated impairments depends upon the site and extent of the brain lesion.

Signs and symptoms of CP range from very mild to severe. Developmental signs include

- *At 2–6 months:* difficulty controlling the head when picked up; lower extremity crossing or "scissoring" when picked up
- *At 6–12 months:* difficulty with head control (an ongoing problem), reaching for an object with only one hand while the other hand forms a fisted position, crawling by pushing off with one hand and leg while the opposite hand and leg drag or lag, inability to sit independently
- *At 12–24 months:* inability to crawl, unable to stand without support
- *Older than 24 months:* inability to walk, unable to push a toy with wheels (Centers for Disease Control and Prevention [CDC], 2011a).

Difficulty with swallowing, movement that seems tight, and decreased spontaneous motor activity may be early indicators of CP (Aisen et al., 2011). The condition might be present before birth or soon after birth. The average prevalence of CP is 3.3–1,000, or 1 in 303 children (CDC, 2011a). No particular ethnic group seems to be at higher risk for CP, but low-income families might be at a higher risk because of poorer access to proper prenatal care and medical services (Rogers et al., 2001).

Sexuality and CP

The impact of CP on appearance, mobility, communication, and task engagement can influence the development of autonomy and sexuality. The majority of youth with CP reside at home with their families. They view nonfamily social interaction (e.g., with peers and friends) as an important component of their lives but may have limited out-of-school contact with peers or friends, negligible participation in organized social activities, and a primary orientation toward sedentary activities. Youth with CP may have friends who date and engage in out-of-home social activities but have limited opportunities themselves to participate in these activities (Blum, Resnick, Nelson, & St. Germaine, 1991).

There is not a great deal of research to date on sexuality and CP. However, one study found that although adolescents with CP seemed less mature and did not have as much sexual experience as their peers without disabilities, they were similar to typically developing peers in terms of how they judged their own bodies (Wiegerink, Roebroeck, Donkervoort, Cohen-Kettenis, & Stam, 2008). The researchers found that adolescents with CP did not have difficulty forming or maintaining close friendships, but they did have difficulty establishing romantic and intimate relationships.

In terms of sexual health, occupational therapy can help adolescents with CP gain occupational awareness, develop socioemotional growth, engage in peer relationships, manage pain and activities of daily living (ADLs), and develop positive self-concept. Occupational therapists can also provide a group venue for youth with CP and other physical disabilities to discuss, problem solve, and share topics related to dating and intimacy. Such groups may also include peers without disabilities.

Muscular Dystrophy

The *MDs*, the most common muscle disorders of childhood, are a group of genetically inherited disorders that are statistically more common in males. MDs cause changes in the biochemistry and structure of the surface and internal membranes of muscle cells and result in progressive degeneration and weakness of various muscle groups (Rogers et al., 2001).

The more common forms of MD appear early in life. Signs and symptoms vary according to the specific types of the disorder. In general, signs of MD include progressive muscle weakness and lack of coordination; as the condition progresses, contractures of joints occur (Mayo Clinic, 2010). There is no cure for MD at this time.

Various forms of MD exist, but all are characterized by muscle weakness and wasting and functional mobility deterioration over time. Forms and symptoms of MD include

- *Duchenne muscular dystrophy (DMD).* DMD occurs in about 1 in every 3,500 male births; a milder version of DMD occurs in a very few female births. DMD affects all voluntary muscles and the heart and breathing muscles. Duchenne presents with generalized weakness and muscle wasting in the hips, pelvis, thighs, and shoulders; the calves are often enlarged. The onset of DMD is between 2–5 years of age. Survival is rare beyond the third decade (Muscular Dystrophy Association [MDA], 2011).

- *Becker muscular dystrophy (BMD).* The symptoms of BMD occur later in life, usually in adolescence or even young adulthood. BMD occurs in about 1 in every 30,000 male births. BMD has presenting symptoms that are similar to those of DMD, but the symptoms are less severe and vary from person to person. BMD might also include significant heart involvement (MDA, 2011).

- *Myotonic muscular dystrophy (MMD).* MMD is the most common disease form and affects more than 30,000 individuals in the United States. MMD might develop after birth, although the more common form might appear during the teenage through young adult years. MMD includes muscle weakness and muscle wasting in the face, lower legs, forearms, hands, and neck. Delayed muscle relaxation after muscle contraction is a common feature of this type of MD. Other symptoms of MMD include gastrointestinal problems, vision deficits, and heart or respiration difficulties. In some cases, learning disabilities are present (MDA, 2011).

- *Limb–girdle muscular dystrophy.* The number of individuals affected by limb–girdle MD is estimated to be in the low thousands. The symptoms begin in later childhood or early adulthood and include weakness evidenced as muscle wasting of the shoulders (limb) and hips (girdle). Disease progression is slow but consistent. Cardiopulmonary complication might occur in the later stages of this type of MD (MDA, 2011).

- *Facioscapulohumeral muscular dystrophy (FMD).* Symptoms of FMD begin by 20 years of age and include muscle weakness and wasting around the eyes and mouth, the upper arms and lower legs, and the shoulders. As this type of MD progresses, weakness and wasting of the abdominal muscles and hip muscles might occur. FMD affects approximately 13,000 individuals in the United States, or 1 of every 20,000 individuals (MDA, 2011).

There are other less common forms of MD, including Emery–Dreifuss MD (fewer than 300 cases reported worldwide), oculopharyngeal MD (most commonly seen in French-Canadian families in Canada and in Spanish-American families in the United States), distal MD (more common in Sweden), and congenital MD (the Fukuyama subtype is most commonly seen in Japan).

Sexuality and MD

The progressive deterioration that is characteristic of MD can cause a variety of physical and psychosocial difficulties for affected individuals. Occupational therapy often focuses on helping individuals to maintain functional interdependence and positive self-concept. There is no cure for MD, and because many affected individuals do not survive into adulthood, there is little research available on sexuality and MD.

However, adolescents with MD have sexual needs that are similar to those of their peers. A recent Danish study of young adult men with DMD found them to have a relatively high self-perceived quality of life (QoL) in spite of their frequent pain and limited social contact, but they often reported that the pain of not having a love life was hardest to bear (Rahbek et al.,

2005). One participant stated, "the absence of love is always somehow present in the mind" (p. 24). The authors exhort professionals and parents to assume that children with DMD will grow into young adults and to include sexuality and intimacy as areas to be addressed.

Spina Bifida

SB refers to the incomplete development of the spine, brain, or meninges and literally translates as "cleft spine" (NIH & National Institute of Neurological Disorders and Stroke [NINDS], 2010). SB occurs early in utero when the neural tube is created from a specialized plate of cells. The top of the neural tube forms the brain, and the remainder of the tube forms the spinal cord. This entire process is completed by the 28th day of gestation. If problems occur during this short period of time (when many women do not realize they are pregnant), neural tube defects can occur, including SB. There are four distinct types of SB:

1. *Occulta.* This is the mildest and most common form, in which one or more vertebrae are malformed. *Occulta* means "hidden." This type of SB rarely causes disability or symptoms.

2. *Closed neural tube defects.* This form of SB is identified by a malformation of fat, bone, or membranes. Incomplete paralysis with associated urinary and bowel dysfunction might be present; however, symptoms might be absent. A tuft of hair, a birthmark, or a small cleft or dimple might mark the site of the malformation.

3. *Meningocele.* This form of SB is characterized by a protrusion of the meninges from the spinal opening. The malformations might be covered by a layer of skin. Some individuals with this type of SB might have few symptoms; others might have symptoms akin to those associated with closed neural tube defects. This form of SB is usually characterized by a protruding, skin-covered sac at the site of the malformation.

4. *Myelomeningocele.* This is the most severe form of the disease and is marked by exposure of the spinal cord through an opening in the spine. Below the spinal opening, there is either partial or complete paralysis with associated bowel and bladder dysfunction. Hydrocephalus might also be present.

Individuals with the milder forms of SB experience few if any symptoms. However, individuals with a more severe form of SB might need assistive devices, crutches, walkers or wheelchairs, along with catheterization and collection bags (NIH & NINDS, 2010). Functional interdependence is the goal, as the individual will depend on family or caregivers for ADLs, including bowel and bladder protocols.

Although the trend in occurrence has decreased since the 1940s, SB is still present worldwide. The highest prevalence rate, about 1 in 200 pregnancies, is reported from the northern provinces in China. Intermediate prevalence rates, about 1 in 1,000, occur in Central and South America. The lowest prevalence rates, <1 in 2,000 births, occur in Europe. In the United States, the highest regional rate for SB occurs in the southeast region, with an incidence of 1 in every 500 births (NIH & NINDS, 2010).

Sexuality and SB

For individuals with severe forms of SB, mobility issues predominate and the use of assistive devices provide a visible sign of disabilities, which may lead to scrutiny by peers. In milder forms, the condition may not be identifiable to others, and limitations may be invisible and less severe. Occupational therapy practitioners may focus on mobility, functional independence or interdependence in self-care (including feminine hygiene), peer socialization, and development of self-esteem and self-concept.

Although not all individuals with SB will reach maturity, recent medical advances in surgical treatment and neurological management allow the possibility of a normal lifespan (Bowman & McLone, 2010; Sawin, Buran, Brei, & Fastenau, 2002). Young people with SB often are, or would like to be, engaged in activities related to sexuality and relationships but rate themselves as having little romantic appeal (Sawin et al., 2002).

Some studies show that young people with SB have knowledge about sexuality and SB-related issues (Sawin et al., 2002). Others demonstrate that adolescents with SB may have knowledge about sex in general but not about how SB affects their sexuality (Shiomi, Hirayama, Fujimoto, & Hirao, 2006). Neurological issues associated with SB, including incontinence and erectile dysfunction (ED), may be perceived as potential obstacles to intimate activities and can cause increased anxiety in young people with SB (Cardenas, Topolski, White, McLaughlin, & Walker, 2008). However, young people with SB can be educated about SB and sexuality to help them gain some sense of control over their symptoms. For example, knowing that research indicates that that penile sensation does not necessarily predict ED (Shiomi et al., 2006) can be helpful. Educating people with SB that emptying bowel and bladder prior to sexual activity might be helpful to address both neurological issues.

Autism Spectrum Disorders

People with developmental disabilities, including ASDs, represent a diverse group with a wide range of functional abilities. Treatment and education about sexuality must be tailored to fit the needs and priorities of individual clients.

The term *ASDs* refers to a group of developmental disabilities that includes autistic disorder, pervasive developmental disorder, and Asperger's syndrome (CDC, 2011c). Individuals on the autism spectrum present with a wide range of functional abilities and can be mildly or severely affected. Young people with ASDs have a higher rate of sensory modulation difficulties (e.g., overresponsivity, underresponsivity, sensation seeking), which can affect participation in activities (Ben-Sasson et al., 2009). ASDs encompass a range of characteristics, but all are marked by difficulties with social interaction.

- *Autistic disorder.* The young child diagnosed with autistic disorder, commonly called *classic autism* (CDC, 2010c), might have achieved developmental, social, and psychosocial milestones, but the developmental progress stops or is thwarted. Typical signs might include poor or limited communication abilities; interest in objects rather than people; presence of stereotypical behaviors (e.g., arms held in high-guard, hand flapping, finger play); significant food preferences and limited diet; limited eye contact or frequent gaze aversion; and failure to achieve developmental milestones from the point of diagnosis. In fact, the child might lose previously attained skills. Individuals with ASDs might also have an ID. The CDC (2007) identified an intelligence quotient (IQ) of 70 or less in 40%–62% of children with ASDs, based on its multisite study in 2000.

- *Asperger's syndrome.* Individuals with Asperger's syndrome (AS) do not have deficits in cognitive or verbal skills. They often have some milder symptoms of an ASD and might have strong special interests (CDC, 2011c). Sensory-processing issues (e.g., hyper- and hyposensitivities) are common (Atwood, 2007). Adolescents who have AS or a high-functioning ASD might strongly want to have relationships with peers but be stymied by difficulty with navigating the social world (Stokes & Kaur, 2005).

- *Pervasive developmental disorder not otherwise specified (PDD–NOS).* Individuals diagnosed with PDD–NOS have some characteristics of ASD but do not meet diagnostic criteria (CDC, 2011c). Symptoms might be mild, and difficulties tend to be mainly in communication or social realms.

The causes of ASDs are still under study and might be linked to a combination of factors, including genetic predisposition, exposure to environmental factors, and disrupted central nervous system development in utero (CDC, 2011c). CDC estimates that 1 out of every 110 children in the United States has an ASD. Boys are four times more likely than girls are to be diagnosed with an ASD (CDC, 2011c).

Sexuality and ASD

Lack of education and knowledge about sex and related issues has been documented for people with ASDs. Stokes and Kaur (2005) found that when compared to neurotypical peers, adolescents with high-functioning ASD and AS demonstrated less awareness about privacy rules and more inappropriate sexual behaviors (e.g., touching their private body parts in public). The researchers suggest that these tendencies might be developmental, as they align with behaviors seen in neurotypical children of a younger age. They also caution that just as sexual behaviors vary widely in the general population, so do they vary among people with ASDs.

Adolescents with AS and high-functioning ASDs experience difficulties in social competencies (e.g., reading social cues, understanding the perspectives of others, understanding the social world). For example, children with ASDs may not be able to distinguish between a friend and an acquaintance and may present as "bossy" or inflexible, which causes peers to turn away from them (Attwood, 2007). Because of their difficulties with social interaction, children with ASDs are at risk of becoming socially isolated. Adolescents with AS have been found to have higher rates of depression and loneliness, which have been associated with poorer quality friendships (e.g., increased betrayal and conflict; Whitehouse, Durkin, Jaquet, & Ziatas, 2009). Not having friends (or having friendships of poorer quality) further prevents children with ASDs from learning the social and relational skills that allow people to become successful relationship partners (Attwood, 2007).

Childhood difficulties with social and friendship skills can transition into adolescent or adult difficulties with behaviors or skills associated with romance, courting, and intimacy. Adolescents and young adults with ASDs have been found to engage in more inappropriate or intrusive courtship behaviors compared to neurotypical peers (Stokes, Newton, & Kaur, 2007). These behaviors are not due to deviant sexuality or aggressive tendencies but rather to a decreased understanding of what is socially appropriate, coupled with a decreased understanding of how such behaviors appear to the objects of their affection. Stokes and colleagues (2007) note that the social disability associated with ASDs may set the stage for an affected person to persist in trying to establish contact with a potential romantic partner in ways that can be construed as stalking behaviors, but the person with the an ASD is not aware that he or she is doing anything wrong. Social functioning predicts romantic functioning for people with ASDs. Stokes et al. found that although people with ASDs learned romantic skills from peers, other sources of potential learning about courtship (e.g., siblings, media, parents, sex education, observation) negatively affected behaviors associated with their romantic functioning.

Developing a positive identity as a loving and loveable potential partner is a challenge for many young people with ASDs. In a case study of identity development, a young man with an ASD stated, "Even if I was capable of having a relationship, it's just too hard to meet somebody. You know, it's like I might have a heart of gold, but there's no way to know that. All they see is the autism" (Bagatell, 2007, p. 424).

However, many young people with ASDs do have fulfilling relationships. Several factors contribute: the partner's understanding of the ASD's "social nearsightedness" and sensory challenges, the person with the ASD's willingness to see things differently and trying to meet partner's needs, and both partners' willingness to communicate and compromise. Jack Robison and Kirsten Lindsmith, both in their early twenties, shared their experiences of being in love and having a fulfilling relationship in the media. Both have an ASD.

> *Robison:* I don't like kissing as much as Kirsten does, but I sort of went along with it. But I don't know. I, the next day, explained my reluctance, sort of, but I tried to play along. . . . I didn't like the sensation of it terribly much, and . . . I was not as enthusiastic as a consequence.

> *Lindsmith:* It wasn't really surprising or confusing that he didn't like kissing, because I'd encountered people before who didn't but who weren't autistic. And he basically explained that it felt to him literally what it was, just two people mashing their mouths together, and that it wasn't—it didn't activate, you know, the kind of romantic inclinations it does in other people who like kissing . . . it felt like pushing faces into another face. And so—sigh. But, alas, it's something that comes with the package. (Donvan, Lindsmith, & Robison, 2012)

Intervention to address social competence, courting behaviors, and sexuality (along with education for law enforcement and legal professionals) is clearly needed. This can be challenging for educators and practitioners alike; sexuality is a complex topic, and ASD is complex, made more so by the wide range of functioning that the autism spectrum encompasses. Given deficits that are social rather than intellectual, adolescents with ASDs may benefit from different curricula and approaches to sexuality than what is offered for adolescents with ID (P. Gerhardt, personal communication, January 30, 2012). Peter Gerhardt, a specialist on adolescents and adults with ASDs and the place of love, romance, and sex in their lives (Donvan et al., 2012), suggested, for example, that movies and television programs can be analyzed for social and romantic content and used in guided discussion (P. Gerhardt, personal communication, January 30, 2012). Social stories might also be helpful in learning expected and healthy romantic behaviors. Additionally, adolescents may benefit from using materials created for typically developing adolescents. Below is a sampling of materials that may be helpful.

- Attwood, S., & Powell, J. (2008). *Making sense of sex: A forthright guide to puberty, sex, and relationships for people with Asperger's syndrome.* Philadelphia: Jessica Kingsley.

- Baxley, D. L., & Zendell, A. (2005). *Sexuality education for individuals and adolescents with developmental disabilities: An instruction manual for educators of individuals with developmental disabilities, sexuality across the lifespan.* Tallahassee: Florida Developmental Disabilities Council.

- Hoertdoerfer, P. (2000). *The parent guide to our whole lives: Grades K–1 and grades 4–6.* Cleveland, OH: United Church Board for Homeland Ministries.

- Wilson, P. M. (1999). *Our whole lives: Sexuality education for grades 7–9.* Cleveland, OH: United Church Board for Homeland Ministries.

Intellectual Disability

ID refers to a group of disorders characterized by decreased cognitive abilities and difficulty with adaptive behaviors, including self-care skills (American Psychiatric Association [APA], 2000; NIH, 2011a). ID is a developmental disorder diagnosed before 18 years of age that may have physical (e.g., CP) or nonphysical (e.g., lack of adult responsiveness) causes (NIH, 2011a). The measure used to determine the level of ID is the IQ score; ID is defined as having an IQ score below 70 (APA, 2000). About 6–7.5 million individuals with ID live in the United States. ID occurs in 2.5%–3% of the general population (Hershey Medical Center, 2010).

Children with ID might present with decreased social abilities, communication problems (both expressive and receptive), and behavior issues. In some cases, children and adolescents with ID might be aggressive toward both others and self. Although their overall development might be delayed, young people with IDs do not stop developing but, more commonly, either reach developmental milestones slower and later than typically developing peers or peak in their abilities at an earlier chronological age.

Sexuality and ID

Adolescents with ID feel the same sexual desires as their peers without disabilities. However, adolescents with ID may not understand how to manage their sexual desires and are at risk of not having the same access to education about sex. Additionally, they might face the obstacle of living with community or family members who are uncomfortable with the idea of people with ID sexually expressing themselves. The American Association on Intellectual and Developmental Disabilities (2012) stated that denying sexual rights and sex education to people with intellectual and developmental disabilities can lead to difficulties with self-esteem, body image, gender identity, personal development, and social interaction.

Education in healthy sexuality is vital for young people with IDs. Because of the cognitive nature of their disability, adolescents with IDs may have difficulty understanding how to manage sexual urges and how to care for their developing bodies. Occupational therapy practitioners can provide intervention targeted toward self-care (e.g., grooming, using deodorant, managing menstruation, determining appropriate places for masturbation, public vs. private behaviors), appropriately socializing (e.g., what it means to be a friend, having a girlfriend or boyfriend, how to appropriately show affection, personal boundaries), and keeping safe (e.g., private parts of body, saying "no," reporting abuse). Collaboration with family and other professionals is recommended.

One challenging sexual behavior for clinicians who work with people who have developmental disabilities is masturbation (Cambridge, Carnaby, & McCarthy, 2003). Education is crucial for these young people, their caregivers, and clinicians to address this issue in a way that promotes adaptive behavior (Cambridge et al., 2003; Murphy & Elias, 2006). For example, educating parents that masturbation is a normal toddler behavior can help them to understand the sexual behaviors of their teenager with ID who is functioning at that developmental level (Murphy & Elias, 2006). The clinician can then guide parents in teaching "public vs. private." Similarly, this concept can be taught to staff who work in residential facilities and to the individuals that they serve (Cambridge et al., 2003). Strategies to address masturbation are included in many education and treatment programs that address sexuality for people with IDs and ASDs (e.g., Cambridge et al., 2003; Tissot, 2009).

Education is essential to help people with IDs and ASDs develop healthy sexuality, and it is important that it cover an array of topics related to sexual development, including social skills training (Stokes & Kaur, 2005). The National Dissemination Center for Children With Disabilities (2011) recommends the inclusion of values, morals, and the subtleties of friendship; dating, love, and intimacy; and education on STDs, pregnancy prevention, and sexual exploitation. Although young people who have disabilities need the same access to education about sexuality as do their peers without disabilities, educational materials might need to be modified so that concepts can be understood (Murphy & Elias, 2006). Murphy and Elias included the following topics as topics for sexuality education for people with IDs or ASDs:

- Anatomy
- Pubertal changes
- Personal care and hygiene
- Medical examinations
- Social skills
- Contraception (including abstinence)
- Sexual expression
- Rights and responsibilities of sexual behaviors.

Many resources are available for clinicians and parents to help address healthy sexual development and adaptive behaviors in people who have IDs or ASDs. Although individual intervention is sometimes needed, group work might often be beneficial. Occupational therapists might play a vital role as part of a team approach by providing education, addressing social and relational skills, and working on ADLs related to sexuality. For example, personal hygiene and menstruation might need to be addressed individually, while concepts such as personal boundaries and appropriate dating conversation might be appropriate to approach in small groups. Social stories have also been found to be a useful approach (Tarnai & Wolfe, 2008). Exhibit 10.2 provides a sampling of the many resources available for clinicians and the families they serve.

It is important to keep in mind that people who have ASDs, IDs, or other developmental disabilities are a very diverse group. Parts of the discussion above might not be relevant for individuals with high-functioning autism and AS because they might have very different needs in developing healthy sexuality and fulfilling relationships. Therapeutic interventions might include support for relational and social skills, activities to develop healthy self-esteem, and opportunities for socialization.

Exhibit 10.2. Sexuality Resources for People With Developmental Disabilities

Alberta Health Services's Web site contains information and lesson plans for teaching sexual health, including lesson plans for young people who have developmental disabilities. For example, see http://www.teaching-sexualhealth.ca/teacher/lessonplans/differingabilities.html

Alberta Health Services. (2009). *Sexuality and disability: A guide for parents*. Available at http://teachingsexualhealth.ca/media/pdf/Sexuality_Developmental_Disability.pdf

Aston, M. (2003). *Aspergers in love: Couple relationships and family affairs*. Philadelphia: Jessica Kingsley.

Couwenhoven, T. (2007). *Teaching children with Down syndrome about their bodies, boundaries, and sexuality: A guide for parents and professionals*. Bethesda, MD: Woodbine House.

Harris, R. (1994). *It's perfectly normal: Changing bodies, growing up, sex, and sexual health*. Cambridge, MA: Candlewick.

Madaras, L., & Madaras, A. (2007a). *My body, my self for boys: What's happening to my body?* (rev. ed.). New York: Newmarket Press.

Madaras, L., & Madaras, A. (2007b). *My body, my self for girls: What's happening to my body?* (rev. 2nd ed.). New York: Newmarket Press.

Schwier, K. M., & Hingsburger, D. (Eds.). (2000). *Sexuality: Your sons and daughters with intellectual disabilities*. Baltimore: Paul H. Brookes.

Walker-Hirsch, L. (Ed.) (2007). *The facts of life . . . and more: Sexuality and intimacy for people with intellectual disabilities*. Baltimore: Paul H. Brookes.

Attention Deficit Hyperactivity Disorder

ADHD is one of the most common neurophysiological disorders in children and adolescents (CDC, 2011b). Data collected from the 2004–2006 National Health Inventory Survey revealed that approximately 9.5% of children ages 6–17 years (an estimated 5.4 million children) were diagnosed with ADHD (CDC, 2011b; Pastor & Reuben, 2008). The disorder is more common in boys than girls, and can occur with or without learning disabilities (Pastor & Reuben, 2008). Both children with ADHD and those with learning disabilities are more likely to have other chronic health conditions when compared with children who do not have either diagnosis (Pastor & Reuben, 2008).

ADHD has three types: (1) predominantly hyperactive–impulsive, (2) predominantly inattentive, and (3) combined type (APA, 2000). For a diagnosis of ADHD to be made, the following criteria must be met:

- Symptoms before 7 years of age
- Impairment in at least two settings (e.g., home, school, play)
- Clinically significant impairment in school, social, or work settings
- Symptoms not only observed during the course of PDD, schizophrenia, or other psychotic disorder, or better accounted for by another mental disorder.

Criteria for the three types of ADHD include

- *Combined type:* Both criteria for hyperactivity–impulsivity and for inattention are met for the past 6 months.
- *Predominantly hyperactive–impulsive type:* Criteria for hyperactivity–impulsivity but not for inattention are met for the past 6 months.
- *Predominantly inattentive type:* Criteria for inattention but not for hyperactivity–impulsivity are met for the past 6 months.

Criteria Symptoms of ADHD

Hyperactivity–impulsivity

Six or more of the following symptoms of hyperactivity–impulsivity be present to an extent that is disruptive and inappropriate for the person's developmental level.

Hyperactivity

- Often fidgets with hands or feet or squirms in seat when sitting still is expected
- Often gets up from seat when remaining in seat is expected
- Often excessively runs about or climbs when and where it is not appropriate (adolescents or adults may feel very restless)
- Often has trouble playing or doing leisure activities quietly
- Often is "on the go" or often acts as if "driven by a motor"
- Often talks excessively.

Impulsivity

- Often blurts out answers before questions have been finished
- Often has trouble waiting turn
- Often interrupts or intrudes on others (e.g., butts into conversations or games).

Inattention

Six or more of the following symptoms of inattention have been present to a point that is inappropriate for the person's developmental level:

- Often does not give close attention to details or makes careless mistakes in schoolwork, work, or other activities
- Often has trouble keeping attention on tasks or play activities
- Often does not seem to listen when directly spoken to
- Often does not follow through on instructions and fails to finish schoolwork, chores, or duties in the workplace (not due to oppositional behavior or failure to understand instructions)
- Often has trouble organizing activities
- Often avoids, dislikes, or does not want to do things that take a lot of mental effort for a long period of time (e.g., schoolwork, homework)
- Often loses things needed for tasks and activities (e.g., toys, school assignments, pencils, books, tools)
- Is often easily distracted
- Is often forgetful in daily activities (APA, 2000; CDC, 2011b).

Stimulant medications are often used to treat ADHD (Hoza et al., 2005). However, researchers have differing theories of ADHD and of the processes by which the condition affects behavior (Barkley, 2003). One view of ADHD purports that inattention and hyperactivity are behavioral manifestations of deficits in executive functions (e.g., working memory, organization) and inhibitory control (Barkley, 2003). However, young people with ADHD have also been found to have difficulty regulating their levels of arousal (Benikos & Johnstone, 2009).

An alternative model is emerging that conceptualizes ADHD as a dysfunction of self-regulation (Martel & Nigg, 2006). This two-path model includes a focus on temperament and considers the developmental path of ADHD. One pathway centers on self-regulation issues of inattention and disorganization, while the other relates to temperament-related issues of emotional reactivity and motivation—links to hyperactivity or impulsivity that are not consciously regulated. The inclusion of temperament in the construct of ADHD allows for the consideration of emotion regulation, which has long been identified as problematic for individuals who have ADHD (Musser et al., 2011).

ADHD is characterized by a deficit in performance rather than of skills (Barkley, 2004; Gumpel, 2007). Performance deficits can impair social participation, but social skills training is often not sufficient or effective (Barkley, 2004; Gumpel, 2007; Hoza et al., 2005). This is because young people with ADHD do not necessarily lack skills or knowledge; a child with ADHD may know what to do but cannot successfully perform at the time that the skill is needed (Barkley, 2004). Therefore, gains made in treatment often do not generalize into natural environments. Although medication helps with some symptoms of ADHD, it has less of an effect on improving positive peer interaction and acceptance by peers (Hoza et al., 2005). Working with young people who have ADHD within the context of social activities can potentially help to ameliorate impaired peer interaction (Gumpel, 2007). Involving typically developing peers in treatment might also be key for young people with ADHD. Children and adolescents with ADHD are involved in peer aggression at a higher rate, and girls with predominantly inattentive type ADHD are at a higher risk of being victimized by peers (Elkins, Malone, Keyes, Iacono, & McGue, 2011).

Sexuality and ADHD

Young people with ADHD are often rejected by their peers and tend to have friendships with others who demonstrate ADHD symptoms or oppositional behaviors (Cordier, Bundy, Hocking, & Einfeld, 2010; Normand et al., 2011).

Children with ADHD have reported more negative and fewer positive features in their friendships (Normand et al., 2011); they have also demonstrated less empathy than typically developing peers (Cordier et al., 2010). Just as with children and adolescents with ASDs, not having close friendships or having friendships of poorer quality can prevent young people with ADHD from developing the relational skills that will be essential for later healthy intimate relationships. Interventions that consider friendship development (e.g., how to choose, make, and keep friends) have been little studied (Mikami, 2010). Treatment programs that target friendship development and integrate social skills and parent involvement hold promise for children with ADHD (Mikami, 2010).

Developing relational skills is important for healthy sexuality in young people with ADHD, and so is refraining from risky sexual behaviors. Young people who have symptoms of ADHD tend to have sexual intercourse for the first time at an earlier age compared to adolescents who do not have ADHD (Price & Hyde, 2009). Adolescents and young adults who were diagnosed with ADHD as children engage in more risky sexual behaviors (e.g., casual sex with infrequent condom use, multiple partners) than typically developing peers (Florey, Molina, Pelham, Gnagy, & Smith, 2006). Given the risk of transmission of sexually transmitted diseases (STDs) and human immuno-deficiency virus (HIV), young people with ADHD who engage in these behaviors may be putting their health at risk. Several factors have been identified as potentially contributing to increased sexual risk-taking behaviors among young people with ADHD, including symptoms of the disorder (e.g., impulsivity), poor parent–adolescent communication, and associations with peers who engage in risky behaviors (Florey et al., 2006). Managing impulsivity, good relationships with caring adults, and positive friendships and peer group interactions can contribute to helping young people with ADHD develop healthy sexuality.

Approach to Sexuality in Adolescents Using the *Occupational Therapy Practice Framework*

The *Framework* (AOTA, 2008) provides a valuable structure with which to address the development of the emergent sexual self of children and adolescents. "Occupational therapy practitioners recognize that health is supported and maintained when clients are able to engage in occupations and activities that allow desired or needed participation in home, school, workplace, and community life" (AOTA, 2008, p. 629). The sexual self is one component of the complete self, and this holistic view of health supports assessment and intervention designed to address sexuality and the development of one's sexual persona. The *Framework* describes all aspects of occupational therapy's domain and is comprehensive in its holistic approach to the psychosocial, physical, emotional, and spiritual health and well-being of individuals.

Occupations

Occupations are activities and participation in activities. Sexual activity is an ADL that falls under the occupational therapy's profession's domain of practice.

Sexuality encompasses much more than the physical act of intimacy or having sex. The scope of sexuality encompasses a wide variety of areas that are commonly addressed by occupational therapists: sensory components, motor input and output, psychosocial engagement with another individual, grooming, hygiene, and so on. Children and adolescents who are developing their sexual personae can benefit by direct or indirect interventions in these tasks.

Client Factors

Client factors include body structures, body functions, and beliefs. Helseth and Misvaer (2010) found *self-image,* which they define as "being one's own best friend" (p. 1457), to be an important factor for QoL in adolescents. Healthy self-image was described by teens in this study as "believing in oneself," but the definition also included one's beliefs about how one appears and is received by others. Younger individuals worry about their physical appearance, physical development and puberty, and being "a part of the group" (Frauman & Sypert, 1979).

Children and adolescents with disabilities might feel that their disabilities set them apart from their peers. During adolescence, a time when individuals want to blend in with the group, a disability might cause an adolescent to stand out from his or her peers. The perception of being different can promote social anxiety, create isolation, thwart the development of a healthy self-esteem, and impede the development of healthy sexual self-image.

Egocentrism

Children and adolescents with chronic impairments might look different and might feel that they are different from their typically developing peers; however, all young people, those with and without disabilities, experience *egocentrism.* The construct of egocentrism was first put forth by Elkind (1967) and consists of the *imaginary audience* and *personal fable.*

Imaginary audience. The construct of the imaginary audience relates to physical appearance and social situations. Adolescents believe that those around them are as concerned and focused on their appearance as they themselves are. Elkind (1967) stated, "The young person believes that he or she will be the focus of attention" (p. 1031) in any situation; this belief is imagination-based and not founded in reality. Egocentrism accounts, for example, for an adolescent's refusal to attend a school dance because of the appearance of a barely noticeable pimple.

The concept of egocentrism might be magnified for an adolescent with a disability. For example, an adolescent who has CP might skip a school dance because he or she is sure that everyone will stare at the joint deformity in his or her hands. Pimples go away, but joint deformities tend to be more stable and visible. Adolescents who have disabilities are vulnerable to negative feedback from peers about their looks and potentially use this feedback to gauge their desirability as a girlfriend or boyfriend (Gordon et al., 2004). The adolescent who has a disability might need support in dealing with the *imaginary audience,* so that he or she can develop a positive body image that sets the foundation for a healthy identity. Body image has an effect on sexual identity and on comfort with intimate relationships (Gordon et al., 2004).

Personal fable. The *personal fable* is the belief that one is special, unique, and invulnerable to harm (Schwartz, Maynard, & Uzelac, 2008). The construct relates to imaginary beliefs and risk-taking behaviors that are commonly seen in adolescents. For example, an adolescent girl might believe that, although a boy in her school has an STD, the disease would *never* happen to her. Personal fables might be perpetuated by the media and dialogue with family, friends, and peers. An adolescent might imagine himself or herself being someone else or perhaps justify feelings and potential behavior by thinking, "A famous person has done this, so why can't I do it?"

The personal fable construct might have another dimension for adolescents with disabilities. For example, a boy with JRA might wrongly believe that most of his peers are sexually active, and that, if he did not have a disability, he too would be sexually active. This belief might prompt him to engage in sexual activity before he is ready or to engage in risky sexual behaviors. A study of adolescents who receive special education services in the United States found that adolescents who have disabilities experience STDs at least at the same rate as their peers without disabilities (Mandell et al., 2008). Similar findings were reported in a study of adolescents with physical disabilites in South Africa (Maart & Jelsma, 2010).

Imagination and fantasy life are important parts of human experience. Although the imaginary audience and personal fable constructs relate to imagined beliefs that might present risks for adolescents who have disabilities, imagination can also serve a protective function. Imagination, including sexual fantasy, can provide an outlet from the everyday experiences of dealing with limitations that might result from disabilities.

Performance Patterns

Performance patterns are the roles and routines one enlists to meet the demands of a particular occupation or task. The occupational therapist considers how a client's pattern of behavior fulfills his or her roles and establishes his or her identity (AOTA, 2008). Thus, regarding sexuality, an adolescent's pattern of activity defines his or her role as boyfriend or girlfriend and contributes to development of his or her sexual identity.

Occupational therapists can work with young clients to help frame the activities and behaviors that constitute healthy sexuality. Authors of the literature on sexuality and adolescents with disabilities suggest that adolescents who have chronic disabilities tend to engage in the same sexual activities as their peers without disabilities (e.g., Cheng & Udry, 2002; Suris, Resnick, Cassuto, & Blum, 1996). Adolescents with disabilities also tend to have intercourse for the first time at about the same age as their peers (Suris et al., 1996). Research also suggests that, similar to individuals without disabilities of the same age group, young people who have disabilities develop gender identity during adolescence, that is, they identify themselves as heterosexual, homosexual, and so on (Suris et al., 1996).

Environment

The environmental interface encompasses a wide constellation of settings (e.g., physical, social, cultural, virtual), each with different contextual demands and requirements for performance. For young people who have chronic disabilities, environmental demands might be greater because of their particular condition or limitations. For example, the physical environment might present challenges for an adolescent with a physical disability who has CP. Her youth group's camping trip would be a great time to hang out with the boy she likes, but the rough terrain might make it difficult for her to go on the trip. The social environment might be daunting for an adolescent who has AS. In his theater group, kids tease each other—that's part of their peer culture. However, he cannot be sure whether the girl he likes is teasing him because she likes him or if she is just being mean.

The virtual environment provides opportunities for young people with disabilities to socialize and explore. However, like their typically developing peers, adolescents with disabilities might need help to navigate Internet culture safely and might be vulnerable to victimization (e.g., cyber bullying).

Social

Social interaction is of particular prominence in the adolescent age group. Children with chronic disabilities might be sheltered or come from protected living settings. When these individuals are thrust into middle or high school, they might have difficulty understanding the subtle interaction styles and nonverbal social cues necessary to be successful in social situations (e.g., classroom, moving from class to class, lunch, study time, physical education, social gatherings like dances).

Young people who have conditions that include difficulty with understanding social interaction might engage in inappropriate sexual behaviors (e.g., uninvited or unwanted kissing or sexual advances, taking clothes off, touching private body parts in public; Stokes & Kaur, 2005). For adolescents who have ASDs, these behaviors might result from emerging sexual urges that are "not accompanied by the socialization and understanding of social norms governing acceptable behaviors that a typical peer will gain" (Sullivan & Caterino, 2008, p. 383).

Family Environment

It is also important to consider the concerns of parents and caregivers. Youth with disabilities tend to be more reliant upon parents or caregivers and have less opportunity for interaction with peers (Murphy, 2005). Parents and caregivers might be uncomfortable discussing sexual issues with their children (Gordon et al., 2004). Parents, and sometimes clinicians, might have the misinterpretation that they are protecting an adolescent from being hurt by not addressing sexuality (Milligan & Neufeldt, 2001), or they might not address the issue because they do not see these individuals as sexual beings (Frauman & Sypert, 1979).

A study of parental approaches to health-related topics for adolescents with disabilities found that some parents were concerned that their children might face obstacles to fulfilling relationships and sexual expression (Antle, Mills, Steele, Kalnins, & Rossen, 2007). Most parents in the study expressed concern about their children's decreased peer interaction and increased social isolation.

Societal Attitudes About Sexuality and Disability

Society has customarily viewed people with disabilities as having no distinct sex role and no sexual desires, or as being *asexual* (Milligan & Neufeldt, 2001; Suris et al., 1996). Although this view is a myth that corresponds to neither the available research nor the reports of people with disabilities, young people who have disabilities are at risk of integrating this view, which might impede the development of a healthy sexual identity (Milligan & Neufeldt, 2001).

Sexuality and disability cannot be discussed without the consideration of social stigma. People who have physical, psychosocial, and cognitive disabilities might be perceived as threatening in some way; some people who do not have disabilities might feel uncomfortable because of their fears, founded or unfounded (Gordon et al., 2004). Stigma can be perceived as an impenetrable barrier to the formation of friendships and relationships that are more intimate.

Societal attitudes about disability can play a role in how an adolescent who has a disability is perceived. In an adult sample, DeLoach (1994) found that, although people might be willing to have a person with a disability as a coworker or acquaintance, they were less likely to accept him or her as a partner. The same might be true of adolescents. In the school environment, for example, there might be a stigma attached to not only *being* an adolescent with a disability but also *dating* an adolescent who has a disability. In other words, it might be considered socially appropriate to have an adolescent with a disability as a casual friend but not as a close friend, girlfriend, or boyfriend.

Activity Demands

Activity demands are the components needed to participate in an activity, including required body functions, social demands, objects and processes involved, and space required. *Space* refers to the physical context of the activity, including elements such as lighting, crowdedness, and noise. Activities related to developing sexuality often require *privacy*, which is, of course, essential for intimate activity. Privacy and autonomy are also normal needs for adolescents as they individuate from their parents and caregivers (Murphy, 2005). However, young people who have disabilities are often not granted the privacy to be alone with a peer or to talk with peers about sex (Jurgens, 2009).

By following the structure of the *Framework* (AOTA, 2008), addressing sexuality and sexual activity with children and adolescents becomes less daunting. It is important to define what is meant by (1) terminology that is related to sexuality and (2) the clients' developmental levels and stated goals. Table 10.2 provides an overview and integration of diagnoses discussed, the *Framework* (AOTA, 2008), and suggestions for interventions related to the development of healthy sexuality.

Occupational Therapy Evaluation

Evaluating children and adolescents with chronic disabilities is a challenging and multifaceted endeavor for occupational therapy practitioners. The

Table 10.2. Potential Occupational Therapy Areas of Intervention Related to Development of Healthy Sexuality in Children and Adolescents With Disabilities

Area of Intervention	Examples of Occupations and Skills	Client Child and Adolescent Population	Considerations, Interventions, and Potential Goals (Group and Individual Treatment)	*Occupational Therapy Practice Framework* Application
Grooming and hygiene	• Manage menstruation • Brush teeth • Use deodorant • Shave face, arms, or legs • Brush hair • Wash hair, face, body	• Physical disabilities (CP, JRA) • ASD, ADHD • ID	• Manage self-care activities with more independence (direct intervention, assistive devices, client–family collaboration). • Establish habits and routines (e.g., checklists, reinforcements) • Skill-based teaching, family or caregiver intervention, environmental supports.	*ADLs* • Bathing and showering, dressing, personal device care, personal hygiene and grooming *Client factors* Body functions— • Neuromusculoskeletal and movement-related • Genitourinary and reproductive functions *Activity demand* • Objects and their properties • Social demands • Required body functions and Structures *Performance skills* • Motor and praxis skills • Cognitive skills • Sensory–perceptual skills *Performance patterns* • Habits, routines
Social skills	• "Read" nonverbal communication • Act according to "rules" of dating, social interaction, and intimacy	• ASD	• Difficulty understanding social world, including social networking, may be a barrier to successful engagement. • May benefit from groups, direct teaching, peer or family coaching	*Social participation* • Peer, friend *Play* • Play participation *Leisure* • Leisure participation

	• Be assertive (rather than passive or aggressive)	• Physical disabilities (CP, MD, JRA)	• Skill deficit may be due to decreased opportunity for social interaction in childhood. • May benefit from support in using social networking.	*IADLs* • Communication management (computers) *Performance skills* • Communication and social skills • Emotional regulation skills • Cognitive skills *Performance patterns* • Habits, routines *Contexts and environments* • Social, virtual, cultural, physical
		ADHD	• Deficit in performance rather than knowledge. Therefore, intervention needs to occur in natural environments after learning of skills. • Impulsivity and tendency toward "approach" behaviors may promote "acting before thinking."	
		ID	• Direct teaching of skills and repeated practice, along with environmental support.	
Relational skills and friendship development	• Empathy; understand others' points of view • Engage in activities with peers with and without disabilities	All disabilities	• For all client populations, having friends with and without disabilities is important for mental health and development of healthy sexual identity. • Occupational therapists may promote friendships through activity groups, peer mentoring, and so on. • Friends are important protective factor for peer victimization. • Clients may need help to understand peer norms.	*Social participation* • Peer, friend—activities at different levels of intimacy, including engaging in desired sexual activity *Play* • Play participation *Leisure* • Leisure participation *Performance skills* • Communication and social skills • Emotional regulation skills • Cognitive skills *Performance patterns* • Roles—friend
		ASD	• Delayed development in understanding POVs of others. Activities may provide increased awareness and practice.	

(*Continued*)

Table 10.2. Potential Occupational Therapy Areas of Intervention Related to Development of Healthy Sexuality in Children and Adolescents With Disabilities (*cont.*)

Area of Intervention	Examples of Occupations and Skills	Client Child and Adolescent Population	Considerations, Interventions, and Potential Goals (Group and Individual Treatment)	*Occupational Therapy Practice Framework* Application
		•ADHD	• Difficulty with cognitive flexibility may promote tendency to "fix" on dating interest.	*Contexts and environments* • Social, virtual, cultural, physical
		•All disabilities	• Delayed development of empathy and difficulty with self-regulation (e.g., managing strong emotions) may interfere with developing close friendships.	
Self-concept and self-esteem	• Active engagement in age-appropriate social activities with peers. • "Dating" behaviors that reflect healthy sense of self. • Awareness of peer norms • Sense of belonging to a social group		Occupational therapists may help clients to: • Develop interests that promote successful engagement, self-efficacy, and positive sense of self • Achieve successes at "just right challenges" • Identify strengths and challenges • Use social and environmental supports • Increase self-advocacy • Analyze media images of masculinity and femininity • Develop a body image that is positive and realistic, which is especially important for clients with physical disabilities.	*Leisure* • Leisure exploration *Client factors* • Values, beliefs, spirituality • Mental functions—experience of self and time (e.g., body image, self-concept, self-esteem) *Performance skills* • Communication and social skills • Emotional regulation skills • Cognitive skills *Performance patterns* • Roles—friend

| Physical development, reproductive health, and sexuality | • Understand puberty and sexual maturation process
• Know reproductive process
• Identify male and female differences
• Understand sexuality as involving more than intercourse | • All disabilities

• ID, ASD | • Approach taken dependent upon client's needs, cognitive level
• Parental consent a consideration when clients are under age 14
• May not be appropriate to broach subject unless client brings up first
• Refer clients to other health professionals as appropriate.
• Occupational therapist may use psychoeducational approach to teach concepts in groups.

Occupational therapy practitioners may work with other healthcare professionals to provide training for staff of residential facilities on sexual development in youth with disabilities. | *ADLs*
• Sexuality—Engaging in activities that result in sexual satisfaction
IADLs
• Informal personal
• Education, participation
Client factors
Body functions—
• Genitourinary and reproductive functions
Body structures—
• Genitourinary and reproductive systems
Performance skills
• Communication and social skills
• Cognitive skills |
| Healthy boundaries | • Self-touch (masturbation)
• Public vs. private behaviors
• Respect the personal physical and emotional space of others
• Protect self from inappropriate or unwanted sexual advances | • All disabilities

• ID, ASD | As young people with disabilities are at higher risk of abuse, clients may need instruction in dealing with unwanted or inappropriate touch and language.
• Practitioners may work with health care professionals and families to help clients learn safe and private ways to engage in self-touch.
• Clients who use self-touch for calming may benefit from learning coping skills. | *ADLs*
• Sexuality—engaging in activities that result in sexual satisfaction
Client factors
Values, beliefs, and spirituality
Performance skills
• Communication and social skills
• Emotional regulation skills
• Cognitive skills
• Motor and praxis skills
• Sensory–perceptual skills
Contexts and environments
• Social, cultural |

(Continued)

Table 10.2. Potential Occupational Therapy Areas of Intervention Related to Development of Healthy Sexuality in Children and Adolescents With Disabilities (*cont.*)

Area of Intervention	Examples of Occupations and Skills	Client Child and Adolescent Population	Considerations, Interventions, and Potential Goals (Group and Individual Treatment)	*Occupational Therapy Practice Framework* Application
			• Practitioners may work with other health care professionals to provide staff training on boundaries, respecting client privacy, reinforcing concepts of public vs. private, laws concerning abuse, and so on. • Young people with developmental disabilities may need help to recognize and understand appropriate vs. inappropriate sexual behaviors.	
STDs and pregnancy prevention	• Understand STDs, their transmission, and associated risks. • Understand pregnancy prevention and readiness for parenthood. • Know safer sex practices (e.g. condoms, abstinence)	• All disabilities • ADHD	• Children and adolescents who have disabilities need the same information about STDs and pregnancy prevention that is provided for young people who do not have disabilities. • Information and teaching must be modified to be appropriate for the age and developmental level of the client. • Youth who have difficulty with impulse control may be at risk of engaging in risky sexual behaviors.	*IADLs* • Health management and maintenance—Decreasing health risk behaviors *Education* • Informal personal education participation *Client factors* • Values, beliefs, and spirituality • Thought (e.g., recognition, categorization, reality-based, logical) *Performance skills* • Communication and social skills • Cognitive skills

| Anxiety and self-regulation | • Concerns about sexuality, being different or stigma
• Participation in social environments
• Relaxation techniques
• Coping skills
• Learning to manage emotions | • All disabilities

• ASD

• ADHD, ASD | • Interacting with other young people with disabilities allows a sense of belonging and to discuss issues related to being different.
• Interactions with peers who do not have disabilities to reinforce social acceptance.
• Coping skills and relaxation techniques may be taught in group or individual sessions.
• Young people with AS, SPD, and high-functioning ASD may need support for dealing with social anxiety.
• Cognitive–behavioral techniques may be helpful.
• Youth with ADHD, ASD, and SPD may need intervention to learn to manage strong emotions. | *Client factors*
Mental functions—
• Emotional (e.g., coping, behavioral regulation)
• Thought (recognition, categorization, reality-based, logical)
• Values, beliefs, spirituality
• Mental functions (e.g., experience of self and time, body image, self-concept, self-esteem)
Performance skills
• Communication and social skills
• Emotional regulation skills
• Cognitive skills
• Sensory–perceptual skills |

Note. ADHD = attention deficit hyperactivity disorder, ADL = activity of daily living, AS = Asperger's syndrome, ASD = autism spectrum disorder, CP = cerebral palsy, IADL = instrumental activity of daily living, ID = intellectual disability, JRA = juvenile rheumatoid arthritis, POV = point of view, SPD = sensory processing disorder, STD = sexually transmitted disease.

following guidelines should be considered in the evaluation process in general, and especially when addressing sexuality.

- *Consider the age and developmental stage of the individual.* Assessing an older child with an evaluation that he or she thinks is "childish" might create assessment and intervention barriers.

- *Understand the disability and underlying issues.* For example, a child with SB might experience motor deficiencies that create problems with personal grooming—a major occupation for older children and adolescents.

- *Understand the extent of the individual's physical and psychological maturation.* Taking into account male or female issues (e.g., late sexual development, stature when compared with peers, interests when compared with peers) and focusing on the physical and psychological needs expressed by the client will make the evaluation process more relevant. This includes puberty, sexual development, secondary sex characteristics, and related physical and psychological issues. For example, is the adolescent a "late bloomer" and somewhat ashamed of his or her lack of sexual development? Is the adolescent more physically mature than his or her chronological age indicates? Is the individual an introvert or extrovert regarding talking and sharing his or her experiences, interests, or fantasies? Does the individual appear older or younger than his or her chronological age?

- *Self-care.* How functional is the individual in dealing with self-care, and to what extent is caregiver involvement necessary? Who is the primary caregiver? (For example, is the caregiver a female for an adolescent boy?) Is there an adult in the adolescent's life who talks with him or her about issues of sexuality, such as dating, physical changes, masturbation, grooming, menstruation, and wet dreams? Although the evaluator would not ask about these issues in an initial evaluation, they are important components of emerging sexuality and might warrant consideration. A good therapeutic relationship with an adolescent's caregiver will facilitate discussion of these issues in therapy. The occupational therapist might be the person to discuss these issues with the adolescent. Helping identify an adult who can address them might be critical to the adolescent's development of a healthy sexual self.

- *Leisure and social interests.* What are the leisure and social interests of the individual? Identifying, exploring, and supporting the young person's interests facilitates the development of a strong identity.

- What are the individual's abilities, skills, strengths, and limitations?

- What is the emotional and psychosocial maturity level of the individual?

These key items will help determine the type of assessment and appropriate venue for administration of the evaluation. In general, assessment should be completed in a one-to-one setting. A one-to-one setting should also be considered for the assessment of sexual development and sexuality within this age group.

The specific assessment tools chosen depend upon the needs and goals of the client. For example, when occupational choice, interests, and future aspirations are considered important treatment focuses, the Adolescent Role Assessment (Black, 1976) might be useful. When overall satisfaction and understanding of how the disabling condition might be affecting a client's life is relevant, a QoL inventory (e.g., Frisch, 1994; Varni, 2011) would be indicated. The Bell Relationship Inventory for Adolescents (BRIA; Bell, 2005) is an appropriate assessment for individuals who have relationship problems or concerns. The Children's Assessment of Participation and Enjoyment (CAPE); Preferences for Activities of Children (PAC; King et al., 2004) are appropriate assessment choices when leisure interests or out of school–time occupations are a target for intervention.

The major focus of any evaluation in occupational therapy is to "identify what obstacles interfere with participation in daily life" (Asher, 2007, p. 12). The assessments discussed in the section that follows represent a sample of tools that contain age-appropriate content and relevancy for children and adolescents who have chronic disabilities. Keep in mind that these assessments are tools and comprise only part of the assessment process. Evaluation will also include learning about the client's needs and wants; the family; client factors and performance skills; and the expectations, affordances, and challenges of the client's occupational environments. Other assessment tools that address these areas might also be useful. Use assessment tools that seem most appropriate for the client as a way to inform goal setting and explore client priorities.

Adolescent Role Assessment

The Adolescent Role Assessment (Black, 1976) aims to identify deficiencies in the occupational choice process and provides content for occupational therapy interventions. It is useful in screening at-risk adolescents to identify those who might have difficulty with the process of occupational choice. Although this is an older assessment, it looks at the social, emotional, leisure, and interpersonal factors that are present for clients 11–18 years of age. This assessment is administered by using a questionnaire.

Black (1976) identified three developmental stages of occupational choice: (1) childhood play, (2) adolescent socialization, and (3) adulthood work. These stages represent a hierarchy in which childhood fantasy, games, interaction, and interests provide the basis for adolescent explored interests, responsibilities, values, goals, and socialization. The adolescent stage becomes the base for adulthood work, occupational choices, and other adult responsibilities.

Adolescents with disabilities are more likely to experience the work arena with fewer or lower aspirations, fewer incentives, and less opportunity than their peers without disabilities. The Adolescent Role Assessment helps to identify deficits in development of occupational choice and related goals to enhance that development. Occupational therapists can then provide goal-directed practice in skills to help children and adolescents with disabilities achieve a greater level of productivity and independence.

Quality of Life Inventories

QoL is an important outcome measure, and QoL inventories can be useful in determining clients' priorities, assessing participation, establishing goals, and measuring progress. Several inventories assess QoL in children and adolescents. Self-report surveys obtain a client's perception of his or her own QoL in many domains: social, academic, leisure, and peer relationships.

Health-related QoL inventories are also available for children and adolescents with specific chronic conditions. For example, the Pediatric Quality of Life (Varni, 2011) has versions for both children and adolescents with diagnoses, including CP, asthma, arthritis, and diabetes. These inventories assess the impact of the condition on the individual's perceived QoL. The Child Health Questionnaire (Landgraf & Ware, 2011) is another QoL assessment; it includes a version for children with ADHD.

Although these assessments do not directly address sexuality, they give the clinician a picture of a client's overall satisfaction and participation that might be related to his or her developing self-esteem and identity. The Quality of Life Inventory (Frisch, 1994) is appropriate for use with clients who are 17 years of age or older and includes items related to health, love, and relationships.

Bell Relationship Inventory for Adolescents

The BRIA (Bell, 2005) was designed to assess object relations in children and adolescents for diagnostic and treatment planning, and for research. It is used with the adolescent age group (11–17 years of age) to address alienation, insecure attachment, egocentricity, social incompetence, and positive attachment. Written statements are answered as *true* or *false* by the responder.

Children's Assessment of Participation and Enjoyment; and Preferences for Activities of Children

The CAPE/PAC (King et al., 2004) are assessments that are woven together to determine enjoyment and preference in out-of-school activities. These tools look at participation and desire for involvement in a picture-based format. Scores are calculated for each of five dimensions (*diversity, intensity, with whom, where,* and *overall enjoyment*). Scores are further analyzed to determine the responder's preference among recreational, physical, social, skill-based, and self-improvement activities (King et al., 2004).

These assessments represent only a sample of assessments available for occupational therapists to use in the evaluation of children and adolescents when sexuality might be addressed. Assessments can be used in conjunction with other occupational therapy assessment tools. Using these assessments, additional information about the individuals' interests, issues, and personal goals can be established. Treatment interventions can be client-centered and based on personal skills, abilities, problems, interests, and concerns.

Occupational Therapy Interventions

In any intervention with children or adolescents, the occupational therapy practitioner must adopt a *therapeutic use of self*, which involves intentionally interacting with a client in a manner that is caring, respectful, and therapeutic (Taylor, 2008). In group treatment with adolescents, therapist bonding has been shown to be the factor that most positively affects successful outcomes in social competence (Schectman & Katz, 2007). Being mindful of the therapist–client relationship is especially important when addressing sexuality and the components of developing a healthy sexual identity. Clinicians who address issues of sexuality with children and adolescents who have disabilities must acknowledge their own personal feelings, as well as any biases they might have (Gordon et al., 2004). For example, a clinician who is uncomfortable discussing masturbation or who believes it to be an inappropriate behavior might be at risk of causing a client for whom this is an issue to feel shame. The clinician and client might benefit from the clinician's seeking help from a colleague to appropriately address the issue.

Therapeutic interventions can be conducted individually or in a group setting. At this time in health care, the one-to-one setting might provide more comfort and confidentiality to some clients than can be achieved in a group treatment setting. If client discomfort or resistance is noted, a one-to-one setting is the most appropriate format. However, most older children and adolescents value peer feedback and use it to estimate their own sense of self and their problem-solving strategies. Additionally, older children and adolescents might feel that "an older person" (yes, that's you, the practitioner) does not truly understand their angst, so the use of peer groups can become very positive, useful, and time efficient.

Groups serve two purposes, called the *dyadic construct* of groups. Groups address (1) the topic or activity and (2) behaviors and interactions that occur within the group context among members and the group leader or therapist. Cole (2008) provided a structured and sequential method of conducting groups using "The Seven Step Method" for conducting groups (Exhibit 10.3).

Conducting groups with this structured sequence of events helps the occupational therapy practitioner appropriately plan and execute a group with any composition of clients, especially children and adolescents. The structure and process help to facilitate communication and feedback when dealing with nonthreatening and difficult subjects. When the therapist addresses the subject of sexuality with this age group, group participant interaction, feedback, and communication are essential to both group success and client learning.

Using groups, many therapeutic interventions can occur. When dealing with adolescents, education, support and friendship, and the development of a healthy and realistic self-esteem are of primary concern. Clients talking about their experiences, fears, and hopes with peers who might share similar experiences and feelings can help to create a stronger sense of self. The clinician who leads such a group plays a valuable role in helping to guide discussion, provide education and resources, and give positive feedback for social and relational skills as they are practiced.

Education

One way to promote healthy habits and routines related to sexuality is through educationally based interventions. Adolescents with disabilities have reported that they have not had sufficient education about sexuality (Berman et al., 1999) and might not have the same knowledge about sex and appropriate behaviors as their peers without disabilities (Stokes & Kaur, 2005). Children and adolescents who have disabilities have the same rights to education about sexuality as their typically developing peers (Murphy, 2005). Murphy (2005) stated that sex education for children who have disabilities should include "body parts, pubertal changes, personal care and hygiene, medical examinations, social skills, sexual expression, and the rights and responsibilities of sexual behavior" (p. 643).

> ## Exhibit 10.3. Cole's Seven-Step Method for Conducting Groups
>
> - *Step 1: Introduction.* The multi-step process of the introduction includes the introduction of the leader and group members; a warm-up to help put clients at ease and to prepare members for the activity; setting the mood for the activity, including the therapist's tone of voice and facial expressions, the environment, and the media to be used for the group; verbally identifying the expectations of the group, including a review of group rules (norms); and a clear explanation or outline of the group to be conducted.
>
> - *Step 2: Activity.* The activity or "bulk" of the group should last no more than 20 to 60 minutes. Activity consideration must relate to the client goals and needs, interests, abilities, and capacities and to the skills and abilities of the group leader. The group topic or focus should be beneficial for the clients.
>
> - *Step 3: Sharing.* After completion of the activity, participants are asked to share their work or experience with the group as a whole. For example, this can involve showing the completed item to the group or talking about the personal experience.
>
> - *Step 4: Processing.* This is considered the most difficult of the seven steps for new group leaders. Processing occurs when group members express how they feel about the group experience, the leader, and each other. This can include both the verbal and non-verbal aspects of members throughout the group.
>
> - *Step 5: Generalizing.* This cognitive-thinking aspect of the session occurs when the leader reviews the group's responses to the activity; the responses are summarized, and general principles are shared with the group.
>
> - *Step 6: Application.* This step occurs when the leader helps the group to understand how the principles learned in the group can be applied to everyday life.
>
> - *Step 7: Summary.* The summary includes a review of the most important aspects of the group to ensure that this will be correctly remembered and understood by the participants.
>
> *Note.* Cole (2008).

Among the public health concerns targeted by the DHHS (2011a) Healthy People 2020 initiative are two concerns that emerge or peak during adolescence: unplanned pregnancies and STDs (DHHS, 2011a). Another goal of the initiative is to include all people with disabilities in health promotion activities (DHHS, 2011b). In its companion statement to the Healthy People 2010 initiative, DHHS's (2010) Office on Disability noted that, although individuals who have disabilities are as sexually active as their peers without disabilities, they often are not included in sexual education; furthermore, individuals who have disabilities might be at a greater risk of rape. That young people with disabilities might be at a higher risk of being taken advantage of sexually is another reason that education about sexuality is important.

A holistic approach to client care—understanding physical, psychosocial, and cognitive factors—makes occupational therapists well suited to provide education to young people with disabilities on topics related to sexuality and intimacy. Education needs to be tailored to include information that can be understood and integrated by the children and adolescents to whom it is targeted. For example, adolescents who have IDs might need to have concepts simplified and behavioral plans and instructions made concrete, whereas clients who function at higher cognitive levels might require less structure and respond better to more creative and interactive approaches when participating in activities and discussions designed to help them integrate concepts.

DHHS (2010) noted barriers to education about contraception and STD transmission, including written materials that are presented at too high of a level for people who have IDs, materials unavailable in Braille or through assistive technology, and the lack of inclusion of people who have disabilities in educational materials. The latter reinforces the myth that people who have disabilities are not sexual or sexually active. Young people who have disabilities need education about pregnancy prevention and STD prevention that is appropriate and understandable.

The differentiation between public and private behaviors is an example of an educational activity that might be appropriate intervention for an occupational therapist. For some clients, sorting picture cards of activities into *public* and *private* categories might be a good way to introduce the concept. For example, a picture of a group eating lunch would be *public*, whereas a person taking a shower is *private*. Adolescents with disabilities might also benefit from occupational therapy interventions that help them gain a better understanding of social dynamics and sexuality. For example, although a boy might want to kiss a girl he is attracted to, there are important social rules about getting to know her first and moving through the stages of acquaintance, friend, good friend, and so on. This type of intervention could be accomplished by role-playing social situations (without the kissing), using puppets, analyzing television or movie clips, or taking "off-ground" trips to public places to observe social behaviors.

The essence of role-plays and observation of others is to illuminate the appropriate continuum of interaction and the development of intimacy. Sex education alone will not be sufficient, in most cases, to change any negative sexual behavior patterns or increase opportunity for fulfilling relationships (Stokes & Kaur, 2005).

Teaching responsible behaviors needs to be part of any education program for adolescents that addresses sexuality. Values can set the stage for discussing privacy and modesty, STDs, sexual orientation, masturbation, abstinence until marriage, pregnancy prevention, and lifestyle choices (e.g., some people have children and some do not). Explicitly making the point that loving sex occurs privately between two consenting, mature adults who are in a loving, committed relationship might be needed (P. Gerhardt, personal communication, January 30, 2012). The concept of respect needs to be explored, including concrete ways in which respect is shown to others and to self. Clinicians need to consider the policies of their workplaces and values of their clients and their families while simultaneously understanding the need for education for adolescents with disabilities about healthy sexuality that is documented in the research and literature.

Collaboration

Keep in mind that sexuality is a topic that is often best addressed with a team approach. Social workers, psychologists, educators, and nurses are examples of professionals who can help occupational therapy practitioners address sexuality with their clients. Parents are also part of the team. Peer mentors—young people with or without disabilities—can work with occupational therapists to help present information, lead discussions, participate in role-plays, and engage in activities. They can serve as role models for young people with disabilities and as safe people to help them get their questions answered.

Support and Social Groups

Decreased peer interaction has been associated with increased social anxiety and decreased self-esteem in adolescents with chronic conditions (McCarroll, Lindsey, MacKinnon-Lewis, Chambers, & Frabutt, 2009). Support and social groups provide an opportunity for young people with disabilities and chronic illnesses to interact in supportive environments. Support groups should be differentiated from "treatment groups"—groups that are prescribed and have therapeutic goals and objectives—in that support groups might be formed by individuals who share a specific condition or a specific personal goal, for example, how to act at a dance, or how to "hang out" at the mall. Support groups might be prescribed or be voluntary in nature but should have an inherent structure.

Adolescents with disabilities benefit from social interaction with both peers who have disabilities and peers who do not (Gordon & Tshopp, 2004). Young people with chronic illnesses have been found to have less interaction with peers and therefore less opportunity to develop social and relational skills (McCarroll et al., 2009). Support groups provide opportunities for youth with disabilities to share experiences with other young people who have disabilities. Such groups can provide a safe haven for sharing feelings and can help young people with disabilities realize that they are not alone. In addition, support and social groups provide an opportunity to develop and refine age-appropriate social and relational skills (Hillier, Fish, Cloppert, & Beversdorf, 2007).

It is often not enough to put young people who have chronic conditions with peers; social skills might have to be taught during peer interactions (McCarroll et al., 2009). As friendship experiences form the template for intimate relationships (Gordon & Tshopp, 2004), guided interaction with friends in support and social groups can be helpful in developing the relational skills that promote healthy romantic relationships. Dating and relationships are topics that are likely to be discussed frequently in support groups with adolescents.

Case Example 10.1 discusses Julia, an adolescent who is ready for the practitioner to address sexuality with her. Many approaches are available that

---

Case Example 10.1. Julia: CP

Julia is a 15-year-old girl who has CP. She experiences tremors in her nondominant hand, and while Julia can walk using a canes or crutches, she usually uses a wheelchair for mobility. Julia also has mild ID and a very mild speech impediment. She participates in the general education environment and works with a special education teacher. Julia works with a school-based occupational therapist and receives occupational, physical, and speech therapies in an outpatient clinic.

While working with her occupational therapist, Julia identified the goal that she wanted to "do all the things that girls do." This provided a springboard for her occupational therapist to discuss with Julia what it meant to be a young woman, and with gentle questioning, what it meant to her to be a young woman with CP. Julia mentioned several things:

(Continued)

Case Example 10.1. Julia: CP (*cont.*)

- She didn't like that her mother kept track of when her periods were due, and she felt like her mother tried to help her too much with managing her periods.

- There was boy in her youth group at church that Julia really liked, and he seemed to like her, too. He had once tried to kiss her when they were both waiting for their rides home. Julia said that she thought they could be boyfriend and girlfriend someday soon.

- She has been spending less time with her friend, Carmen, since Carmen began dating. Julia said that, other than her church youth group, she didn't have many activities aside from school, and she gets lonely. She didn't think that Carmen understood how she felt.

- Julia said that Carmen is very pretty and that many boys like her. Although the boy in youth group seems to like Julia, she didn't think a boy would ever fall in love with her in the same way that a boy would love Carmen.

- Other girls at school were involved in many things, Julia said. When asked what kinds of things she liked, Julia said that she enjoyed being on the computer (e.g., gaming, social networking), movies, and animals.

The occupational therapist working with Julia needs to consider Julia's developmental stage, how her chronic disability affects her occupations and participation, and her goals and priorities.

Questions to Consider

1. For Julia, how do the developmental challenges of adolescence interact with the challenges of managing her disability and her emerging sexuality?

2. How can Julia be supported in developing a healthy sexual identity and a positive sense of self?

3. How can Julia's mother be included in the therapeutic process while simultaneously respecting Julia's need for privacy and promoting her desire for increased independence?

4. How much education has Julia had about sexuality and reproduction, and what does she need to know?

5. What are the risks to Julia in not addressing sexuality with her?

---

an occupational therapist working with Julia might take. The following are considerations for interventions that might be useful in helping Julia to develop healthy sexuality and positive sense of self.

- The occupational therapist might consider approaching the clinic about setting up a support group or an educational group about sexuality and dating for adolescents with disabilities. Julia might benefit from sharing with other teenagers who also have disabilities, so that she feels that she is not alone.

- Julia might benefit from education about relationships and the development of intimacy. It is not clear that the boy in her youth group is interested in her as a girlfriend, and it might be important for Julia to understand that his attempting to kiss her might not be appropriate. Learning that she does not have to be "physical" with a boy early in a relationship, especially if it is a response to low self-esteem, might be important for Julia.

- The occupational therapist might need to talk with Julia and her mother about privacy to establish boundaries that are agreeable to all of them.

- Julia's self-care abilities in managing menstruation might need to be assessed. The occupational therapist might work with Julia on problem-solving physical strategies for self-care and cognitive strategies for being ready for menstruation. For example, a calendar that Julia uses to keep track of her periods might help her mother to feel she can give Julia more independence. The concept of "interdependence" might be a useful one to discuss with Julia and her mother.

- Julia might benefit from working with her occupational therapist on identifying and exploring activities that she likes and can further develop. For example, her interests in computers and movies might be encouraged and evolve into movie-making using computer technology. Julia's interest in animals might lead to consideration for having a pet or for volunteering at the local zoo. Participation in and mastery of meaningful activities sets the stage for healthy self-concept and identity.

Other Considerations

Social and Other Media

Although a complete discussion of social media and adolescents with disabilities is beyond the scope of this chapter, social media needs to be mentioned for several reasons. First, children and adolescents with disabilities and chronic illnesses are at a higher risk of being bullied than their peers without disabilities (Rose, Monda-Amaya, & Espelage, 2011). *Cyberbullying,* the use of technology (e.g., computers, Internet, cell phones) to hurt another person, is an increasingly common form of peer aggression. The Internet can be a media through which young people with disabilities can have greater connection to peers (Bagatell, 2007). However, social media also pose risks for adolescents with disabilities who may long for a romantic connection and may be vulnerable to cyberbullying or sexual predation.

For adolescents who have difficulty understanding the social world (e.g., young people with ASD), the risks may be magnified. Additionally, an adolescent with ASD may be accused of viewing pornography (or *sexting,* i.e., sending or receiving sexually provocative images) when he or she may have no idea that this is inappropriate or illegal. (P. Gerhardt, personal communication, January 30, 2012). In a related circumstance, the author heard of a case in a school in which a boy with ASD was told by a group of so-called friends to kiss a girl that he liked. The friends knew this was wrong; the boy did not. The boy with ASD was suspended from school; no action was taken against the friends, whose set-up was a form of bullying. The Cyberbullying Resource Center (www.cyberbullying.us) provides information on social media and bullying, including some information related to AS.

Along with social media, entertainment media must be considered when addressing sexuality with young people who have disabilities. In one study of teenagers with and without ADHD, only one factor emerged as being related to early sexual debut when all other factors were controlled: watching sexually provocative television (McNamara, Vervaecke, & Willoughby, 2008). Watching television and movies that have provocative sexual content or whose characters interact inappropriately (including wearing inappropriate clothing) can give young people with disabilities the impression that what they are viewing represents expected social norms. This is especially problematic for adolescents whose disabilities include a preference for visual learning, as in ASD.

As noted earlier, television and movies can be used as teaching content by viewing clips and discussing them with young people (P. Gerhardt, personal communication, January 30, 2012). Students can then learn that what they see around them does not necessarily represent expected and healthy sexual behavior. Young people with ASD may need to be taught the difference between fantasy and reality. Practicing appropriate social and romantic behaviors might be the next step. Some examples might include how to ask someone on a date, how to respond to being asked, where to go on a date, appropriate dating behaviors and boundaries, how to say no to sexual advances, and so on.

Consent and Confidentiality

All medical providers, including occupational therapy practitioners, are required to follow privacy regulations and their state and federal laws. Occupational therapy practitioners need to be aware that the age at which a child can consent to medical and mental health care varies from state to state. For example, according to the Guttmacher Institute (2012), all states allow minors at 12 years of age to give consent to services for STDs; 18 states allow physicians to inform parents if the physicians feel that to do so is in the minor's best interest. The age at which young people may consent to sexual intercourse also varies from state to state. Occupational therapy practitioners are often mandated reporters and must report to the appropriate authorities any suspicion or mention of abuse or danger involving a child or adolescent.

Consent and *confidentiality* do not mean the same thing. Generally speaking, the age at which young people can consent to medical care is the age at which they may keep medical documents confidential; however, as shown above, this is not always the case. Additionally, special circumstances (e.g., legal proceedings) may bring medical records out into the open. Occupational therapy practitioners are advised to keep abreast of privacy regulations and the laws in their states governing consent and confidentiality.

The following resources may be helpful. However, they should not be used as a substitute for legal counsel or direct sources of the legal code.

- Guttmacher Institute State Center (http://www.guttmacher.org/statecenter)
- National Center for Youth Law (http://www.youthlaw.org).

Along with being aware of the laws within their states, occupational therapy practitioners need to know the policies of the workplace that are implemented to ensure confidentiality and uphold state, federal, and local laws.

Summary

The development of the sexual self in children and adolescents with chronic disabilities provides the therapist with many challenges. The therapist must first determine the child or adolescent's functional status regarding diagnosis. Age-appropriate goals must be formulated, followed by meaningful and purposeful therapeutic interventions. Older children and adolescents face not only the maturation process, including puberty, but they also must deal with the ebb and flow of sex hormones, physical body changes, and psychological changes, including the beginning of autonomy and increased importance of peer group relationships. Addressing the maturation processes and providing therapeutic interventions with the "just-right fit or challenge" (e.g., avoiding interventions that are "too childish" or "too adult") is especially important. The therapeutic use of self—the therapist's intentional, compassionate, professional, and therapeutic manner—is essential to helping the young person who has a chronic disability develop a healthy sexual identity and a positive sense of self.

The development of the sexual self in children and adolescents might be addressed by using groups. Groups provide an opportunity for social interaction and promote function through education, skill building, and feedback. Children and adolescents with chronic disabilities who participate in therapeutic and support groups gain some assurance that they are not alone, that their physical and psychological changes due to maturation are normal, and that support and security can be achieved through interaction and engagement with others. Groups can provide a powerful and meaningful format for helping younger individuals develop healthy and realistic sexual personae.

References

Aisen, M. L., Kerkovich, D., Mast, J., Mulroy, S., Wren, T. A., & Rethlefsen, S. A. (2011). Cerebral palsy: Clinical care and neurological rehabilitation. *Lancet Neurology, 10*(9), 844–852.

Alberta Health Services. (2009). *Sexuality and disability: A guide for parents.* Retrieved February 15, 2012, from http://teachingsexualhealth.ca/media/pdf/Sexuality_Developmental_Disability.pdf

American Academy of Pediatrics Council on Children With Disabilities. (2010). Policy statement: AAP publications retired and reaffirmed. *Pediatrics, 125*(2), e444–e445. doi:10.1542/peds.2009-3160.

American Association on Intellectual and Developmental Disabilities. (2012). *Sexuality and intellectual disability.* Retrieved March 5, 2012, from http://www.aamr.org/content_198.cfm

American Diabetes Association. (2007). *Signs and symptoms.* Retrieved August 1, 2010, from http://www.diabetes.org

American Diabetes Association. (2011). *Diabetes statistics.* Retrieved March 1, 2012, from http://www.diabetes.org/diabetes-basics/diabetes-statistics/

American Occupational Therapy Association. (2008). Occupational therapy practice framework: Domain and process (2nd ed.). *American Journal of Occupational Therapy, 62,* 625–683. doi: 10.5014/ajot.62.6.625

American Psychiatric Association. (2000). *Diagnostic and statistical manual of mental disorders* (4th ed., text rev.). Washington, DC: Author.

Antle, B. J., Mills, W., Steele, C., Kalnins, I., & Rossen, B. (2007). An exploratory study of parents' approaches to health promotion in families of adolescents with physical disabilities. *Child: Care, Health, and Development, 34*(2), 185–193.

Asher, I. (Ed.). (2007). *Occupational therapy assessment tools: An annotated index* (3rd ed.). Bethesda, MD: AOTA Press.

Aston, M. (2003). *Aspergers in love: Couple relationships and family affairs.* Philadelphia: Jessica Kingsley.

Attwood, T. (2007). *The complete guide to Asperger's syndrome.* Philadelphia: Jessica Kingsley.

Attwood, S., & Powell, J. (2008). *Making sense of sex: A forthright guide to puberty, sex, and relationships for people with Asperger's syndrome.* Philadelphia: Jessica Kingsley.

Bagatell, N. (2007). Orchestrating voices: Autism, identity, and the power of discourse. *Disability and Society, 22*(4), 413–426.

Barkley, R. A. (2003). Issues in the diagnosis of attention deficit hyperactivity disorder in children. *Brain and Development, 25*(2), 77–83.

Barkley, R. A. (2004). Adolescents with attention deficit hyperactivity disorder: An overview of empirically based treatments. *Journal of Psychiatric Practice, 10*(1), 39–56.

Ballard, K. (2008). Children and adolescents. In P. O'Brien, W. Kennedy, & K. Ballard (Eds.), *Psychiatric mental health nursing: An introduction to theory and practice* (pp. 457–479). Sudbury, MA: Jones & Bartlett.

Baxley, D., & Zendell, A. (2005). *Sexuality education for children and adolescents with developmental disabilities: An instruction manual for educators of individuals with developmental disabilities, sexuality across the lifespan.* Tallahassee: Florida Developmental Disabilities Council.

Ben-Sasson, A., Hen, L., Fluss, R., Cermak, S. A., Engel-Yeger, B., & Gal, E. (2009). A meta-analysis of sensory modulation symptoms in individuals with autism spectrum disorders. *Journal of Autism and Developmental Disorders, 39*, 1–11.

Bell, M. D. (2005). *Bell Relationship Inventory for Adolescents (BRIA).* Los Angeles: Western Psychological Services.

Benikos, N., & Johnstone, S. J. (2009). Arousal-state modulation in children with ADHD. *Clinical Neurophysiology, 120*(1), 30–40.

Berman, H., Harris, D., Enright, R., Gilpin, M., Cathers, T., & Bukovy, G. (1999). Sexuality and the adolescent with a physical disability: Understandings and misunderstandings. *Issues in Comprehensive Pediatric Nursing, 22*(4), 183–196.

Black, M. M. (1976). Adolescent role assessment. *American Journal of Occupational Therapy, 30*(2), 73–79.

Blum, R. W., Resnick, M. D., Nelson, R., & St. Germaine, A. (1991). Family and peer issues among adolescents with spina bifida and cerebral palsy. *Pediatrics, 88*(2), 280–285.

Bowman, R. M., & McLone, D. G. (2010). Neurosurgical management of spina bifida: Research issues. *Developmental Disabilities Research Review, 16*, 82–87.

Cambridge, P., Carnaby, S., & McCarthy, M. (2003). Responding to masturbation in supporting sexuality and challenging behaviour in services for people with learning disabilities: A practice and research overview. *Journal of Intellectual Disabilities, 7*(3), 251–266.

Cardenas, D. D., Topolski, T. D., White, C. J., McLaughlin, J. F., & Walker, W. O. (2008). Sexual functioning in adolescents and young adults with spna bifida. *Archives of Physical Medicine and Rehabilitation, 89*(1), 31–35.

Centers for Disease Control and Prevention. (2007). *Prevalence of autism spectrum disorders: Autism and developmental disabilities monitoring network, six sites, United States, 2000.* Retrieved August 15, 2010, from http://www.cdc.gov/mmwr/preview/mmwrhtml/ss5601a1.htm

Centers for Disease Control and Prevention. (2011a). *Cerebral palsy: Signs and causes.* Retrieved September 12, 2011, from http://www.cdc.gov/features/cerebralpalsy

Centers for Disease Control and Prevention. (2011b). *Facts about ADHD.* Retrieved February 28, 2012, from http://www.cdc.gov/ncbddd/adhd/facts.html

Centers for Disease Control and Prevention. (2011c). *Facts about ASDs.* Retrieved from http://www.cdc.gov/ncbddd/autism/facts.html

Cheng, M. M., & Udry, J. (2002). Sexual behaviors of physically disabled adolescents in the United States. *Journal of Adolescent Health, 31*(1), 48–58.

Cole, M. B. (2008). *Group dynamics in occupational therapy* (3rd ed.). Thorofare, NJ: Slack.

Cole, M. B. (2011). Adolescent social development and participation. In M. B. Cole & M. V. Donohue (Eds.), *Social participation in occupational contexts in schools, clinics, and communities* (pp. 109–126). Thorofare, NJ: Slack.

Cordier, R., Bundy, A., Hocking, C., & Einfeld, S. (2010). Empathy in the play of children with attention deficit hyperactivity disorder. *OTJR: Occupation, Participation and Health, 30*(3), 122–132.

Couwenhoven, T. (2007). *Teaching children with Down syndrome about their bodies, boundaries, and sexuality: A guide for parents and professionals.* Bethesda, MD: Woodbine House.

DeLoach, C. P. (1994). Attitudes toward disability: Impact on sexual development and forging of intimate relationships. *Journal of Applied Rehabilitation Counseling, 25*(1), 18–25.

Donvan, J. (Interviewer), & Gerhardt, P. (Interviewee). (2012). *Learning to love, and be loved, with autism* [Interview transcript]. Retrieved February 27, 2012, from http://www.npr.org/2012/01/18/145405658/learning-to-love-and-be-loved-with-autism

Donvan, J. (Interviewer), Lindsmith, K., & Robison, J. (Interviewees). (2012). *Learning to love, and be loved, with autism* [Interview transcript]. Retrieved February 27, 2012, from http://www.npr.org/2012/01/18/145405658/learning-to-love-and-be-loved-with-autism

Dorland's Medical Dictionary. (2007). Sexuality. Retrieved August 2, 2010, from http://www.dorlandonline.com

Elkind, D. (1967). Egocentrism in adolescence. *Child Development, 38*, 1025–1034.

Elkins, I. J., Malone, S., Keyes, M., Iacono, W. G., & McGue, M. (2011). The impact of attention deficit hyperactivity disorder on preadolescent adjustment may be greater for girls than for boys. *Journal of Clinical Child and Adolescent Psychology, 40*(4), 532–545.

Erikson, E. H. (1964). *Childhood and society* (2nd ed.). New York: W. W. Norton.

Erikson, E. H. (1968). *Identity: Youth and crisis.* New York: W. W. Norton.

Florey, K., Molina, B. S., Pelham, W. E., Gnagy, E., & Smith, B. (2006). Childhood ADHD predicts risky sexual behavior in young adulthood. *Journal of Clinical Child and Adolescent Psychology, 35*(4), 571–577.

Frauman, A., & Sypert, N. (1979). Sexuality and illness: Impact on sexual development and forging of intimate relationships. *Journal of Applied Rehabilitation Counseling, 25*(1), 18–25.

Frisch, M. B. (1994). *Manual and treatment guide for the Quality of Life Inventory (QOLI).* Minneapolis, MN: National Computer Systems.

Gordon, P. A., & Tschopp, M. K. (2004). Dating considerations for adolescents with disabilities. In C. A. Bowman & P. T. Jaeger (Eds.), *A guide to high school success for students with disabilities* (pp. 70–82). Westport, CT: Greenwood Press.

Gordon, P. A., Tschopp, M. K., & Feldman, D. (2004). Addressing issues of sexuality with adolescents with disabilities. *Child and Adolescent Social Work Journal, 215,* 513–527.

Gumpel, T. P. (2007). Are social competence difficulties caused by performance or acquisition deficits? The importance of self-regulatory mechanisms. *Psychology in the Schools, 44*(4), 351–372.

Guttmacher Institute. (2012). *State policies in brief: An overview of minors' consent law.* Retrieved February 28, 2012, from http://www.guttmacher.org/statecenter/spibs/spib_OMCL.pdf

Harris, R. H. (1994). *It's perfectly normal: Changing bodies, growing up, sex, and sexual health.* Cambridge, MA: Candlewick Press.

Haydon, A. A., McRee, A. L., & Halpern, C. T. (2011). Unwanted sex among young adults in the United States: The role of physical disability and cognitive performance. *Journal of Interpersonal Violence, 26*(17), 3476–3493.

Helseth, S., & Misvaer, N. (2010). Adolescent's perceptions of quality of life: What it is and what matters. *Journal of Clinical Nursing, 19,* 1454–1461.

Hershey Medical Center. (2010). *Health and disease information: Mental retardation.* Retrieved June 14, 2010, from http://www.hmc.psu.edu/childrens/healthinfo/m/mentalretardation.htm

Hillier, A., Fish, T., Cloppert, P., & Beversdorf, D. Q. (2007). Outcomes of a social and vocational skills support group for adolescents and young adults on the autism spectrum. *Focus on Autism and Other Developmental Disabilities, 22*(2), 107–115. doi: 10.1177/10883576070220020201

Hoertdoerfer, P. (2000). *The parent guide to our whole lives: Grades K–1 and grades 4–6.* Cleveland, OH: United Church Board for Homeland Ministries.

Howland, C. A., & Rintala, D. H. (2001). Dating behaviors of women with physical disabilities. *Sexuality and Disability, 19,* 41–70.

Hoza, B., Gerdes, A. C., Mrug, S., Hinshaw, S. P., Bukowski, W. M., Gold, J. A., et al. (2005). Peer-assessed outcomes in the multimodal treatment study of children with attention deficit hyperactivity disorder. *Journal of Clinical Child and Adolescent Psychology, 34*(1), 74–86.

Jones, S. E., & Lollar, D. J. (2008). Relationship between physical disabilities or long-term health problem and health risk behaviors or conditions among U.S. high school students. *Journal of School Health, 78*(5), 252–257.

Jurgens, M. (2009). Sexuality and disability. In F. Chan, E. Cardoso, & J. Chronister (Eds.), *Understanding psychosocial adjustment to chronic illness and disability: A handbook for evidence-based practitioners in rehabilitation* (pp. 443–478). New York: Springer.

Juvenile Diabetes Research Foundation. (2010). *Type I diabetes.* Retrieved June 15, 2010, from http://www.jdrf.org

Juvenile Diabetes Research Foundation. (2011). *Juvenile diabetes fact sheet.* Retrieved September 13, 2011, from http://www.jdrf.org/index.cfm?page_id = 102585

Kidshealth.org. (2010). *Juvenile rheumatoid arthritis.* Retrieved August 1, 2010, from http://www.kidshealth.org

King, G., Law, M., King, S., Hurley, P., Rosenbaum, P., Hanna, S., et al. (2004). *Children's Assessment of Participation and Enjoyment.* San Antonio, TX: Harcourt Assessment.

Landgraf, J. M., & Ware, J. E. (2011). *Child Health Questionnaire (ECHQS).* Cambridge, MA: HealthActCHQ.

Maart, S., & Jelsma, J. (2010). The sexual behavior of physically disabled adolescents. *Disability and Rehabilitation, 32*(6), 438–443.

Madaras, L., & Madaras, A. (2007a). *My body, my self for boys: What's happening to my body?* (rev. ed.). New York: Newmarket Press.

Madaras, L., & Madaras, A. (2007b). *My body, my self for girls: What's happening to my body?* (rev. 2nd ed.). New York: Newmarket Press.

Mandell, D. S., Eleey, C. L., Cederbaum, J. A., Noll, E., Hutchinson, M. K., Jemmott, L. S., et al. (2008). Sexually transmitted infection among adolescents receiving special education services. *Journal of School Health, 78,* 382–388.

Martel, M. M., & Nigg, J. T. (2006). Child ADHD and personality/temperament traits of reactive and effortful control, resiliency, and emotionality. *Journal of Child Psychology and Psychiatry, 47*(11), 1175–1183. doi:10.1111/j.1469-7610.2006.01629.x

Mayo Clinic. (2010). *Muscular dystrophy signs and symptoms.* Retrieved June 17, 2010, http://www.mayoclinic.com

McCarroll, E. M., Lindsey, E. W., MacKinnon-Lewis, C., Chambers, J. C., & Frabutt, J. M. (2009). Health status and peer relationships in early adolescence: The role of peer contact, self-esteem, and social anxiety. *Journal of Child and Family Studies, 18,* 473–485. doi:10.1007/s10826-008-9251-9

McNamara, J. K., Vervaecke, S. L., & Willoughby, T. (2008). Learning disabilities and risk-taking behavior in adolescents: A comparison of those with and without comorbid attention deficit hyperactivity disorder. *Journal of Learning Disabilities, 41*(6), 561–574.

Mikami, A. Y. (2010). The importance of friendship for youth with attention deficit hyperactivity disorder. *Clinical Child and Family Psychology Review, 13(2)*, 181–198.

Milligan, S., & Neufeldt, A. H. (2001). The myth of asexuality: A survey of social and empirical evidence. *Sexuality and Disability, 19(2)*, 91–109.

Mosby's Medical Dictionary. (2009). Sexuality. Retrieved August 2, 2010, from http://www.mosbysonline.com

Murphy, N. (2005). Sexuality in children and adolescents with disabilities. *Developmental Medicine and Child Neurology, 47*, 640–644.

Murphy, N., & Elias, P. (2006). Sexuality of children and adolescents with developmental disabilities. *Pediatrics, 118*, 398–403. doi:10.154/peds.2006-1115

Muscular Dystrophy Association. (2011). *Diseases*. Retrieved June 20, 2011, from http://www.mda.org/disease

Musser, E. D., Backs, R. W., Schmitt, C. F., Ablow, J. C., Measelle, J. R., & Nigg, J. T. (2011). Emotion regulation via the autonomic nervous system in children with attention-deficit/hyperactivity disorder (ADHD). *Journal of Abnormal Child Psychology, 39(6)*, 841–852.

National Dissemination Center for Children with Disabilities. (2011). *Intellectual disability* [NICHCY Fact Sheet 8]. Available from http://nichcy.org/disability/specific/intellectual#char

National Institutes of Health. (2011a). *Intellectual and developmental disabilities*. Retrieved from http://report.nih.gov/NIHfactsheets/ViewFactSheet.aspx?csid=100

National Institutes of Health. (2011b). *Juvenile rheumatoid arthritis*. Retrieved June 18, 2011, from http://www.ncbi.nlm.nih.gov/pubmedhealth/PMH0001487

National Institutes of Health, & National Institute of Neurological Disorders and Stroke. (2010). *Spina bifida signs and symptoms*. Retrieved August 1, 2010, from http://www.ninds.nih.org

Normand, S., Schneider, B. H., Lee, M. D., Maisonneuve, M. F., Kuehn, S. M., & Robaey, P. (2011). How do children with ADHD (mis)manage their real-life dyadic friendships? A mulit-method investigation. *Journal of Abnormal Child Psychology, 39*, 293–305.

Ostlie, I. L., Dale, O., & Moller, A. (2007). From childhood to adult life with juvenile idiopathic arthritis: A pilot study. *Disability and Rehabilitation, 29(6)*, 445–452.

Pastor, P. N., & Reuben, C. A. (2008). Diagnosed attention deficit hyperactivity disorder and learning disability: United States, 2004–2006. *Vital and Health Statistics, 10(237)*. Washington, DC: National Center for Health Statistics.

Price, M. N., & Hyde, J. S. (2009). When two isn't better than one: Predictors of early sexual activity in adolescence using a cumulative risk model. *Journal of Youth and Adolescence, 38*, 1059–1071.

Rahbek, J., Werge, B., Madsen, A., Marquardt, J., Steffensen, B. F., & Jeppesen, J. (2005). Adult life with Duchenne muscular dystrophy: Observations among an emerging and unforeseen patient population. *Pediatric Rehabilitation, 8*(1), 17–28.

Rogers, S. L., Gordon, C. Y., Schanzenbacher, K. E., & Case-Smith, J. (2001). Common diagnosis in pediatric occupational therapy practice. In J. Case-Smith (Ed.), *Occupational therapy for children* (4th ed., pp. 136–187). St. Louis, MO: Mosby/Year Book.

Rose, C., Monda-Amaya, L. E., & Espelage, D. (2011). Bullying perpetration and victimization in special education: A review of the literature. *Remedial and Special Education, 32,* 114–130.

Sawin, K. J., Buran, C. F., Brei, T. J., & Fastenau, P. S. (2002). Sexuality issues in adolescents with a chronic neurological condition. *Journal of Perinatal Education, 11*(1), 22–34.

Schectman, Z., & Katz, E. (2007). Therapeutic bonding in group as an explanatory variable of progress in the social competence of students with learning disabilities. *Group Dynamics: Theory, Research, and Practice, 11*(2), 117–128.

Schwartz, P. D, Maynard, A. M., & Uzelac, S. M. (2008). Adolescent egocentrism: A contemporary view. *Adolescence, 43*(171), 441–448.

Schweier, K. M., & Hingsburger, D. (Eds.). (2000). *Sexuality: Your sons and daughters with intellectual disabilities.* Baltimore: Paul H. Brookes.

Shiomi, T., Hirayama, A., Fujimoto, K., & Hirao, Y. (2006). Sexuality and seeking medical help for erectile dysfunction in young adults with spina bifida. *International Journal of Urology, 13,* 1323–1326.

Stokes, M. A., & Kaur, A. (2005). High-functioning autism and sexuality: A parental perspective. *Autism, 9,* 266–289.

Stokes, M., Newton, N., & Kaur, A. (2007). Stalking and social and romantic functioning among adolescents and adults with autism spectrum disorder. *Journal of Autism and Developmental Disorders, 37*(10), 1969–1986.

Sullivan, A. L., & Caterino, L. C. (2008). Addressing the sexuality and sex education of individuals with autism spectrum disorders. *Education and Treatment of Children, 31*(3), 381–384.

Suris, J., Resnick, M. D., Cassuto, N., & Blum, R. W. (1996). Sexual behavior of adolescents with chronic disease and disability. *Journal of Adolescent Health, 19,* 124–131.

Taylor, R. (2008). *The intentional relationship: Occupational therapy and use of self.* Philadelphia: F. A. Davis.

Tarnai, B., & Wolfe, P. S. (2008). Social stories for sexuality education for persons with autism/pervasive developmental disorder. *Sex and Disability, 26,* 29–36.

Tissot, C. (2009). Establishing a sexual identity: Case studies of learners with autism and learning difficulties. *Autism, 13,* 551–566.

U.S. Department of Health and Human Services. (2010). *Fact sheet on sexually transmitted diseases and disability: A companion document to Healthy People 2010.* Retrieved August 20, 2010, from http://www.hhs.gov/od/about/fact_sheets/std-chapter25.html

U.S. Department of Health and Human Services. (2011a). *Healthy People: 2020 topics and objectives: Adolescent health*. Retrieved August 20, 2011, from http://www.healthypeople.gov/2020/topicsobjectives2020/overview.aspx? topicid=2

U.S. Department of Health and Human Services. (2011b). *Healthy People: 2020 topics and objectives—Disability and health*. Retrieved August 20, 2011, from http://www.healthypeople.gov/2020/topicsobjectives2020/overview.aspx? topicid=9

Varni, J. W. (2011). *Pediatric Quality of Life Scales (Peds–QL)*. Retrieved August 18, 2011, from www.pedsql.org. (See also http://www.mapi-trust.org/services/ questionnairelicensing/cataloguequestionnaires/84-pedsql)

Walker-Hirsch, L. (Ed.). (2007). *The facts of life . . . and more: Sexuality and intimacy for people with intellectual disabilities*. Baltimore: Paul H. Brookes.

Whitehouse, J. O., Durkin, K., Jaquet, E., & Ziatas, K. (2009). Friendship, loneliness, and depression in adolescents with Asperger's syndrome. *Journal of Adolescence, 32*, 309–322.

Wiegerink, D. J., Roebroeck, M. E., Donkervoort, M., Cohen-Kettenis, P. T., & Stam, H. J. (2008). Social, intimate, and sexual relationships of adolescents with cerebral palsy compared with able-bodied age-mates. *Journal of Rehabilitation Medicine, 40*, 112–118.

Wilson, P. M. (1999) *Our whole lives: Sexuality education for grades 7–9*. Cleveland, OH: United Church Board for Homeland Ministries.

Worley, G., Houlihan, C. M., Herman-Giddens, M. E., O'Donnell, M. E., Conaway, M., Stallings, V. A., et al. (2002). Secondary sexual characteristics in children with cerebral palsy and moderate to severe motor impairment: A cross-sectional survey. *Pediatrics, 110*(5), 897–902.

Appendix A

Illustrations of Positions for Sexual Intercourse

The following illustrations show various positions for sexual intercourse.

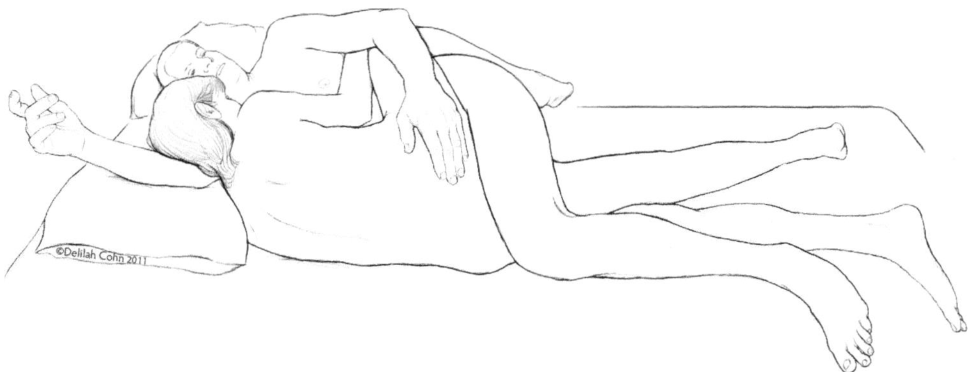

Figure A.1. Side-lying position.

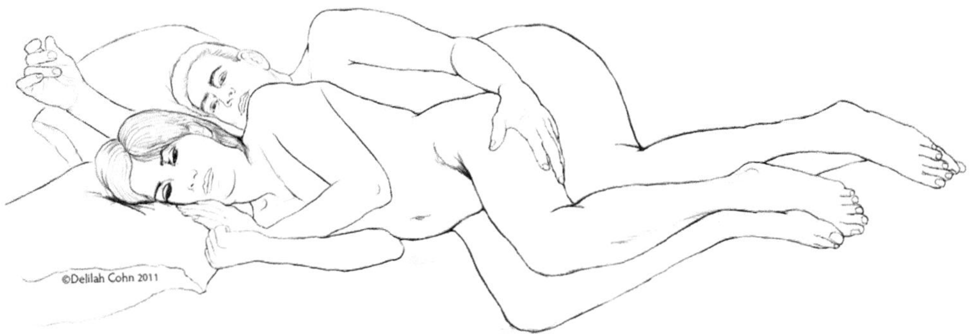

Figure A.2. Variation of the side-lying position, with the man behind the woman.

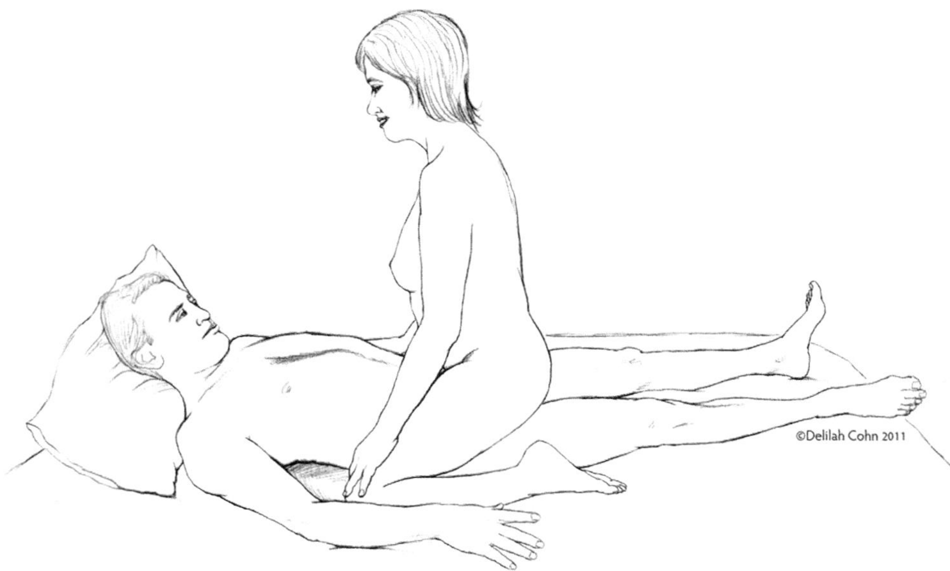

Figure A.3. Woman-on-top position.

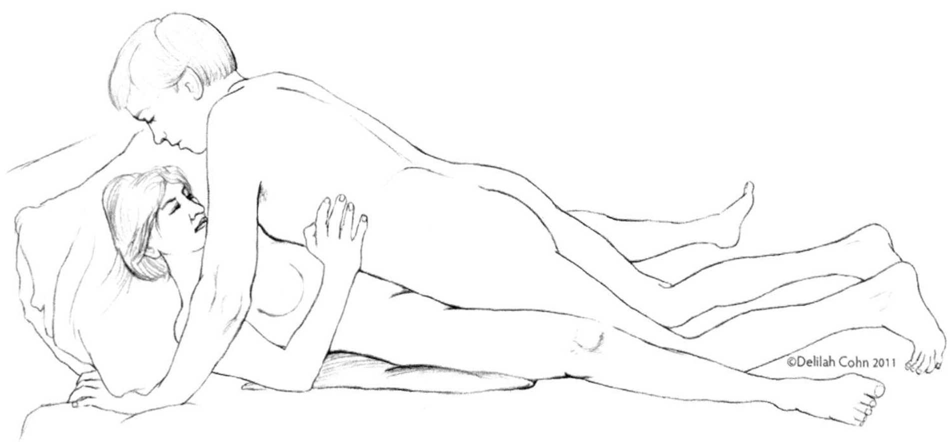

Figure A.4. Man-on-top position.

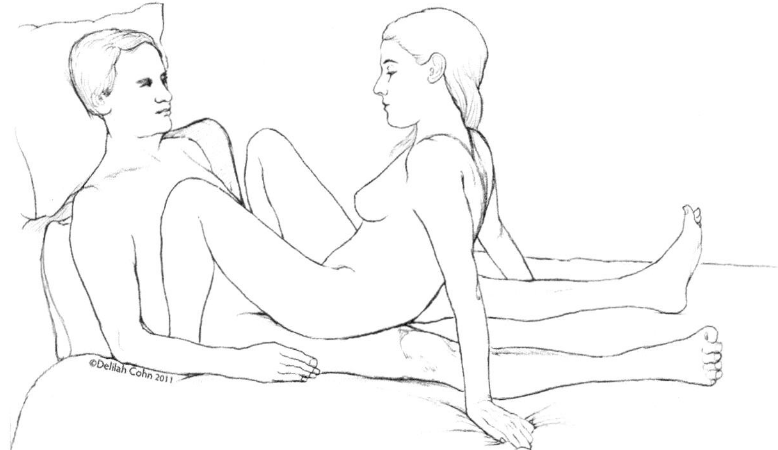

Figure A.5. Sexual intercourse with pillow support.

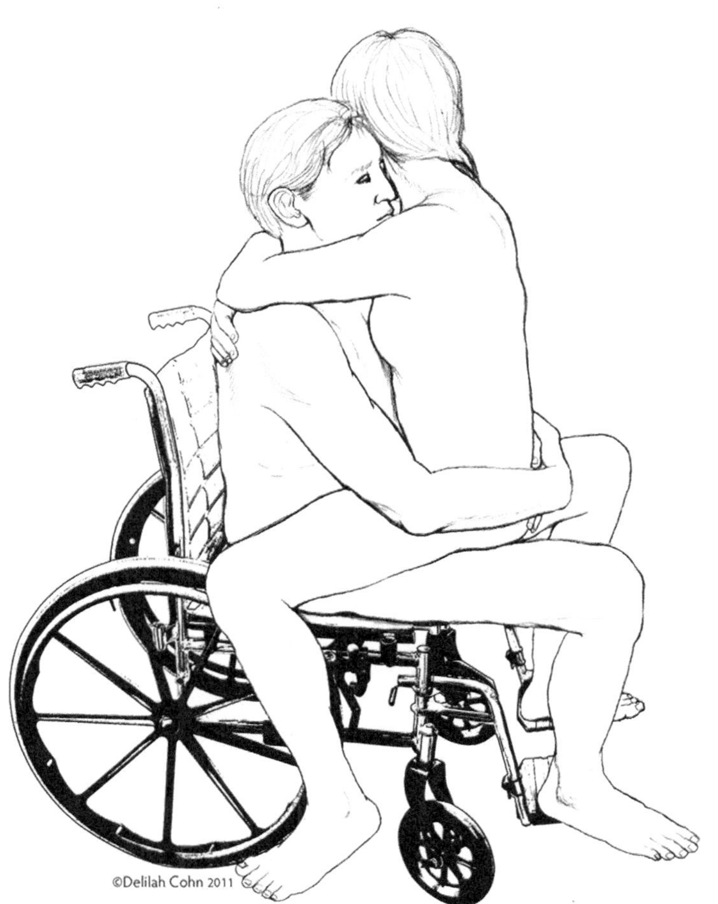

Figure A.6. Couple positioned with wheelchair.

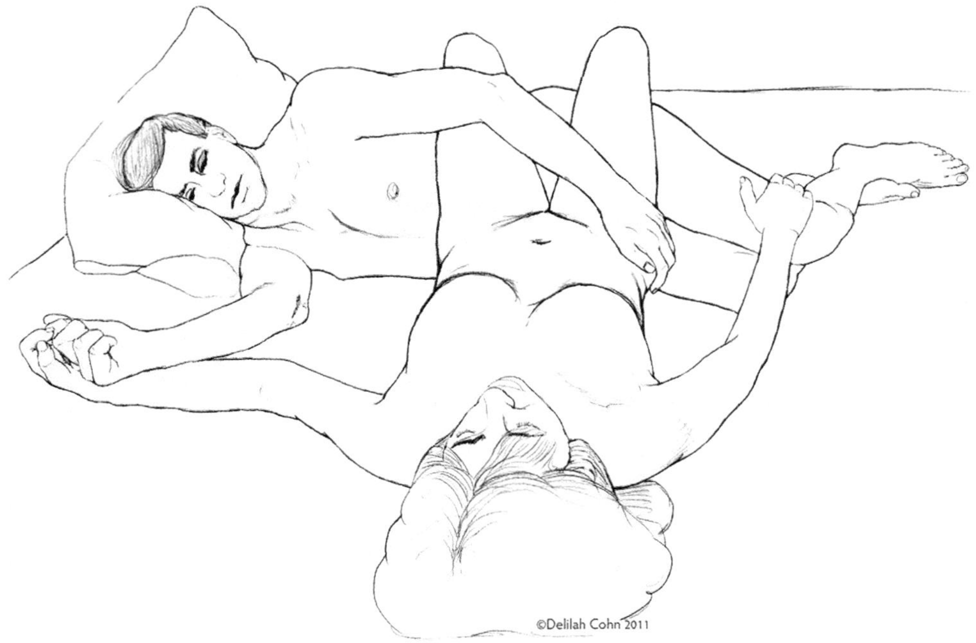

Figure A.7. Couple perpendicular.

Appendix B

Sexuality Questionnaire

To realistically address the subject of sexual activity with a client, the use of this questionnaire may reduce anxiety and facilitate more open communication in the therapist–client relationship. If the therapist is not comfortable with broaching the subject of sexual activity, a referral to another health care professional is strongly recommended.

This questionnaire can be given to a client who indicates interest in discussing sexuality. The therapist can then use it to direct interventions. The questions also address potential intervention methods that can be used by the occupational therapist, including pain reduction, range of motion, self-esteem, and communication issues.

Please circle an answer to the following statements.

1. I believe that I will not be able to have sex because of my symptoms.

    Y   N

2. My pain or discomfort level will make it difficult for me to engage in sex.   Y   N

3. Please identify where you are having pain: _______________________

4. I have spoken with my partner about my concerns about having sex.

    Y   N

5. I do not have a partner, and this concerns me.   Y   N

6. I do not feel attractive or appealing.   Y   N

Note. Courtesy of Bernadette Hattjar. Used with permission.

7. I do not believe that I will be able to enjoy intimacy because of my limitations.   Y   N

8. Sexual activity is not an important consideration for my daily life.

    Y   N

9. I do not want to address this topic in therapy.   Y   N

10. I want to address this topic in therapy.   Y   N

11. I would like my partner to be included when dealing with sexual activity in therapy.   Y   N

12. I would like to investigate other methods of getting sexual pleasure other than intercourse.   Y   N

13. I would like to investigate methods for decreasing my pain or discomfort.   Y   N

14. I currently use a form of contraception.   Y   N

15. Rather than talking about sexual activity, I'd rather receive handouts or brochures about this subject.   Y   N

16. I'd prefer to talk about this subject *and* receive handouts or brochures about this subject.   Y   N

Index